FIRST AID

Q&A
for the
NBDE
PART II

JASON E. PORTNOF, DMD, MD

Attending Oral and Maxillofacial Surgeon
Beth Israel Medical Center
Jacobi Medical Center
Assistant Professor
Departments of Dentistry and Otorhinolaryngology, Head and Neck Surgery
Albert Einstein College of Medicine
Bronx, New York

TIMOTHY LEUNG, DMD, MHSc, MD

Private Practice
Oral and Maxillofacial Surgery
Toronto, Ontario, Canada
Oral and Maxillofacial Surgery Residency Program
Department of Dentistry, Oral and Maxillofacial Surgery
Jacobi Medical Center
Bronx, New York

MELVYN S. YEOH, DMD, MD

Resident, Department of Oral and Maxillofacial Surgery
New York Presbyterian Hospital
Weill Cornell Medical College
New York, New York

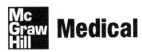 **Medical**

New York / Chicago / San Francisco / Lisbon / London / Madrid / Mexico City

Milan / New Delhi / San Juan / Seoul / Singapore / Sydney / Toronto

First Aid™ Q&A for the NBDE Part II

NOTICE

Medicine is an ever-changing science. As new research and clinical experience broaden our knowledge, changes in treatment and drug therapy are required. The authors and the publisher of this work have checked with sources believed to be reliable in their efforts to provide information that is complete and generally in accord with the standards accepted at the time of publication. However, in view of the possibility of human error or changes in medical sciences, neither the authors nor the publisher nor any other party who has been involved in the preparation or publication of this work warrants that the information contained herein is in every respect accurate or complete, and they disclaim all responsibility for any errors or omissions or for the results obtained from use of the information contained in this work. Readers are encouraged to confirm the information contained herein with other sources. For example and in particular, readers are advised to check the product information sheet included in the package of each drug they plan to administer to be certain that the information contained in this work is accurate and that changes have not been made in the recommended dose or in the contraindications for administration. This recommendation is of particular importance in connection with new or infrequently used drugs.

This book was set in Electra LH by Aptara Inc.
The editors were Catherine A. Johnson and Brian Kearns
The production supervisor was Sherri Souffrance.
Project management was provided by Indu Jawwad, Aptara Inc.
Quad/Graphics was printer and binder.

This book is printed on acid-free paper.

Library of Congress Cataloging-in-Publication Data
Portnof, Jason E.
  First aid Q&A for the NBDE part II / Jason E. Portnof, Timothy Leung, Melvyn S. Yeoh.
     p. ; cm.
  Other title: First aid Q&A for the National Board Dental Exam part II
  ISBN-13: 978-0-07-161372-9 (pbk. : alk. paper)
  ISBN-10: 0-07-161372-2 (pbk. : alk. paper)   1. Dentistry–Examinations, questions, etc.
2. Dentists–Licenses–United States–Examinations–Study guides.   I. Leung, Timothy.
II. Yeoh, Melvyn S.   III. Title.   IV. Title: First aid Q&A for the National Board Dental Exam part II.
     [DNLM: 1.   Dentistry–Examination Questions.   2. Emergencies–Examination Questions.
3. Emergency Treatment–Examination Questions. WU 18.2 P853f 2010]
  RK57.P67 2010
  617.60076–dc22   2010023051

McGraw-Hill books are available at special quantity discounts to use as premiums and sales promotions, or for use in corporate training programs. To contact a representative, please e-mail us at bulksales@mcgraw-hill.com.

JEP would like to dedicate this book to his two best friends: his beautiful wife, Courtney, and his amazing son, Justin. Thank you for making life wonderful!

TL would like to dedicate this book to his wife Josephine and new baby daughter Evelyn.

MSY would like to dedicate this book to his wife, Sophia, and son, Max, who tolerate his mood swings and behavior and still love him in spite of it and to his parents, who have been supportive in all his pursuits.

CONTENTS

CONTRIBUTORS

Anayo O. Adachie, DMD, MD
Resident, Oral and Maxillofacial Surgery
Beth Israel Medical Center, Jacobi Medical Center,
    Albert Einstein College of Medicine
Bronx, New York

Jose Ignacio Alamo, Jr., DMD
Resident, Senior General Practice
Department of Dentistry & Oral and Maxillofacial Surgery
New York Presbyterian Hospital—Weill Cornell Medical College
New York, New York

David M. Alfi, DDS, MD
Resident, Oral and Maxillofacial Surgery
Division of Oral and Maxillofacial Surgery
New York Presbyterian Hospital
New York, New York

Will R. Allen, DMD
Resident, Oral and Maxillofacial Surgery
Beth Israel Medical Center/Jacobi Medical Center/
    Albert Einstein College of Medicine
Bronx, New York

LoanAnh Bui
Student
Class of 2010
SUNY Stony Brook School of Dental Medicine
Stony Brook, New York

Margaret LeeAnn Clark
Student
Class of 2009
New York University College of Dentistry
New York, New York

Jennifer Frangos, DDS
Intern, Department of Oral and Maxillofacial Surgery
Baltimore College of Dental Surgery
University of Maryland
Baltimore, Maryland

Daniel Fruchter DMD
Resident, General Practice
Department of Dentistry
Jacobi Medical Center
Bronx, New York

Evan Hershkowitz, DDS
Resident, Pediatric Dental
Department of Dentistry
Jacobi Medical Center
Bronx, New York

Jamie J. M. Hwang, DMD
Private Practice, General Dentistry
New York, New York

James A. Kraus, DMD
Chief Resident, Oral and Maxillofacial Surgery
Tufts Medical Center
Boston, Massachusetts

Lindsey J. Krecko, DDS
Chief Resident, General Practice Dentistry
Illinois Masonic Medical Center Department of Dentistry
Chicago, Illinois

Andrew W. C. Lee, MSc, DDS, MD
Resident, Oral and Maxillofacial Surgery
Department of Dentistry & Oral and Maxillofacial Surgery
New York Presbyterian Hospital—Weill Cornell Medical College
New York, New York

Katherine Lee, DDS
Intern, Oral and Maxillofacial Surgery
Department of Dentistry
Jacobi Medical Center
Bronx, New York

Won Sang Lee, DDS
Resident, Oral and Maxillofacial Surgery
Department of Dentistry
Beth Israel Medical Center, Jacobi Medical Center,
    Albert Einstein College of Medicine
Bronx, New York

Avi Malkis, DDS
Student
Class of 2010
New York University College of Dentistry
New York, New York

Mariya Mamkin, DDS
Attending Dentist, Department of Dental and Oral Medicine
New York Hospital of Queens
Queens, New York

Pankti Mehta, DDS
Private Practice, General Dentistry
Danbury, Connecticut

Keith Murtagh, DDS, FAAOMP
Resident, Oral and Maxillofacial Surgery
Brookdale University Hospital and Medical Center
Brooklyn, New York

Nona Naghavi, DDS
Resident, Orthodontics
Jacksonville University
Jacksonville, Florida

Niral N. Parikh, DDS, BDS
Resident, Oral and Maxillofacial Surgery
Department of Dentistry
Beth Israel Medical Center, Jacobi Medical Center,
    Albert Einstein College of Medicine
Bronx, New York

Debbie M. Parnes, DMD
Resident, Department of Orthodontics
Temple University
Philadelphia, Pennsylvania

Clifford Salm, DMD
Beth Israel Medical Center
Private Practice, Oral and Maxillofacial Surgery
New York, New York

Dara J. Sandler, MS, RD, CDN
Private Practice, Registered Dietitian
New York, New York

Jonathan W. Shum, DDS, MD
Resident, Oral and Maxillofacial Surgery
Department of Dentistry & Oral and Maxillofacial Surgery
New York Presbyterian Hospital—Weill Cornell Medical College
New York, New York

Robert M. Spriggel, DDS, Capt., USAF, DC
Clinical Dentist
1st Special Operations Medical Group, Dental Squadron
Hurlburt Field, Florida

David E. Webb, DDS, Capt, USAF
Resident, Oral and Maxillofacial Surgery
Wilford Hall Medical Center
Lackland Air Force Base
San Antonio, Texas

Marta Williams, DDS
Intern, Oral and Maxillofacial Surgery
Department of Dentistry
Jacobi Medical Center
Bronx, New York

Stacy B. Wolf, DDS
Student
Class of 2009
New York University College of Dentistry
New York, New York

Victor M. Badner, DMD, MPH
North Bronx Healthcare Network
Chairman, Department of Dentistry/OMFS
Dental Public Health Residency—Site Director
Jacobi Medical Center
Bronx, New York

Daniel Buchbinder, DMD, MD
Chief, Division of Oral and Maxillofacial Surgery
OMFS Residency Program Director
Head and Neck Institute
Department of Otolaryngology
Beth Israel Medical Center
New York, New York

Stuart A. Caplan, DDS, MS
Assistant Professor, Diagnostic Sciences
Nova Southeastern University
College of Dental Medicine
Fort Lauderdale, Florida

Kenneth B. Cooperman, DMD
Private Practice, Orthodontics
New York, New York
Assistant Professor of Dentistry
Albert Einstein College of Medicine
Jacobi Medical Center
Bronx, New York

Dennis Davis, DMD, MS
Adjunct Professor, Department of Periodontology
University of Florida College of Dentistry
Gainesville, Florida
Private Practice
Lady Lake, Florida

Jennifer Blake Eli, DMD
Private Practice, General Dentistry
Lake Forest, California

Francisco Eraso, DMD, MS, ABO
Radiologist, Oral & Maxillofacial
Adjunct Associate Professor of Orthodontics
Department of Orthodontics and Oral Facial Development
Indiana University School of Dentistry
Oral & Maxillofacial Imaging Center—Indianapolis
Indianapolis, Indiana

Andrew Forrest, DMD, MS
Clinical Assistant Professor
Department of Periodontics
College of Dental Medicine
University of Florida
Gainesville, Florida

Andrew A. C. Heggie, MBBS, MDSc, FFDRCS, FACOMS, FRACDS (OMS)
Section Chief, Oral and Maxillofacial Surgery
Department of Plastic and Maxillofacial Surgery
Royal Children's Hospital
Associate Professor
Department of Pediatrics
University of Melbourne
Melbourne, Victoria, Australia

Christine Heng, DDS, MPH
Captain, United States Public Health Service
Federal Correctional Institution
Danbury, Connecticut
Department of Dentistry/OMFS
Jacobi Medical Center
Bronx, New York

Marcela Herrera, DMD
Clinical Assistant Professor
Department of Preventive and Restorative Sciences
University of Pennsylvania School of Dental Medicine
Philadelphia, Pennsylvania

Jason P. Hirsch, DMD MPH
Private Practice, Pediatric Dentistry
Plantation, Florida

Laurance Jerrold, DDS, JD, ABO
Dean and Program Director
Jacksonville University School of Orthodontics
Jacksonville, Florida

Kevin Kohler, DMD
Private Practice, Family and Cosmetic Dentistry
Boise, Idaho

Keith S. Margulis, DDS
Diplomate, American Board of Pediatric Dentistry
Assistant Director—Advanced Education in Pediatric Dentistry
North Bronx Healthcare Network
Jacobi Medical Center
Bronx, New York

Christopher Phelps, DMD
Private Practice, General Dentistry
Charlotte, North Carolina

Gol Pourkhomami, DMD
Family and Cosmetic Dentistry
Adjunct Faculty
Arizona School of Dentistry and Oral Health
A.T. Still University
Mesa, Arizona

Morton Rosenberg, DMD
Professor of Oral and Maxillofacial Surgery
Tufts University School of Dental Medicine
Associate Professor of Anesthesia
Tufts University School of Medicine
Tufts Medical Center
Boston, Massachusetts

Michelle Segal, DMD
Private Practice, General and Cosmetic Dentistry
Miami, Florida

Robert M. Sorin, DMD
Clinical Instructor in Surgery
Attending Dentist
Division of Dentistry, Oral and Maxillofacial Surgery
New York Presbyterian Hospital—Cornell Campus
New York, New York

James D. Toppin DDS, MBA
Clinical Assistant Professor, Oral and Maxillofacial Pathology,
   Radiology and Medicine
New York University College of Dentistry
New York, New York

Robert A. Uchin, DDS
Dean, College of Dental Medicine
Health Professions Division
Nova Southeastern University
Fort Lauderdale, Florida

Farhad Yeroshalmi, DMD, FAAPD
Diplomate, American Board of Pediatric Dentistry
Program Director, Pediatric Dentistry Residency Program
Jacobi Medical Center
Bronx, New York

Preparation advice from Dara Sandler, MS, RD who is a Clinical Nutritionist in New York, New York:

Although the anticipation and uncertainty of stepping into the testing center to take the Dental Board Exam can be taxing on the mind, it can also take its toll physically. You should regard nourishment, hydration, and rest equally as important as being academically prepared. You will enhance and sustain your ability to focus and perform by providing your body with the necessary vitamins and minerals. Eating a balanced meal that consists of protein, complex carbohydrates, fat, and B vitamins prior to sitting down for the test improves your memory function and increases your mood.

Proteins—such as eggs, milk products, and nuts—keep your blood sugar steady, a function of both keeping your brain alert and your hunger satisfied over long periods of time. Complex carbohydrates (3 g or more per serving) that exist in foods such as whole grains, oatmeal, legumes, fruits, and vegetables will also help to sustain your energy. Fats, such as Omega-3 fatty acids, are important to include in your pretest meal because they help with blood circulation, memory, and your immune system. Nuts and seeds, vegetable oil, avocado, and different types of fish are good sources of Omega-3s. Foods that contain B vitamins, such as whole grains, eggs, and milk products, are extremely important in maintaining your mental energy.

Combining all these nutrients into a well-balanced meal will allow you to sustain your energy and keep you sharp and focused. A breakfast of eggs, cheese, whole-grain toast, and yogurt will meet all the criteria and carry you through the test; cottage cheese, fruit, and whole-grain crackers, or a protein smoothie made with peanut butter, milk, and fruit are also great choices.

During the test, smart snacking will supplement your balanced meal and allow you to maintain focus. Small snacks containing protein and complex carbohydrates are your best options: peanut butter on a banana, whole-wheat crackers with cheese, or cottage cheese and nuts.

Finally, hydration is a key factor in rounding out your day. Stress can cause mild dehydration; make sure to drink plenty of water before and during the test. It is recommended that adults drink eight 8-ounce glasses of fluid each day.

Following these simple guidelines will help your mind stay razor sharp and enable you to concentrate on your exam rather than on your stomach. Take a break from studying and take a trip to your local market to plan your exam-day diet. You owe it to yourself!

CHAPTER 1

Pharmacology

1. A 63-year-old male patient with a history of infrequent dental visits reports to your office with the complaint of swollen gums. He has a history of high blood pressure, high cholesterol, and was in the hospital 2 years ago after suffering a silent myocardial infarction. He also has a history of asthma. He is currently taking lisinopril, nifedipine, atenolol, simvastatin, and albuterol as needed. Which of the following medications is the most likely cause of his hyperplastic gingiva?

   A. Lisinopril
   B. Nifedipine
   C. Atenolol
   D. Simvastatin
   E. Albuterol

2. A 52-year-old overweight male patient presents to your office with erosion of the lingual surfaces of all his maxillary teeth. The patient also says he suffers from heartburn, dysphagia, and a chronic cough. The patient's physician has prescribed him cimetidine and told him to take over-the-counter antacids. Which of the following is the most likely mechanism of the therapeutic effect of cimetidine?

   A. Eradicates *Helicobacter pylori*
   B. Neutralizes stomach acid
   C. Reduces GI motility and acid secretion
   D. Blocks histamine-2 receptors on parietal cells
   E. Blocks proton pumps on parietal cells

3. A female patient presents to your office with facial and torso obesity, facial hair growth, and a deepened voice. The patient explains these changes occurred when she started taking a common drug to treat Crohn's disease, and subsequently she recently discontinued the drug use. While performing a surgical extraction, the patient suddenly starts breathing at a fast rate, sweating, and complains of nausea and chills. You recognize that the patient is experiencing a crisis and reach for your Emergency Kit. Which of the following contents of your Emergency Kit would be most appropriate to alleviate this crisis?

   A. Oxygen
   B. Epinephrine
   C. Nitroglycerin
   D. Sugar
   E. Hydrocortisone

4. A 15-year-old male patient presents to your office for an initial dental visit. While reviewing the patient's medical history with him and his parents, he reveals that during a recent basketball game he suffered from chest pain and fainted. After several tests, including an echocardiogram, he was diagnosed with hypertrophic cardiomyopathy. He also has a history of exercise-induced asthma. He has an albuterol inhaler but cannot remember the name of the medication he was recently put on for his heart condition. Which of the following beta-blockers is he most likely taking?

   A. Propranolol
   B. Labetalol
   C. Metoprolol
   D. Nadolol
   E. Timolol

5. A 55-year-old female patient was referred to your office by her physician because she is preparing to receive an infusion of zoledronic acid. Her physician told her to see a dentist to determine if she has any teeth that may need to be extracted in the near future. If so, these should be extracted prior to the infusion because of the risk of poor bone healing (osteonecrosis) that sometimes occurs in patients receiving infusions of zoledronic acid. Prior to the infusion, the patient was taking an oral form of this type of drug. What is another major side effect of the oral form that her physician may have warned her about?

   A. Anemia
   B. Xerostomia
   C. Edema
   D. Esophageal perforation
   E. Orthostatic hypotension

6. In rats, a new anticonvulsant drug has an lethal dose $(LD)_1$ of 20 mg, and LD_{50} of 30 mg, an effective dose $(ED)_{50}$ of 5 mg, and an ED_{99} of 10 mg. What is the experimental drug's therapeutic index and safety index, respectively?

    A. 2 and 1.5
    B. 1.5 and 2
    C. 6 and 2
    D. 2 and 6
    E. 3 and 4
    F. 4 and 3

7. A 40-pound child presents to your office for a pulpotomy and placement of a stainless steel crown on tooth #L. What would be the approximate maximum recommended dose of 2% lidocaine?

    A. 1 carpule
    B. 2 carpules
    C. 3 carpules
    D. 4 carpules
    E. 5 carpules

8. Your 55-year-old male patient is scheduled for three quadrants of periodontal surgery. Each surgical procedure is scheduled 4 weeks apart. This patient is allergic to penicillin and has a history of a mitral valve prolapse. On the basis of the current guidelines, which prescription would be most appropriate to adequately premedicate this patient for all of his visits?

    A. Amoxicillin 2-g tablets; Disp: 3 tablets; Sig: take 1 tablet 30–60 minutes prior to dental procedure
    B. Amoxicillin 2-g tablets; Disp: 6 tables; Sig: take 2 tablets 30–60 minutes prior to dental procedure
    C. Clindamycin 600-mg tablets; Disp: 3 tablets; Sig: take 1 tablet 30–60 minutes prior to dental procedure
    D. Clindamycin 600-mg tablets; Disp: 6 tablets; Sig: take 2 tablets 30–60 minutes prior to dental procedure
    E. No prescription necessary

9. Your patient presents to your office and reports that he recently completed a 2-month course of the following medications: isoniazid, rifampin, ethambutol, and pyrazinamide. He states that a few months back, he acquired an infection while working at a homeless shelter in the nearby city and was admitted to the hospital after developing pneumonia. His most recent chest x-ray was negative, but he still has a positive skin test. On the basis of the disease, this patient has been treated for and the intraoral image taken during the examination, what oral mucosal lesion does this patient have?

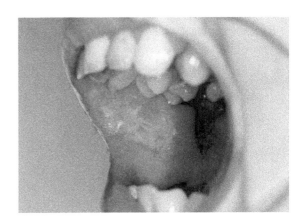

    A. Linea alba
    B. Nonhealing ulcer
    C. Perioral vesicles
    D. Hairy leukoplakia
    E. Lichen planus

10. An elderly patient presents to your office with a long list of medications that she is currently taking to treat the following conditions: history of stroke, depression, arthritis, and glaucoma. In the clinical examination, you note multiple cervical caries and severe dry mouth. Which of the following medications is the most likely cause of xerostomia in this patient?

    A. Amitriptyline
    B. Aspirin
    C. Pilocarpine
    D. Nabumetone
    E. Physostigmine

11. An emergency patient presents to your office with trismus, fever, and a swelling on one side of his lower face. The patient questionnaire he filled out in the waiting room states that he has no medical issues, takes no medications, and has a history of alcohol abuse but has been sober for one month. During the examination, you observe extensive decay on #18 and a small abscess in the apical region of #18. The tooth is hopeless, but before extraction, you decide to place the patient on an antibiotic to clear up the acute intraoral infection. Which of the following antibiotics would you want to avoid because of the patient's social history and the potential disulfiram-like effect?

    A. Clarithromycin
    B. Metronidazole
    C. Clindamycin
    D. Doxycycline
    E. Rifampin

12. One of your friends, who is also a patient, is in your office for a routine visit. While in your office, she asks if you can write a prescription for one of the drugs her primary care physician normally prescribes for an existing condition. Your friend, the patient, says she does not have much time to make an appointment with her primary care physician so she would really appreciate if you could write a script for the pharmacist. When faced with this question, as a practicing dentist, it is important to keep in mind that you can legally write prescriptions for which of the following drugs?

    A. Oral contraceptives
    B. Blood pressure lowering drugs
    C. Analgesic agents
    D. Antidiabetic agents
    E. Amphetamines
    F. Antiasthmatics

13. A patient presents to your office for an initial visit. When reviewing the patient's medical history, the patients tells you that she is taking 81 mg of aspirin once a day and several alternative medications. She does not specify which alternative medications she is taking because she assumes they are not necessary for you to know. In fact, it is important for dentists to know about all medications and supplements to protect patients from possible substance interactions. When planning for a surgical procedure, which of the following alternative medications might you want to discontinue to prevent excessive bleeding in this patient?

    A. Ginseng
    B. Echinacea
    C. St. John's Wort
    D. Ginkgo Balboa
    E. Capsaicin

14. During a routine medical history interview, your patient tells you he is taking celecoxib for osteoarthritis. He has been on this medication for the past year. Compared to traditional non-steroidal anti-inflammatory drugs (NSAIDs) like ibuprofen, celecoxib:

    A. Is a more effective analgesic for acute post-surgical pain
    B. Produces greater anti-inflammatory responses in osteoarthritis patients
    C. Produces less water and sodium retention
    D. Produces less gastrointestinal ulcers and bleeds with chronic use
    E. Is more effective at fever reduction

15. You received a call from the emergency department at your local hospital concerning a pediatric patient that you recently treated. The patient is a 6-year-old boy who was brought to the emergency department in a comatose state. His parents state that he recently visited your office for extraction of a grossly decayed primary tooth. The parents state that they had given him a few pain pills to help with the discomfort following the extraction. Physical examination of the boy revealed "comatose, hepatomegaly, and yellow sclera." A computerized tomography (CT) scan revealed cerebral edema. Laboratory results showed elevated alanine aminotransferase (ALT), aspartate aminotransferase (AST), and prothrombin time (PT). The emergency department physician believes that treatment with the antidote N-acetylcysteine is necessary but has called you to confirm whether you prescribed any medications. What agent is most likely involved in the symptoms of this patient?

    A. Aspirin
    B. Acetaminophen

C. Codeine
D. Celecoxib
E. Ibuprofen

16. A patient presents to your office with the following current medication list: warfarin, aspirin, and clotrimazole. Before beginning the procedure you had planned, you decide it is worthwhile to look up further information on these drugs. Warfarin is metabolized in the liver and has a volume of distribution of approximately 0.14 L/kg. You are slightly concerned that this patient may experience increased bleeding because of these properties along with the concomitant medications he is taking. Which of the following properties of a drug is the *least* likely to contribute to a significant adverse interaction with another drug?

A. The drug has a low therapeutic index
B. The drug has minimal protein binding
C. The drug undergoes extensive cytochrome P450 metabolism
D. The drug is an enzyme inducer
E. The drug has a low volume of distribution

17. Many people use herbal supplements as alternate therapy for a variety of conditions. It is important for physicians and dentists to know what medications their patients are taking, including herbal supplements. St. John's Wort is an example of a supplement commonly used to relieve depression. The simultaneous ingestion of the herbal St. John's Wort has been shown to decrease the half-life of oral contraceptives because St. John's Wort:

A. Blocks the active secretion of oral contraceptive
B. Induces CYP-3A4 in the gut and liver
C. Increases stomach acidity
D. Blocks both estrogen and progesterone receptors
E. Decreases serotonin levels in the brain

18. After taking Drug X for 5 days, steady free blood levels average about 20 ug/mL. Drug Z is then introduced while the patient continues to take Drug X, and the free blood levels of Drug X increase to 100 ug/mL. What could have accounted for this?

A. Drug Z is a liver microsomal enzyme inducer
B. Drugs X and Z formed a chelation product in the intestine
C. Drug Z increased the glomerular filtration rate
D. Drug Z has a positive inotropic and chronotropic effect
E. Drugs X and Z are highly bound to plasma proteins

19. A patient presents to your office for a surgical extraction. Following the procedure, you prescribe the patient tylenol #3 (acetaminophen + codeine). The patient is taking several other drugs concurrently. Which of the following drugs is most likely to inhibit the effectiveness of codeine?

A. Terazosin
B. Glipizide
C. Lisinopril
D. Fluoxetine
E. Lithium

20. A patient with uncontrolled asthma may be taking multiple medications to attempt to control the disease. Which of the following best describes the mechanism of action of montelukast?

A. Beta-2 adrenergic agonist
B. Leukotriene receptor antagonist
C. Lipoxygenase pathway inhibitor
D. Muscarinic receptor antagonist
E. Corticosteroid used to reduce inflammation
F. Suppresses the cough reflex

21. A patient presents to your office with complaints of a burning tongue. She is overweight and says her average fasting blood glucose level is 326 mg/dL. She also states that her most recent HbA1c was 9%. The patient was prescribed several medications by her physician but claims that most of them she does not take because she forgets. Which of the following medications should the patient be taking?

A. Levothyroxine
B. Hydrocortisone
C. Insulin
D. Omeprazole
E. Ranitidine

22. A patient presented to your office for an emergency visit. One side of the patient's face was swollen, and on examination, a small abscess was present apical to tooth #3. The abscess was incised and drained, penicillin was prescribed, and root canal treatment was recommended. The next day, the patient calls your office and complains of swollen lips and a developing rash. The best response to this situation is to:

    A. Tell the patient not to worry; this is a normal reaction
    B. Prescribe epinephrine
    C. Instruct the patient to discontinue the penicillin and prescribe amoxicillin instead
    D. Instruct the patient to discontinue the penicillin and prescribe clindamycin instead

23. A pediatric patient is scheduled to have multiple restorative procedures carried out in the operating room under anesthesia. The drug chosen for anesthesia is fentanyl. Should this patient show signs of respiratory depression, what would be the appropriate reversal agent?

    A. Epinephrine
    B. Naloxone
    C. Flumazenil
    D. Clonidine
    E. Hydrocortisone

24. Which drug is most appropriate to treat oral candidiasis?

    A. Penicillin
    B. Amphotericin B
    C. Nystatin
    D. Tetracycline
    E. Valacyclovir

25. Which of the following local anesthetics is most likely to cause an allergic reaction?

    A. Lidocaine
    B. Propoxycaine
    C. Prilocaine
    D. Mepivicaine
    E. Bupivacaine

26. Accidental ingestion of warfarin can lead to elevated PT and PTT. Which one of the following is the most appropriate treatment?

    A. Vitamin A
    B. Vitamin B
    C. Vitamin C
    D. Vitamin D
    E. Vitamin K

27. A 50-year-old man complains of heartburn. Which one of the following medications will help prevent acid secretion in the stomach?

    A. Omeprazole
    B. Cimetidine
    C. Famotidine
    D. Ketoconazole
    E. Ranitidine

28. Which one of the following benzodiazepines does not require Phase I metabolism by the liver?

    A. Alprazolam
    B. Oxazepam
    C. Midazolam
    D. Triazolam
    E. Diazepam

29. Continuous infusion of medication A is given to a 65-kg patient. The pharmacokinetic parameters are as follows: clearance = 9 mL/min/kg, volume of distribution = 65 L, half-life = 4 hours. How long will it take for the medication level to reach 93.75% of steady state?

    A. 8 hours
    B. 10 hours
    C. 14 hours
    D. 16 hours
    E. 18 hours

30. Which one of the following is an ester local anesthetics?

    A. Bupivacaine
    B. Lidocaine
    C. Mepivacaine
    D. Tetracaine
    E. Prilocaine

31. A 75-year-old smoker with history of chronic obstructive disease presents to clinic with blood pressure of 160/96 mm Hg. Which one of the

following medications is contraindicated in this patient?

A. Atenolol
B. Metoprolol
C. Propranolol
D. Esmolol
E. Acebutolol

32. A new antibiotic is being tested in a clinical trial. The following pharmacokinetic parameters are listed as follows: Clearance = 200 mL/min, volume of distribution (Vd) = 50 L, half-life = 6 hours. Assuming that the drug is being administered intravenously, what loading dose (LD) should be given to the patient to reach a plasma concentration (Cp) of 5 mg/L?

A. 50
B. 100
C. 150
D. 200
E. 250

33. A 60-year-old female patient with history of hypertension was recently put on antihypertensive medications. She is now reporting recent onset of polyuria and polydipsia. The patient does not appear to have any other medical conditions. Which one of the following medication is most likely of what the patient is taking?

A. Hydrochlorothiazide
B. Enalapril
C. Terazosin
D. Methyldopa
E. Diltiazem

34. A 20-year-old man with no prior significant medical history visits his oral surgeon for wisdom tooth extraction with IV sedation. He was given IV midazolam during the procedure. Midway through the surgery, he suddenly becomes agitated and combative and exhibits involuntary movements. The surgeon determines that this is likely due to disinhibition reaction to the benzodiazepine. Which one of the following medication can be used to reverse the effect of midazolam?

A. Naloxone
B. Naltrexone

C. Protamine
D. Flumazenil
E. Insulin

35. Which one of the following is true regarding paroxetine?

A. It specifically inhibits scrotonin reuptake
B. It is used to treat mania
C. It can be safely taken with monoamine oxidase inhibitor (MAOI)
D. GI upset is not a common side effect
E. Sexual dysfunction is rarely reported

36. Which one of the following beta-lactam antibiotics has antipseudomonal properties?

A. Penicillin V
B. Penicillin G
C. Piperacillin
D. Amoxicillin
E. Ampicillin

37. Which one of the following statements is true regarding heparin?

A. Its effect cannot be reversed with protamine sulfate
B. It can bind and activate antithrombin III, resulting in the inactivating thrombin and factor Xa
C. It can lead to decrease in PTT, which is a clinical measure used to follow the anticoagulant effect caused by heparin
D. It decreases the synthesis of vitamin K coagulation factors
E. There are no applications of heparin in pulmonary embolism

38. Which one of the following statements is true regarding warfarin?

A. Follow PTT in determining its clinical effect
B. It inhibits the synthesis of vitamin K-dependent clotting factors (III, VIII, XI, XII)
C. It is teratogenic
D. Protein C and S levels are not affected
E. It is false that warfarin is found in rat poison

39. What do prazosin, doxazosin, and terazosin have in common?

    A. They are all alpha-2 receptor blocker that causes a decrease in peripheral vascular resistance
    B. They are diuretics used to control hypertension
    C. Side effects of the drugs include orthostatic hypotension
    D. They are noncompetitive alpha-receptor blockers.
    E. They rarely cause headache or dizziness

40. A 50-year-old patient with recent diagnosis of hypertension presents to your clinic complaining of a sudden increase in the size of his tongue and slight difficulty in breathing. He was recently started on an antihypertensive medication. Which one of the following drug classes may have caused the patient's presentation?

    A. Beta-blocker
    B. Alpha 1-blocker
    C. Thiazide diuretic
    D. Angiotensin-converting enzyme (ACE) inhibitor
    E. Calcium channel blocker

41. Which one of the following is true regarding tricyclic antidepressants (TCAs)?

    A. They include phenelzine, isocarboxazid, and tranylcypromine
    B. They inhibit reuptake of norepinephrine and serotonin into presynaptic nerve terminals
    C. They are only used in depression
    D. Arrhythmias are a concern with TCA overdose
    E. Orthostatic hypotension rarely occurs

42. Which one of the following anticonvulsants is known to cause neural tube defects in unborn fetus?

    A. Phenytoin
    B. Carbamazepine
    C. Gabapentin
    D. Benzodiazepines
    E. Valproic acid

43. Which one of the following statements is true regarding sulfonylureas?

    A. They include glipizide and glyburide
    B. They stimulate insulin release from alpha cells of pancreas and binding of insulin to target tissue and inhibit release of glucagons
    C. It can decrease hepatic gluconeogenesis
    D. It is the first-line medication for type I diabetes mellitus
    E. Lactic acidosis is a concern for sulfonylureas overdose

44. Which one of the following is not an antifungal?

    A. Nystatin
    B. Amphotericin B
    C. Ketoconazole
    D. Esomeprazole
    E. Griseofulvin

45. N-acetylcysteine is used as an antidote for overdose of which of the following medications?

    A. Acetaminophen
    B. Ibuprofen
    C. Celecoxib
    D. Indomethacin
    E. Naproxen

46. All of the following statement is true regarding NSAIDs, *except*:

    A. Aspirin irreversibly inhibits cox-1 and cox-2 cyclooxygenases
    B. All NSAIDs, except aspirin, are reversible inhibitors of cox-1 and cox-2 cyclooxygenases
    C. Prostaglandin synthesis is rarely affected
    D. They are used for inflammation, analgesia, and antipyrexia
    E. Side effects include dyspepsia, GI ulcers, and renal failure

47. Which one of the following is true about H1 antihistamines?

    A. They include cimetidine and diphenhydramine
    B. They are rarely used for allergy
    C. Some are more sedating than others
    D. loratadine is a first-generation H1 antihistamine
    E. They can be used for motion sickness

48. All of the statements below about glucocorticoids are true, *except*:

A. They function by binding to an extracellular receptor
B. They decrease the production of leukotrienes and prostaglandins
C. Inhibition of phospholipase A2 is a key to their mechanism of action
D. They are contraindicated in Cushing syndrome
E. They are commonly used in inflammation and immunosuppression

49. Which one of the following is true about opioids?

A. They can interact with μ, δ, and/or κ opioid receptor in PNS and enteric nervous system
B. They can cause respiratory depression
C. They can cause diarrhea
D. All can cause mydriasis
E. Naloxone is an example of an opioid

50. Misoprostol can be used for the following, *except*:

A. Abortion
B. Induction of labor
C. Prevention of NSAID-induced peptic ulcer disease
D. Rheumatoid arthritis
E. Maintenance of patent ductus arteriosus (PDA) in newborns with certain congenital cardiovascular defects

51. All of the following statements are true regarding bioavailability, *except*:

A. Route of administration is important in determining bioavailability
B. High hepatic first pass effect decreases bioavailability
C. Degradation of drug prior to absorption increases bioavailability
D. Hydrophilic drugs are less able to cross lipid-rich cell membranes than hydrophobic drugs
E. IV administration yields 100% bioavailability

52. After 0.6 g of Drug A was administered intravenously, the plasma concentration is 100 g/L. What is the correct volume of distribution of Drug A in liters?

A. 6
B. 60
C. 0.167
D. 166.67
E. 0.006

53. Which of the following is correct regarding side effects of angiotensin-converting enzyme (ACE) inhibitors?

A. Hypertension
B. Hyperkalemia
C. Cough
D. Cerebral edema
E. Depression

54. The plasma concentration of drug X is 150 mg/L, and it is eliminated from the body at a rate of 3 mg/min. Which of the following is the clearance rate of drug X?

A. 0.2 L/min
B. 0.02 L/min
C. 2 L/min
D. 50 L/min
E. 200 L/min

55. All of the following statements are correct regarding penicillin, *except*:

A. Penicillin is a bactericidal antibiotic that works by binding to penicillin-binding protein, and blocking transpeptidase from crosslinking peptidylglycine in bacterial cell wall
B. Not all penicillins are effective against *Pseudomonas aeruginosa*
C. Amoxicillin can cover both *Escherichia coli* and *Haemophilus influenzae*
D. Combined with clavulanic acid or tazobactam, penicillins possess anti-beta lactamase activity
E. Penicillin is a bacteriostatic antibiotic that works by inhibiting bacterial protein synthesis

1. **The correct answer is B.** Nifedipine is an example of a calcium channel blocker (CCB). These drugs work by blocking calcium entry into smooth muscle cells of the heart and its associated arteries. Calcium is responsible for heart contraction and narrowing of the arteries, and its inhibition results in vasodilation of coronary and peripheral blood vessels and decreased contraction force (negative inotropic effect) and rate (negative chronotropic effect). CCBs are used for treating hypertension, angina, and arrhythmias. Side effects of CCBs include gingival hyperplasia and orthostatic hypotension. Other drugs that cause gingival hyperplasia include phenytoin and cyclosporine.

Lisinopril is an example of an ACE inhibitor; is used for treating hypertension and heart failure, prevention of strokes, and kidney failure; and improves survival after heart attacks. ACE inhibitors work by inhibiting the enzyme ACE, which catalyzes the conversion of angiotensin I to angiotensin II, a potent vasoconstrictor and stimulant of aldosterone. As a result, blood vessels dilate and sodium and water retention is reduced. In addition, ACE inhibition blocks the breakdown of bradykinin, a vasodilator. The side effects of ACE inhibitors can be remembered using the mnemonic "CAPTO-PRIL" (another example of an ACE inhibitor), which stands for: cough, angioedema, potassium excess, taste changes, orthostatic hypotension, pregnancy contraindication, rash, indomethacin inhibition, liver toxicity. Gingival hyperplasia is not on this list.

Atenolol is an example of a beta adrenergic receptor blocker. Beta blockers inhibit beta adrenergic substances from affecting the sympathetic nervous system. In the heart, their effect is to lower cardiac output and decrease the workload of the heart, resulting in reduced peripheral pressure. These drugs are used for hypertension, angina, arrhythmias, and migraine headaches. Side effects include orthostatic hypotension and difficulty breathing, particularly in asthmatics.

Simvastatin is an example of HMG-CoA reductase inhibitors (statins) that block the rate-limiting step in cholesterol synthesis. This class of drugs is used to control hypercholesterolemia and coronary artery disease. Adverse effects of statins include muscle pain, with an increased risk of muscle toxicity (rhabdomyolysis) when these drugs are taken concomitantly with drugs that inhibit the CYP3A4 enzyme system, including erythromycin and azole antifungals.

Albuterol is an example of a beta-2 adrenergic agonist, meaning that it stimulates beta-2 receptors located on the muscles surrounding the airways. Stimulation of these receptors induces bronchodilation. It is taken via inhalation to treat acute asthmatic attacks. Side effects include anxiety, tremors, fast heart rate, and throat irritation.

2. **The correct answer is D.** Based on the signs and symptoms that the patient described above is experiencing, he is most likely suffering from a gastrointestinal (GI) problem. All of the answer choices are mechanisms of drugs that are used to treat GI upset (i.e., duodenal ulcers, gastroesophageal reflux disease (GERD), or Zollinger–Ellison syndrome) and choice D best describes the mechanism of cimetidine, an antihistamine H2 blocker. H2 receptor blockers complete with histamine only in the GI tract and consequently interrupt the signal for the parietal cell to secrete acid, resulting in overall decreased acid secretion. When a patient is on cimetidine, it is also important to be aware of potential drug interactions that may occur because it is a CYP3A4 inhibitor and can increase levels of drugs metabolized in the liver by the CYP3A4 enzyme. Other H2 blockers (i.e., ranitidine, famotidine) are not associated with these potential interactions.

Helicobacter pylori is a bacterium that is associated with gastritis, duodenal or stomach ulcers (especially recurrent ulcers), and stomach cancer, including MALT lymphoma. Infection with this bacterium is most likely acquired from contaminated food or water and must be treated with antibiotics. Because *H. pylori* is capable of developing resistance to commonly used antibiotics, usually two or more antibiotics are prescribed along with a proton pump inhibitor (PPI) and/or bismuth-containing compound to eradicate this bacterium.

Antacids are used to treat GI upset associated with heartburn (dyspepsia) and acid indigestion. Antacids work by neutralizing excess stomach acid (increasing pH). Antacids work relatively quickly and are meant for short-term relief. The differences in how fast antacids work and for how long they provide relief depends on what ingredients (aluminum, calcium, magnesium, sodium bicarbonate) they contain.

Antimuscarinic drugs (i.e., atropine) are responsible for decreased gastric secretions and decreased GI motility. Because of these effects, in addition to being used to treat heartburn and acid indigestion, they may also be used to treat diarrhea, to prevent secretions (gastric and salivary) preoperatively, and to prevent/reduce motion sickness.

Proton pump inhibitors (i.e., omeprazole) are also used to treat acid-related GI conditions and work by blocking the H^+/K^+ ATPase pumps on parietal cells that are directly responsible for secreting H^+ ions into the stomach. By targeting the terminal step in acid secretion, PPIs are more potent than H2 blockers at reducing acid secretion.

3. **The correct answer is E.** Crohn's disease is a chronic inflammatory condition that can affect the entire digestive system. There is no cure for this disease; its symptoms can be minimized and sent into remission with anti-inflammatory medications and immune modulators. On the basis of the symptoms this patient has experienced as a side effect of taking a drug to treat her Crohn's disease, it is likely that she had been taking a systemic corticosteroid to reduce inflammation. Long-term use of corticosteroids can suppress the ability of the adrenal glands to produce natural cortisol and as a result when these drugs are discontinued abruptly, the body can display symptoms of adrenal insufficiency (adrenal crisis), like the patient above did during the dental procedure, because of a lack of natural cortisol. To prevent the above scenario, gradually taper the dose when discontinuing corticosteroids and take an extra dose prior to stressful situations for up to 2 years after discontinuing the drug. The best answer choice would be Hydrocortisone (2-mL dose), an artificial corticosteroid,

which would temporarily relieve the symptoms of adrenal insufficiency.

Oxygen is useful in every emergency, with the exception of hyperventilation. Oxygen would have been helpful to get the patient through the symptoms of the adrenal crisis; however, it would not have been sufficient to alleviate the crisis.

Epinephrine is the drug of choice to treat anaphylaxis in the dental chair. Signs of anaphylaxis would include flushing and itching of the skin, feelings of anxiety, rapid pulse, and difficulty breathing. Epinephrine is typically given intramuscularly and has a very rapid onset and short duration of action. Epinephrine can also be used to treat an asthma attack that does not initially respond to a beta-2 agonist such as albuterol.

Nitroglycerine is used in the case of acute angina attack or myocardial infarction in the dental office. It is given sublingually, as a tablet or spray, and has a rapid onset. When a patient experiences signs of angina, one dose should be given. If relief does not occur, second and third doses can be given at 5-minute intervals. It is also useful to have an automated external defibrillator (AED) available in the office in the case of cardiac arrest.

Sugar, either in an oral form or injectable form, is indicated for the management of hypoglycemia. Conscious patients will be able to take an oral source of sugar, such as fruit juice, whereas unconscious patients will require IM glucagon or IV dextrose. When treating diabetic patients, it is important to ask about their most recent HBA1c and daily blood glucose levels and to be aware of their risk of hypoglycemia, as often times patients will take their medications for diabetes and then skip a meal prior to their dental visits.

4. **The correct answer is C.** Beta-blockers inhibit endogenous catecholamines (i.e., epinephrine) from stimulating beta adrenergic receptors, part of the sympathetic nervous system. There are two types of beta receptors, beta-1 and beta-2, located mainly in the heart and the lungs, respectively. When beta-1 receptors are blocked, the result is reduced cardiac output and decreased workload of the heart because of negative chronotropic and inotropic effects. When beta-2 receptors are

blocked, the result is bronchoconstriction. On the basis of the cardiac effects, beta blockers are indicated for the treatment of hypertrophic cardiomyopathy, a condition in which the cardiac muscle is hypertrophic without any obvious cause. All of the answer choices are examples of beta blockers; however, because this patient also has asthma, it would be advisable to use a cardioselective beta blocker, specific for beta-1, which will not cause the unwanted side effect of bronchospasm, sometimes observed when non-selective beta blockers are taken. The only example above of a cardioselective beta blocker is metoprolol.

Propranolol is a nonselective beta blocker, also referred to as a beta-adrenergic blocking agent, beta-adrenergic antagonist, or a beta-antagonist. In general, beta blockers are used for hypertension, cardiac arrhythmias, chest pain (angina), migraine headaches, and glaucoma.

Labetalol is a mixed alpha-1 and beta blocker. By also blocking alpha-1, there is an additional vasodilation effect. Because of the additional alpha-1 blockade, it is important to be aware of the risk of orthostatic hypotension when the patient leaves the dental chair. Labetalol is used to treat hypertension and is specifically indicated to treat pregnancy-induced hypertension. Pregnancy-induced hypertension (HTN) is often associated with pre-eclampsia, a condition in which there is increased protein in the urine (proteinuria).

Nadolol and timolol are nonselective beta blockers.

5. **The correct answer is D.** Zoledronic acid is an example of a bisphosphonate used to treat conditions of the bones, such as osteoporosis, osteopenia, Paget disease, or hypercalcemia of malignancy. Bisphosphonates are antibone resorbers that work by inhibiting the actions of osteoclasts. Side effects of bisphosphonates include: irritation of the esophagus (potentially causing perforations), headaches, muscle and joint pain, constipation, diarrhea, flatulence, dysphagia, and risk of osteonecrosis. Choice D is therefore the best answer. To best reduce the incidence of esophageal perforation, it is recommended to take the oral drugs in the morning with a full glass of water at least 30 minutes prior to intake of any other substance and to sit or stand for at least 30 minutes after ingestion of the drug.

Drug-induced hemolytic anemia may occur when a drug causes the immune system to react against its red blood cells. Drugs that may have this effect include: cephalosporins and penicillins, levodopa (used to treat Parkinson disease), methyldopa (an alpha-2 agonist used to treat hypertension), quinidine, and some anti-inflammatory drugs.

Xerostomia, or dry mouth, is not a disease, rather a symptom of other medical conditions or a side effect of numerous medications. The major classes of drugs that cause xerostomia are antihistamines, antidepressants, anticholinergics, antihypertensives, antipsychotics, anti-Parkinson agents, diuretics, sedatives, and anorexiants.

Edema is defined as the retention of fluid in an organ or in the body that results in swelling. Drugs that may cause edema include chemotherapy agents (such as rituximab that is also used for rheumatoid arthritis) and corticosteroids (such as prednisone).

Orthostatic hypotension (or postural hypotension) occurs when there is a sudden drop in blood pressure. This side effect is often seen in patients taking drugs that have an alpha-1 blocking effect. Drugs with this effect include those used to treat hypertension, such as alpha-blocking agents (i.e., terazosin), mixed alpha- and beta-blocking agents (i.e., carvedilol, labetalol), calcium channel blockers (i.e., nifedipine, verapamil), and antidepressants, both tricyclics (i.e., amitriptyline) and monoamine oxidase inhibitors (i.e., phenelzine).

6. **The correct answer is C.** The therapeutic index (TI) is defined as a number, LD_{50}/ED_{50}, the ratio comparing the lethal dose of a drug for 50% of the population to the effective dose of a drug for 50% of the population. A drug with a high (or broad) index can typically be given with greater safety than one with a low (or narrow) index. Digoxin, for example, has a very low TI and requires close monitoring of the patient's blood levels to minimize the occurrence of adverse reactions. The therapeutic index is usually calculated from data obtained from experiments

with animals. The comparison of the LD_{50} and ED_{50} is most significant when the dose-effect curves from which these median doses are inferred are parallel (see graph below). The therapeutic index can also be calculated using data that does not include lethal effects and instead applies the median dose causing minimally toxic effects (TD_{50}). The safety index is defined as a number, LD_1/ED_{99}, the ratio comparing the lethal dose of a drug in 1% of the population to the effective dose in 99% of the population. The safety index indicates by what percentage of itself a dose must be exceeded to produce a lethal effect in just 1% of the population. Clinically, the safety index is more practical than the therapeutic index, and unlike the therapeutic index, the determination of the safety index does not depend on the parallelism of the dose-effect curves from which the LD_1 and ED_{99} are inferred. On the basis of the following calculations, choice C is correct. TI = LD_{50}/ED_{50} = 30 mg/5 mg = 6. Safety index = LD_1/ED_{99} = 20 mg/10 mg = 2.

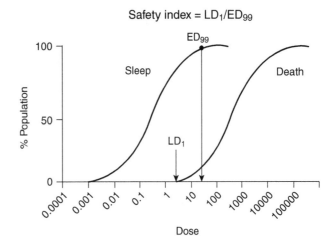

In choice E, these values were determined by calculating LD_{50}/ED_{99} and LD_1/ED_{50}, of which neither are the correct formulas for therapeutic index and safety index.

Answer choice F is the reverse of those in choice E and again, neither of the formulas used are representative of therapeutic index or safety index.

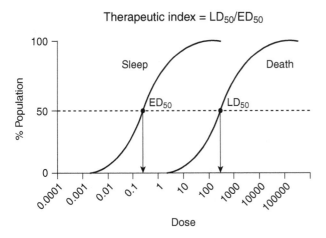

In answer choice A, these values were determined by calculating the ED_{99}/ED_{50} and LD_{50}/LD_1, of which neither are the correct formulas for therapeutic index and safety index.

In answer choice B, these values are the reverse of those in choice A and again, neither of the formulas used are representative of therapeutic index and safety index.

Answer choice D is incorrect because the values are determined by reversing the formulas for therapeutic index and safety margin.

7. **The correct answer is C.** The first step is to determine the local anesthetic concentration of 2% lidocaine present in one carpule on the basis of one carpule containing 1.8 mL of fluid. The following formula is used: 2% = 2 g/100 mL = 2,000 mg/100 mL = 20 mg/mL; 20 mg/mL × 1.8 mL/carpule = 36 mg/carpule. There are 36 mg/carpule in a 2% solution of lidocaine. The next step is to take into account the maximum recommended dosage (MRD) for lidocaine, which is 2.0 to 3.2 mg/lb (or 4.5–7.0 mg/kg). For a 40-pound child, 40 lb × 2.0 to 3.2 mg/lb = 80 to 128 mg. On the basis of this range and the knowledge that there are 36 mg/carpule in a 2% lidocaine solution, the following formulas are used: 80 mg/36 mg/carpule = 2.2 carpules and 128 mg/36 mg/carpule = 3.5 carpules. The high end of the acceptable range is 3.5 carpules; therefore, three carpules would be an acceptable volume to administer.

One and two carpules would be acceptable amounts of anesthetic to give; however, it would not be the *maximum* recommended dose.

Four and five carpules are greater than the acceptable range for the maximum recommended dose.

8. **The correct answer is E.** The American Heart Association guidelines for antibiotic prophylaxis were revised in April 2007. According to the new guidelines, patients requiring prophylaxis include those with a history of prosthetic cardiac valve, history of previous infective endocarditis, history of congenital heart disease, and history of cardiac transplantation resulting in cardiac valvulopathy. It is no longer recommended to prescribe antibiotics for those patients with a history of mitral valve prolapse. The guidelines also define which procedures do and do not require antibiotic prophylaxis. Periodontal surgery would require antibiotic prophylaxis, along with any procedure that involves manipulation of gingival tissue, the periapical region of teeth, and the perforation of the oral mucosa. Procedures that do not require antibiotic prophylaxis include: routine anesthetic, injections through noninfected tissue, taking dental radiographs, placement of removable prosthodontic or orthodontic appliances, adjustment of orthodontic appliances, placement of orthodontic brackets, shedding of deciduous teeth, and bleeding from trauma to the lips or the oral mucosa. The guidelines did not change for those patients with a history of prosthetic joint replacement.

In the case that a patient has one of the four conditions requiring antibiotic prophylaxis and had no allergy to penicillin, 2 g of amoxicillin would be an appropriate prescription to cover the patient for the three different surgical procedures.

Four grams of amoxicillin would be more than necessary to give for antibiotic prophylaxis prior to each procedure.

Patients who have one of the four conditions requiring antibiotic prophylaxis and who are also allergic to penicillin require 600 mg of clindamycin 1 hour prior to their surgical procedures. Twelve hundred milligram of clindamycin would be more than necessary to give for antibiotic prophylaxis prior to each procedure.

9. **The correct answer is B.** The patient described above was taking antitubercular medications to treat tuberculosis (TB), a bacterial infection caused by *Mycobacterium tuberculosis*. It is caused by inhalation of the bacteria and can easily be spread in crowded areas such as homeless shelters. The medications listed above are typically given together for 2 months in the case of active infection, and after 2 months, only two drugs are continued. Active infection is determined by a positive skin test, an abnormal chest x-ray, and sputum containing TB bacteria. Treatment can continue for months or years depending on the patient. If a patient has TB in an inactive state, an antibiotic, typically isoniazid, may be given alone. Rifampin is metabolized largely in the liver by the CYP450 enzyme system, and it is, therefore, important to be aware of the effect it can have on the metabolism of other drugs metabolized by CYP450 enzymes, including oral contraceptives, warfarin, and azole antifungals. One of the oral signs of TB is a chronic nonhealing ulcer, most commonly on the dorsum of the tongue, which occurs following lung infection. The differential diagnosis of a tuberculosis ulcer should also include: aphthous ulcers, traumatic ulcers, syphilitic ulcers, and malignancy. The diagnosis can be confirmed by the presence of acid-fast bacilli in the specimen.

Linea alba is an example of a mucosal lesion caused by trauma, typically cheek biting. It appears as a raised white line in the buccal mucosa, usually along the plane of occlusion. Under a microscope, it appears as hyperkeratosis. It is a variation of normal and therefore requires no pharmacologic treatment.

Perioral vesicles are associated with the herpes simplex virus. Primary infection is predominant among children. The virus cannot be cured with medications and remains latent in the trigeminal ganglion. Pharmacologic treatment for herpes virus is aimed at treating the symptoms. Topical agents to treat the vesicles include 1% penciclovir cream. In addition, antiviral medications, such as acyclovir (mechanism: inhibits viral DNA synthesis), valacyclovir, and famciclovir, can be effective when given systemically and when initiated early; however, the symptoms usually resolve on their own in 10 to 14 days.

Hairy leukoplakia is associated with the Epstein–Barr virus and occurs mostly in people infected with HIV. Hairy leukoplakia is an opportunistic infection that presents as a nonpainful white plaque along the lateral borders of the tongue. Hairy leukoplakia does not always require treatment. When it is treated, the following medications may be used: systemic antivirals (to slow down EBV), and topical agents such as podophyllum resin solution and tretinoin (retinoic acid).

Lichen planus is thought to be caused by cytotoxic cell-mediated hypersensitivity and is sometimes associated with hepatitis C. Lichen planus appears as a white, lacy rash (Wickham's striae) on the buccal mucosa. Certain drugs, such as those containing arsenic, bismuth, or gold, can cause a response in the oral mucosa that is indistinguishable from lichen planus. In addition, long-term use of antimalaria drugs, such as quinidine, may produce lichen planus. No treatment is required for asymptomatic lesions. If symptomatic (itchiness, unpleasant appearance), topical steroid creams, antihistamines, or systemic steroids can be used. If the question above described a patient with hepatitis C, he may have been taking the following antiviral medications: interferon (peginterferon) or ribavirin.

10. **The correct answer is A.** Amitriptyline is an example of a tricyclic antidepressant (TCA). TCAs work by inhibiting the reuptake of norepinephrine and serotonin at nerve terminals. Their application is based on the theory that abnormal levels of these neurotransmitters may relate to depression in some patients. TCAs in general have an anticholinergic effect, and therefore adverse reactions may include: xerostomia, urinary retention, constipation, increased ocular pressure, and mydriasis. Other classes of drugs associated with xerostomia include: anticholinergics, anticonvulsants, antihistamines, antihypertensives, antiparkinsonians, antipsychotics, antispasmodics, appetite suppressants, barbiturates, bronchodilators, decongestants, diuretics, hypnotics, muscle relaxants, and opioid analgesics.

Aspirin is the most popular antiplatelet drug and is available over-the-counter. Doses range from 81 to 325 mg/day to prevent myocardial infarctions and occlusive strokes in high-risk people. Aspirin works by irreversibly inhibiting platelet aggregation. Because of its irreversible nature, it needs to be discontinued for 5 to 7 days to allow for normal clotting following the synthesis of new platelets. Other applications of aspirin are: (1) an analgesic for minor aches and pains, (2) an antipyretic to reduce fever, and (3) an anti-inflammatory medication. Adverse effects of aspirin include GI ulcers, stomach bleeding, prolonged bleeding, tinnitus, and an increased risk of Reye syndrome (characterized by acute encephalopathy and fatty liver) in children with viral diseases.

Pilocarpine is a nonselective cholinergic agonist. It has a direct effect on muscarinic acetylcholine receptors and can be applied topically. It produces rapid miosis and contraction of ciliary muscles and is used by patients with glaucoma. It also stimulates the secretion of large amounts of saliva and sweat and is used to treat xerostomia, rather than cause xerostomia. Adverse effects of pilocarpine relate to its nonselective nature and include: excessive sweating and salivation, bronchospasm and increased bronchial mucous secretion, bradycardia, hypotension, and diarrhea.

Nabumetone is an example of a nonsteroidal anti-inflammatory drug (NSAID). NSAIDs work by inhibiting the enzyme cyclooxygenase, resulting in lower concentrations of prostaglandins, chemicals produced by the body that are responsible for inflammation, pain, and fever. Nabumetone may be taken once a day for long term by patients with osteoarthritis and rheumatoid arthritis. The most common side effects of nabumetone affect the GI system. To reduce the incidence of GI ulceration with chronic use of this drug, a prostaglandin analog (i.e., misoprostol) may also be prescribed. Prostaglandin analogs must be used with caution because of their potential as an abortive agent or labor inducer. Other drugs used to treat osteoarthritis include: aspirin or acetaminophen, selective COX-2 inhibitors, prednisone injections, and topical capsaicin.

Physostigmine is an indirect acting cholinergic agonist that exerts its effect by reversibly inhibiting cholinesterase from breaking down acetylcholine, thereby increasing the level and duration of action of acetylcholine in the neuromuscular junction. It has several clinical applications, including glaucoma, urinary retention, reversal of neuromuscular junction blockage, and myasthenia gravis. Researchers have also found some potential for its use in treating depression and Alzheimer disease. Adverse reactions include the potential to cause SLUDGE, an acronym for a cholinergic syndrome with the following characteristics: salivation, lacrimation, urination, diarrhea, GI cramping, and emesis.

11. **The correct answer is B**. Disulfiram is used in the treatment of chronic alcoholism by causing an acute sensitivity to alcohol. The underlying mechanism is the accumulation of acetaldehyde in the blood because of inhibition of hepatic aldehyde dehydrogenase by disulfiram. Acetaldehyde is one of the major causes of the symptoms of a "hangover." Within minutes of its accumulation, the individual can become acutely ill with a severe "hangover," experiencing generalized flushing, nausea, vomiting, headache, and more serious symptoms, such as accelerated heart rate and circulatory collapse. There are several other drugs that can produce this disulfiram-like effect including: phenacetin, antibiotics, such as nitrofurantoin, cephalosporins, and metronidazole, anti-angina medication (nitrates), and first-generation sulfonylureas, such as chlorpropamide and tolbutamide. Metronidazole works by inhibiting DNA bacterial synthesis, exclusively against strict anaerobic infections.

Clarithromycin is in the class of macrolide antibiotics that exert their effects by inhibiting bacterial protein synthesis. Clarithromycin should be prescribed with caution to patients taking other drugs that interact with the CYP3A4 enzyme, found largely in the liver. Because clarithromycin is a CYP3A4 substrate, it may cause increased serum levels of other drugs that are CYP3A4 substrates, including several benzodiazepines, calcium channel blockers, immunosuppressants, statins, SSRIs, TCAs, azole antifungals, and others such as mirtazapine, nefazodone, venlafaxine, terfenadine, cisapride, theophylline, and warfarin. It is also possible for other drugs, CYP3A4 inhibitors and CYP3A4 inducers, to cause increased or decreased levels of clarithromycin, resulting in adverse reactions or ineffectiveness, respectively.

Clindamycin is an antibiotic that works by inhibiting bacterial protein synthesis. The most severe common adverse effect of clindamycin is *Clostridium difficile*-associated diarrhea (the most frequent cause of pseudomembranous colitis, a potentially lethal condition). This side effect can occur with other antibiotics as well but most commonly occurs with clindamycin use. Because clindamycin concentrates in bone, it is often used in dentistry to treat periapical bony infections.

Doxycycline is a member of the tetracycline class of antibiotics, another group of antibiotics that works by inhibition of bacterial protein synthesis. Significant adverse effects of doxycycline include photosensitivity and discoloration of teeth and inhibition of bone growth when taken during development in infants and children.

Rifampin is antituberculosis drug. The most serious adverse effect of rifampin is related to its hepatotoxicity.

12. **The correct answer is C**. Analgesic agents, such as narcotics, are commonly prescribed by dentists to treat emergencies and preoperative and postoperative pain. Dentists may prescribe medications and controlled substances only for dental-related conditions. The ADA defines dentistry as follows: "... the evaluation, diagnosis, prevention and/or treatment (nonsurgical, surgical or related procedures) of diseases, disorders and/or conditions of the oral cavity, maxillofacial area and/or the adjacent and associated structures and their impact on the human body; provided by a dentist, within the scope of his/her education, training and experience, in accordance with the ethics of the profession and applicable law." Any medication that falls within the scope of this definition can be prescribed by a dentist. Under no circumstances may a dentist prescribe anything outside the course of his/her practice of dentistry. To do so is a serious violation of the laws and regulations, and a dentist may be disciplined by the Board. A dentist must avoid self-prescribing, and any medications prescribed for office staff or family members must be solely for dental-related conditions and must be clearly and specifically documented in the patient's file.

Oral contraceptives, antihypertensives, antidiabetic agents, amphetamines, and antiasthmatics do not fall within the scope of dentistry and therefore should not be prescribed by a dental practitioner.

13. **The correct answer is D.** Ginkgo balboa is mainly used as a memory and concentration enhancer and to treat circulatory disorders. Like many alternative medications, there is much conflicting research on its effectiveness. Some laboratory studies have shown that ginkgo balboa improves blood circulation by dilating blood vessels and blocking the effects of platelet-activating factor. Because of its potential effect to improve blood flow, ginkgo balboa is often taken by patients with intermittent claudication (pain caused by inadequate blood flow to the legs). Because ginkgo balboa decreases the aggregation ability of platelets, there is some concern that its use, particularly when combined with other anticoagulants, such as aspirin, puts patients at increased risk of bleeding. Of special concern is the increased risk of intracranial hemorrhage.

Ginseng has multiple traditional uses including: improving recovery from illness and well-being, treating erectile dysfunction, hepatitis C, and symptoms associated with menopause, lowering blood sugar, and controlling blood pressure. Given the diversity of its uses, it may be taken by many patients who believe in the use of complementary medicine. The most common side effects of ginseng are headaches and GI upset. An important precaution in the use of ginseng should be given to patients with diabetes because of its potential to lower blood sugar.

Echinacea is traditionally used to treat or prevent colds or the flu by boosting the immune system. Side effects include allergic reactions or GI upset.

St. John's Wort is one of the most commonly used herbal supplements in the United States. It is used to help mild-to-moderate depression. It can enhance the effects of anesthesia, and because St. John's Wort induces CYP3A4 in the gut and liver, it may decrease the metabolism of other CYP3A4 substrates, which includes at least half of marketed medications, including some anesthetics.

Capsaicin is the active ingredient in chili peppers. It is usually used in a topical cream form to relieve pain and itching. For instance, a dental practitioner may recommend it to patients

with postherpetic neuralgia. Capsaicin works by depleting substance P, a neurotransmitters that signals pain. Side effects of capsaicin include a burning sensation in the area it is applied, redness, and skin blisters.

14. **The correct answer is D.** Celecoxib is an example of a selective COX-2 inhibitor. This class of drugs works by blocking the facultative COX-2 isoenzyme but sparing the constitutive COX-1 isoenzyme. Both cyclooxygenase enzymes are responsible for the conversion of arachidonic acid to prostaglandins. The main distinction is that prostaglandins whose production requires the COX-1 isoenzyme are responsible for protection of the gastric mucosa, whereas the prostaglandins whose synthesis involves COX-2 are responsible for inflammation and pain. Traditional NSAIDs work by inhibiting both COX-1 and COX-2, thereby decreasing inflammation and pain and decreasing cytoprotection of the GI tract. Selective COX-2 inhibitors work only to decrease inflammation and pain. Chronic use of traditional NSAIDs (6–12 months) in the treatment of osteoarthritis and rheumatoid arthritis is associated with approximately 1% to 3% yearly incidence of clinically significant GI ulcers. With chronic dosing, celecoxib reduces the incidence of GI perforations, ulcerations, and bleeds by approximately 50% to 60% compared with conventional NSAIDs. An area of concern when taking selective COX-2 inhibitors is the implication that COX-1 is working unopposed, which means it is continually contributing to the synthesis of thromboxane, involved in platelet aggregation, thereby increasing the risk of thrombotic events.

Traditional NSAIDs and celecoxib are equally effective as analgesics for acute postsurgical pain than celecoxib since both drugs inhibit the desired target—COX-2 prostaglandins. Some sources states that traditional NSAIDs are actually more effective and are comparable to narcotics as an analgesic without the CNS-mediated side effects.

Traditional NSAIDs and celecoxib also produce equal anti-inflammatory responses in osteoarthritis patients, although celecoxib may be preferred because of the tendency for osteoarthritis patients to use these drugs for long term.

Traditional NSAIDs and celecoxib have similar effects on renal function as measured by glomerular filtration rate, creatinine clearance, and urinary and serum sodium and potassium values. Selective COX-2 inhibition may transiently increase sodium retention.

Traditional NSAIDs and celecoxib have similar antipyretic qualities.

15. **The correct answer is B**. The most likely cause of these symptoms is an overdose of acetaminophen (APAP). APAP is used as an analgesic and antipyretic. Its exact mechanism is unknown. APAP is metabolized in the liver by CYP2E1 to N-acetyl-benzoquinoneimine (NAPQI), a toxic by-product, which is later inactivated by glutathione. In the case of an overdose, glutathione stores are depleted and NAPQI damages hepatocytes. Signs of liver toxicity include hepatomegaly, jaundice, GI bleeding, and encephalopathy. Death may occur because of cerebral edema, sepsis, or multiorgan failure. Treatment may include the ingestion of activated charcoal or the antidote, N-acetylcysteine. These are best given within 12 hours before the liver damage becomes irreversible. If treatment is not initiated quickly enough, liver failure may ensue requiring a liver transplant. It is important for parents to pay close attention to the dosages of medications that they provide to their children. For children younger than 12 years and/or less than 50 kg in weight, the maximum daily dosage of acetaminophen is 80 mg/kg (not to exceed a cumulative daily dose of 2.6 g). Weight-based oral dosing for children is 10 to 15 mg/kg every 4 to 6 hours with a maximum of five doses per 24-hour period.

Aspirin is an irreversible inhibitor of COX-1. It serves as an analgesic, antipyretic and, anti-inflammatory agent and inhibits platelet aggregation. Adverse effects of aspirin include: GI irritation, tinnitus, vertigo, hypersensitivity, and bleeding complications. An additional adverse effect that many parents may not be aware of is its ability to serve as a trigger for Reye syndrome, a highly lethal disease. To avoid Reye syndrome, aspirin (and its derivatives) should not be given to children with chicken pox or influenza B infection. Reye syndrome may be misdiagnosed as a drug overdose and blood work would be helpful to confirm the diagnosis. The treatment for Reye syndrome should include: hypertonic IV glucose solutions and mechanical ventilation.

Codeine is an example of a narcotic used as an analgesic agent and sometimes for its antitussive and antidiarrheal properties. Narcotics are centrally acting drugs that work by binding to opiate receptors (opiate agonist). In the case of codeine, which is a prodrug, its active metabolites, including morphine, bind to the opiate receptors. Codeine is converted to morphine via the CYP2D6 enzyme, and because of its interaction with the CYP450 enzyme system, its serum levels are susceptible to changes by interactions with other drugs (i.e., CYP2d6 inducers). A potentially serious side effect of codeine toxicity is respiratory depression, and in the case of a codeine overdose, the reversal agent, naloxone, should be given. Codeine, like other narcotics, can cause a physical or psychological dependence as well as tolerance to the drug to develop.

Celecoxib is a variation of an NSAID and is classified as a selective COX-2 inhibitor. It is used in patients with gastric ulcers when the inhibition of COX-1 should be avoided. It has similar anti-inflammatory effects as traditional NSAIDs. According to some research, when celecoxib is used for long term, it is capable of producing cardiotoxicity.

Ibuprofen is a traditional NSAID that works by nonselectively inhibiting COX-1 and COX-2. Ibuprofen has analgesic, antipyretic, and anti-inflammatory effects. The major concern with the overuse of ibuprofen is the increased risk of GI ulcerations and GI bleeding and nephrotoxicity.

16. **The correct answer is B**. A drug with minimal protein binding is *least* likely to contribute to a significant adverse drug interaction. On the other hand, drugs that are highly protein bound can be displaced by other drugs that are highly protein bound when taken simultaneously. For instance, warfarin is typically 99% plasma protein bound, meaning that only 1% of the drug

is free and therefore only 1% is active. Drugs like aspirin or other salicylates will compete for the protein receptor sites that warfarin has a tendency to bind to. This competition will cause displacement of warfarin, resulting in greater availability of the drug and therefore an increased effect, which in warfarin's case can result in increased bleeding.

Therapeutic index (TI) represents the margin of safety of a drug. Drugs with a low (or narrow) TI have a small margin of safety. TI is equivalent to LD_{50}/ED_{50}, or the lethal dose in 50% of patients compared with the effective dose in 50% of patients. If a drug has a low TI, such as a TI of 3, this means that if only three times as much as the effective dose is taken, there is a 50% chance for a lethal effect.

Drugs that are metabolized by the CYP450 enzyme system in the liver are subject to changes in metabolism when taken concomitantly with other drugs that modify the activity of the CYP450 system. Many drugs may increase or decrease the activity of CYP450 by acting as an inducer or inhibitor, respectively, and resulting in depletion or accumulation of the drug in question, respectively.

Drugs that are enzyme inducers, as in those associated with the CYP450 system, have the potential to speed up metabolism of a drug, thereby depleting the presence of the drug.

The volume of distribution is used to describe the quantity of medication in the plasma and the rest of the body. Drugs with a low volume of distribution have a higher concentration in the plasma and the potential for greater activity.

17. **The correct answer is B**. St. John's Wort is a CYP3A4 inducer. As an inducer, St. John's Wort causes the CYP3A4 enzyme (part of the CYP450 enzyme system) to become more active. Drugs that are substrates of CYP3A4 are therefore metabolized more rapidly, and their blood levels are reduced. In the case of oral contraceptives, if inadequate amounts of hormone are present, the overall effectiveness of the oral contraceptive may be reduced. Patients taking St. John's Wort may require increased dosages of other drugs. Other examples of CYP3A4 substrates include calcium channel blockers, cyclosporine, ben-

zodiazepines, azole antifungals, erythromycin and clarithromycin, antiretrovirals, statins, and SSRIs.

St. John's Wort does not block active secretion of the oral contraceptive, does not affect stomach acidity, does not block estrogen and progesterone receptors, and does not decrease serotonin levels in the brain. The exact mechanism by which St. John's Wort functions to decrease depression is unclear. However, it is believed that one way the herbal product is thought to exert its effect is by inhibiting the reuptake of serotonin, thereby increasing levels of serotonin in the brain.

18. **The correct answer is E**. If Drugs X and Z both have a tendency to be highly bound to plasma proteins, then when Drug Z is introduced there would be an increased competition for protein binding sites. This would cause displacement of Drug X from plasma proteins, and the result would be increased free Drug X in the plasma, resulting in increased free blood levels of Drug X. An example of this interaction occurs when aspirin is introduced in a patient who is currently taking warfarin.

Drugs that induce liver microsomal enzymes increase their activity. If Drug Z was an inducer, and assuming that Drug X was a substrate of liver microsomal enzymes, then increasing the activity of the enzymes would speed up the metabolism of Drug X. If Drug X was metabolized more rapidly, decreased blood levels of Drug X would be expected.

If Drugs X and Z formed a chelation product in the intestine, this would result in decreased free levels of Drug X. For example, when a patient taking tetracycline also takes an antacid (or ingests any food product containing divalent and trivalent cations), the components of the antacid will form a chelation product with tetracycline. When tetracycline is bound to another molecule through chelation, this translates to decreased free levels of tetracycline, resulting in decreased absorption of tetracycline and decreased effectiveness.

If Drug Z increased the glomerular filtration rate, and it was assumed that Drug X was excreted via the kidneys, this would result in more rapid excretion of Drug X. If the elimination of

Drug X is increased, then the free blood levels of Drug X are decreased.

If Drug Z has a positive inotropic and chronotropic effect, this would have little effect on the blood levels of Drug X. Positive inotropic drugs (examples include digoxin, epinephrine, and amrinone) increase the strength of muscle contraction of the heart. Positive chronotropic drugs (examples include atropine, dopamine, and epinephrine) increase heart rate. While both of these types of agents may increase blood flow through the body, they have no effect on the concentration of drugs in the blood.

19. **The correct answer is D.** Codeine is a narcotic with analgesic, antidiarrheal, and antitussive properties. It is classified as a Schedule III drug and has the potential for drug abuse and dependence. Codeine is readily absorbed from the GI tract, is not bound to plasma proteins, is eliminated primarily through the kidneys, reaches its peak analgesic effect within 2 hours, and persists between 4 and 6 hours. Codeine is considered a prodrug. In the liver, codeine is converted to the active compounds morphine and codeine-6-glucuronide, which exert their effects by binding to opiate receptors. This reaction is catalyzed by the cytochrome P450 enzyme, CYP2D6. Drugs that inhibit CYP2D6 prevent this conversion to active compounds from occurring, thereby reducing the overall effectiveness of codeine. Examples of strong CYP2D6 inhibitors include selective-serotonin reuptake inhibitors (SSRIs), such as fluoxetine (choice D) and paroxetine, other antidepressants, such as bupropion, terbinafine, and quinidine.

Terazosin is an alpha-adrenergic blocker. By blocking the alpha-1 receptor, terazosin causes vasodilation, thereby lowering blood pressure, and smooth muscle relaxation, particularly in the prostate. Terazosin is indicated for hypertension and benign prostate hyperplasia. The most important drug interactions to be aware of in a patient taking terazosin is if the patient is taking additional antihypertensives or vasodilators as this will increase risk of hypotension and orthostatic hypotension. Terazosin has no effect on codeine.

Glipizide belongs to the class of sulfonylurea drugs used by patients with type II diabetes. Sulfonylureas work by increasing the amount of insulin release from beta cells of the islets of Langerhans of the pancreas. These drugs are ineffective if there is no insulin available, as in type I diabetes. Some sulfonylureas are metabolized by the CYP450 enzyme system in the liver, and their metabolism, like codeine, can be influenced by inducers and inhibitors of this system. Some sulfonylureas are bound to plasma proteins and can be displaced by other drugs, resulting in increased free blood levels of sulfonylureas. Glipizide has no effect on codeine.

Lisinopril inhibits angiotensin-converting enzyme (ACE) that catalyzes the conversion of angiotensin I to angiotensin II. Effects include vasodilation, decreased aldosterone secretion, decreased water and sodium retention, and increased bradykinin. Drugs that interact with lisinopril include diuretics and NSAIDs, resulting in hypotension and renal damage, respectively. Lisinopril has no effect on codeine. Angiotensin II receptor antagonists ("sartan" drugs) are an improvement on this class of drugs; by directly blocking angiotensin II, they eliminate the unwanted bradykinin-induced side effects associated with ACE inhibitors.

Lithium is an antipsychotic commonly used by patients with bipolar disorder. Lithium has a narrow therapeutic index and can cause serious renal and CNS toxicity. Metronidazole inhibits lithium clearance from the kidneys, resulting in high lithium blood levels. Renal toxicity can occur when diuretics and lithium are taken concurrently because of excessive sodium depletion. Lithium has no effect on codeine.

20. **The correct answer is E.** Montelukast (singulair) is a leukotriene receptor antagonist used for the prophylactic and chronic treatment of asthma and seasonal allergies. Leukotrienes are released by inflammatory cells and cause the following symptoms in asthma: hypersecretion of mucus, decreased mucus transport and mucosal accumulation, bronchoconstriction and airway narrowing, and infiltration of inflammatory cells in the airway wall. These symptoms are decreased by drugs that competitively inhibit the binding of leukotrienes to their receptors.

Montelukast is not useful for the treatment of acute asthma attacks.

Albuterol is an example of a short-acting beta-2 adrenergic agonist, which causes smooth muscle relaxation resulting in bronchodilation. It can be used for acute asthma attacks. Albuterol is most often given in the inhaled form using a nebulizer.

Zileuton is an example of a lipoxygenase pathway inhibitor. This drug blocks leukotriene synthesis by competitively inhibiting 5-lipooxygenase, an enzyme that catalyzes the formation of leukotrienes from arachidonic acid via oxygenation. Zileuton is not useful for the treatment of acute asthma attacks. Zileuton is a weak inhibitor of CYP1A2 and therefore has significant drug interactions with CYP1A2 substrates such as warfarin and theophylline. Zileuton also causes elevations of liver enzymes (AST, ALT).

Ipratropium is an anticholinergic agent. By blocking muscarinic receptors, this drug inhibits bronchoconstriction and mucus secretion. It does not diffuse through the blood, preventing any potential systemic side effects, including cardiac effects and is therefore safe to use in patients with heart disease. It is not as powerful as the beta-2 adrenergic agonists but can be used along with a beta-2 agonist in the case of acute asthma attacks. It is sometimes associated with dry mouth.

Triamcinolone is an example of a glucocorticoid. Glucocorticoids are effective in treating asthma because of their anti-inflammatory effects. Inhaled forms of glucocorticoids eliminate systemic side effects, but occasional reports of local candidiasis do occur.

Benzonatate is an antitussive agent that works by depressing the medullary cough center and exerting an anesthetic action on the respiratory mucosa. It is unrelated to narcotic antitussive agents such as codeine.

21. **The correct answer is C**. On the basis of the symptoms described and the laboratory values provided, this patient is suffering from diabetes and malnutrition. The patient is not taking the appropriate medications to treat these conditions and therefore has higher than normal HbA1c and glucose values. The best answer choice would therefore be insulin. Insulin is taken subcutaneously by patients type I diabetes who lack endogenous insulin. Other antidiabetic drugs that are effective only in patients with type II diabetes include: sulfonylureas (increases insulin release), biguanides, such as metformin and glitazones (increase sensitivity to insulin), and alpha-glucosidase inhibitors (slow digestion of starch).

22. **The correct answer is D**. The symptoms that patient describes are representative of an allergic reaction to a drug, in this case, penicillin. Clindamycin is a lincosamide antibiotic, typically used to treat anaerobic infections. In patients with hypersensitivity to penicillins, clindamycin may be used to treat infections caused by susceptible aerobic bacteria as well. It is also used to treat bone and joint infections, particularly those caused by *Staphylococcus aureus*. Amoxicillin would be an inappropriate alternative as it is from the same family of antibiotics as penicillin.

23. **The correct answer is B**. Naloxone is the drug of choice for the treatment of opioid overdose. Naloxone is a μ-opioid receptor competitive antagonist. Naloxone has a high affinity for the μ-opioid receptor in the central nervous system and is capable of competitively displacing opioids from the receptor. Flumazenil is used to treat benzodiazepine overdose. It reverses the effects of benzodiazepines by competitively inhibiting the GABA$_A$ receptor. Clonidine treats high blood pressure by stimulating the α$_2$ receptors in the brain, which results in a decrease in sympathetic tone. Clonidine has also been used to ease withdrawal symptoms associated with the long-term use of substances, such as narcotics, alcohol, and nicotine, but not for acute reversal of narcotic overdose. It is mainly used to address the sympathetic nervous system response to opiate withdrawal, like hypertension and tachycardia, in the initial days of withdrawals.

24. **The correct answer is C**. Nystatin is a polyene antifungal effective against molds and yeasts including the *Candida* spp. The drug has minimal mucosal absorption and is thus used as a topical treatment for oral candida. The other answer

choices are ineffective against yeast organisms. Amphotericin B is also a polyene antifungal but is used intravenously to treat systemic fungal infections.

25. **The correct answer is B.** Allergic reactions to local anesthetics typically involve the ester anesthetics. The sensitivity is usually because of a reaction against the preservative found in ester local anesthetics called para-aminobenzoic acid (PABA). Among the answer choices, only propoxycaine is an ester anesthetic. The others are amide local anesthetics.

26. **The correct answer is E.** Warfarin interferes with synthesis of vitamin K-dependent coagulation factors (II, VII, IX, X). This could lead to increased clotting time for both extrinsic (PT) and intrinsic (PTT) coagulation pathways. Vitamins A, B, C, and D are not directly involved in the coagulation cascade.

27. **The correct answer is A.** Omeprazole is an irreversible inhibitor of H^+/K^+ ATPase of the parietal cells used to treat peptic ulcer disease. Cimetidine, famotidine, and ranitidine are H2-receptor antagonists that block histamine-induced acid secretion. Ketoconazole is an antifungal medication.

28. **The correct answer is B.** Oxazepam is a benzodiazepine that does not require phase I metabolism by the liver. Therefore, it can be useful in patients with liver failure. Phase I reactions occur via oxidation, reduction, hydrolysis cyclization, or decyclization reactions to either inactivate or activate drugs. Phase II reactions involve methylation, syphation, acetylation, and glucuronidation. The smooth endoplasmic reticulum of the liver cell in the principal location of drug metabolism. Lorazepam and temazepam are the two other benzodiazepines whose levels are not significantly affected by the liver. Alprazolam, midazolam, triazolam, and diazepam all require phase I metabolism by the liver.

29. **The correct answer is D.** It takes one half-life to get to 50% of steady state, two to reach 75%, and four to reach 93.75%. Therefore, four half-lives are 4 × 4 hours, which is a total of 16 hours. Each successive half-life brings the level of medication A closer to 100%.

30. **The correct answer is D.** Tetracaine is a long-acting ester local anesthetics. The rest of the options are all amides.

31. **The correct answer is C.** Propranolol is a nonselective beta blocker that is contraindicated in patients with COPD or asthma. It can cause bronchoconstriction by blocking the beta 2 receptors. Acebutolol, atenolol, esmolol, metoprolol, and betaxolol are all beta 1 selective blockers that are safer to use for this patient.

32. **The correct answer is E.** The loading dose (LD) is a function of the volume of distribution (Vd) and the desired drug level in the plasma. In this case, LD = Vd × Cp = 50 L × 5 mg/L = 250 mg.

33. **The correct answer is A.** Hydrochlorothiazide is a thiazide diuretic that can lead to increase in urination. The rest of the options are all antihypertensives that work through different mechanisms. Diltiazem is a calcium channel blocker. Enalapril is an ACE inhibitor. Methyldopa is a centrally acting alpha receptor agonist. Terazosin is a peripherally acting alpha receptor blocking agent.

34. **The correct answer is D.** Flumenazil is a benzodiazepine antagonist used to treat in the case of overdose. Naloxone and naltrexone are opioid receptor antagonists. Protamine is an antidote for heparin overdose. Insulin is used to treat hyperglycemia.

35. **The correct answer is A.** Paroxetine is a selective serotonin reuptake inhibitor that is used commonly in the management of depressive disorders. It is preferred over other antidepressants because of less severe side effects. Common side effects include GI upset, decreased libido, and sexual dysfunction. Taking SSRI in combination with MAOi can increase the risk of having life-threatening serotonin syndrome (autonomic instability, somatic, and cognitive symptoms).

36. **The correct answer is C.** Piperacillin along with carbenicillin and ticarcillin are beta-lactamase resistant antibiotics. They have extended spectrum against many Gram-negative bacilli, including *Pseudomonas aeruginosa*. The remaining antibiotics are all penicillin or its derivatives that do not have antipseudomonal effects.

37. **The correct answer is B:** Heparin can bind and activate antithrombin III, resulting in the inactivating thrombin and factor Xa. This leads to increase in PTT, a marker for the heparin's anticoagulant effect. It is not related to synthesis of vitamin K coagulation factors, unlike warfarin.

    Clinical applications of heparin include pulmonary embolism, ischemic myocardial infarction, and deep venous thrombosis. Overdose of heparin can be reversed with protamine sulfate.

38. **The correct answer is C.** Warfarin has been used as a rat poison. However, it also has clinical application in humans for long-term anticoagulation. It acts by inhibiting the synthesis of vitamin K-dependent clotting factors (II, VII, IX, X), as well as proteins C and S. This affects the extrinsic coagulation pathway; thereby, one can follow the PT or INR levels for its clinical effect. Warfarin is known to be teratogenic; therefore, a pregnancy test should be performed on patients with childbearing potential. Vitamin K is used as a treatment for warfarin overdose.

39. **The correct answer is C.** Prazosin, doxazosin, and terazosin are competitive alpha-1 receptor antagonists that are used to lower peripheral vascular resistance. They can be used to control hypertension and urinary retention. Side effects of these medications commonly include postural hypotension, headache, and dizziness.

40. **The correct answer is D.** Patient here presents with angioedema, a side effect of ACE inhibitors such as captopril, enalapril, and lisinopril. ACE inhibitors decrease the conversion of angiotensin I into angiotensin II, thereby preventing vasoconstriction and resultant increase in aldosterone. It is commonly used in the treatment of hypertension, especially in the context of other comorbidities such as diabetes mellitus. Other adverse effects of ACE inhibitors include cough, hyperkalemia, rash, taste changes, orthostatic hypotension, and liver toxicity. ACE inhibitors are contraindicated during pregnancy because of their potential for teratogenicity.

41. **The correct answer is B.** TCAs (e.g., amitriptyline, imipramine, nortriptyline, desipramine, trimipramine, doxepin, and clomipramine) can inhibit reuptake of norepinephrine and serotonin into presynaptic nerve terminals. Besides usage in depression, TCAs can be used in the treatment of neuropathy and panic disorders. Its side effects include antimuscarinic, antiadrenergic, and antihistamine effects such as dry mouth, orthostatic hypotension, and sedation. Serious adverse effects include coma, convulsion, and cardiotoxicity (arrhythmias).

42. **The correct answer is E.** Valproic acid is an anticonvulsant that blocks sodium channels and increases GABA concentration. It is also used for rapid cycling and mixed affective disorders as mood stabilizer. Side effects include hepatotoxicity, hemorrhagic pancreatitis, thrombocytopenia, and neural tube defects.

43. **The correct answer is A.** Sulfonylureas include glipizide, glyburide, tolbutamide, and chlorpropamide. They stimulate insulin release from beta cells of the pancreas and binding of insulin to target tissues. They also inhibit release of glucagon. Metformin is a biguanides that can decrease hepatic gluconeogenesis. Lactic acidosis is a concern for metformin overdose. Both types of medications are used commonly in the treatment of type II diabetes mellitus.

44. **The correct answer is D.** Esomeprazole (nexium) is an H^+/K^+ ATPase inhibitor that is used in the treatment of GERD or peptic ulcer disease. The rest are all antifungal that work through various different mechanisms.

45. **The correct answer is A.** Acetaminophen is used as an analgesic and antipyretic. Its mechanism is not fully known, possibly related to inhibition of cyclooxygenases in the CNS. Hepatotoxicity is a great concern with the use of acetaminophen in context of overdosing or patients with hepatic failure. N-acetylcysteine allows an increase in

supply of intracellular glutathione via elevated intracellular cysteine, thereby decreasing the formation toxic metabolites.

46. **The correct answer is C.** Nonselective NSAIDs are commonly used for inflammation, analgesia, and antipyrexia. They can inhibit both cox-1 and cox-2 cyclooxygenases (aspirin irreversibly, others reversibly). This can lead to a decrease in prostaglandin synthesis. Common side effects include dyspepsia, GI ulcers, and renal failure. Aspirin is also associated with Reye syndrome.

47. **The correct answer is C.** There are two generations of H1 antihistamine (first generation: diphenhydramine, dimenhydrinate; second generation: fexofenadine, loratadine). They are commonly used for allergies. Second-generation medications are less sedating than the ones from the first-generation. Toxicities include anticholinergic and antiadrenergic effects.

48. **The correct answer is A.** Glucocorticoids (e.g., prednisone, triamcinolone, dexamethasone, and hydrocortisone) are used in many different clinical situations, including inflammation, immunosuppression, Addison disease, and asthma. They function by binding to intracellular cytoplasmic receptor, phospholipase, thereby indirectly inhibiting production of leukotrienes and prostaglandins.

49. **The correct answer is B.** Opioids (e.g., morphine, heroin, codeine, and fentanyl) interact with opioid receptor in the CNS and GI. They are used to treat for pain, cough, and diarrhea. Side effects include respiratory depression, constipation, miosis, and CNS depression. Opioid use can lead to abuse and dependence. Naloxone is an opioid receptor antagonist.

50. **The correct answer is D.** Misoprostol is a synthetic prostaglandin E1 analog that can be used for abortion, labor induction, prevention of NSAID-induced gastric ulcers, and maintenance of PDA in certain cardiac congenital defects.

51. **The correct answer is C.** Degradation of drug prior to absorption decreases bioavailability. Bioavailability is a measure of how much drug reaches the circulatory system and is available at the site of action. Factors influencing the bioavailability of a drug include: route of administration (IV > oral), degradation of drug prior to absorption (decreases bioavailability), efficient gastrointestinal absorption (increases bioavailability), drug solubility (hydrophobic better absorbed than hydrophilic), hepatic first pass effect (decreases bioavailability), and drug chemistry.

52. **The correct answer is A.** Volume of distribution (Vd) is defined as total amount of drug in the body/plasma drug concentration = 600 mg ≈ 100 mg/L = 6 L.

53. **The correct answer is C.** ACE inhibitors, such as captopril, enalapril, and lisinopril, block angiotensin-converting enzyme, resulting in the decrease in conversion of angiotensin I into angiotensin II, hence a potent vasoconstrictor. Adverse effects of ACE inhibitors include cough, angioedema, proteinuria, hyperkalemia, taste changes, orthostatic hypotension, fetal toxicity, and rash.

54. **The correct answer is B.** Clearance is defined as rate of elimination/plasma drug concentration = 3 mg/min/150 mg/L = 0.02 L/min.

55. **The correct answer is E.** Penicillin is a bactericidal antibiotic (not bacteriostatic) that works by binding to penicillin-binding protein and blocking transpeptidase from crosslinking peptidylglycine in bacterial cell wall. Not all penicillins are effective against *Pseudomonas aeruginosa*. Antipseudomonal penicillins include piperacillin, carbenicillin, and ticarcillin. Amoxicillin has an extended spectrum that is able to cover *E. coli*, *Haemophilus influenza*, *Proteus mirabilis*, *Listeria monocytogenes*, and *Salmonella*. By adding clavulanic acid or tazobactam to penicillins, the antibiotics are rendered beta-lactamase resistant.

CHAPTER 2

Operative Dentistry and Prosthodontics

1. A 13-year-old female patient presents with yellow, pitted enamel on all permanent teeth. Her mother reports that all of the patient's baby teeth had a similar appearance. The patient has excellent hygiene and no caries but is concerned about her appearance. What is the best treatment to address this patient's chief complaint?

   A. Composite bonding
   B. Facial veneers
   C. Full crown coverage
   D. No dental treatment, but refer to a clinic for treatment of an eating disorder
   E. No treatment is necessary

2. A 27-year-old female presents with pain on the lower right side in the area of the second premolar. The HIV-positive patient has smoked two packs of cigarettes per day for 15 years and is not interested in quitting smoking. She has multiple amalgam and composite restorations in all quadrants. Clinically, the tooth resembles a primary mandibular second molar and has a large occlusal composite with open margins. Radiographic examination reveals widely divergent mesial and distal roots and radiolucency in the furcation. What is the most appropriate treatment for this patient?

   A. Extract the tooth and place an implant
   B. Root canal therapy, post and core, full coverage crown
   C. Removal of existing composite, direct pulp cap, and composite restoration
   D. Extract the tooth and replace with three-unit fixed partial denture
   E. No treatment is necessary

3. A 25-year-old male patient presents to your office for a routine checkup. He has no significant medical history. Dental history includes orthodontic treatment 10 years ago and several occlusal amalgam restorations that which are 15- to 17-years old.

   You notice white spots on the facial surfaces of teeth #8 and #9. Which of the following diagnostic tools would best aid in differentiating the white lesions as incipient caries versus hereditary enamel hypocalcification?

   A. Radiograph
   B. Fully or partially disappears when wet
   C. Caries detector
   D. Transillumination
   E. Sharp explorer

4. As caries progresses from enamel to dentin and toward the pulp interproximally, the radiographic appearance resembles which of the following?

   A. V shape in the enamel with the apex toward the DEJ and V shape in dentin with apex toward the pulp
   B. V shape in enamel with apex toward the proximal surface and V shape in dentin with the apex toward the pulp, resulting in a diamond appearance
   C. V shape in enamel with the apex toward the DEJ and V shape in dentin with the apex toward the DEJ, resulting in a bowtie appearance
   D. V shape in enamel with the apex toward the proximal surface and V shape in dentin with the apex toward the DEJ

5. In a carious lesion in which caries has extended into dentin, which of the following zones contains infected dentin and is not capable of remineralization?

   A. Normal dentin
   B. Subtransparent dentin
   C. Transparent dentin
   D. Turbid dentin
   E. Eburnated dentin

6. Which of the following is NOT a parafunctional movement?

   A. Swallowing
   B. Bruxism
   C. Nail biting
   D. Clenching

7. A 28-year-old asymptomatic male patient presents with active caries and active periodontal disease. What is the best treatment for a posterior endodontically treated premolar?

A. Veneer
B. Metal–ceramic crown
C. MO amalgam
D. Extraction
E. Fixed partial denture
F. Partial-coverage restoration

8. A patient moves his mandible in a right lateral excursion. To which direction will the nonworking condyle move?

A. Down, forward, and medially
B. Down, forward, and laterally
C. Up, back, and down
D. Up, back, and out
E. None of the above

9. At the wax try-in, the maxillary plane appears to be correct, yet when the patient closes lightly in centric relation, the mandibular teeth appear to show too much. The patient's lips do not contact unless the patient forces them to do so. What is the most likely error that has occurred?

A. Excessive vertical dimension of occlusion
B. Inaccurate face-bow transfer
C. Over closed vertical dimension of occlusion
D. Excessive amount of freeway space

10. During the insertion of a complete lower denture, you observe that there is a lift in the denture. You observe the denture becomes dislodged with constriction of the genioglossus muscle. What portion of the denture lifted from position because of contraction of the genioglossus muscle?

A. Entire denture lifts
B. Entire denture dislodges
C. Anterior portion lifts
D. None of the above

11. A 44-year-old male presents with missing teeth #6 to #9. After being presented with many treatment options including rockets power dancers (RPD), dental implants, and bridge, the patient elects for the fabrication of an RPD. Where is the path of insertion going to allow for the best esthetics minimizing space between artificial and natural teeth?

A. Parallel to the most distal maxillary molar or most posterior tooth

B. Extracting remaining anterior teeth and then fabricating RPD would be best for esthetics
C. Parallel to the proximal surfaces of the abutment teeth adjacent to the space
D. Parallel to the mandibular anterior teeth due to occlusion
E. An RPD should not be considered

12. A patient with a 22-mm working length (WL) will need a post after the endodontic treatment is completed. Which of the following statement is true concerning post placement?

A. A 3-mm apical seal must be maintained
B. As post length increases, retention decreases
C. Endodontically treated tooth should not be treated with posts
D. A 5-mm apical seal must be maintained
E. A post less than 3-mm long is acceptable

13. A 68-year-old male presents with severe loss of tooth structure on an abutment for an existing removable partial denture. A crown is indicated for the tooth. Which of the following are important considerations when preparing a removable partial denture abutment to receive a crown?

A. Path of draw
B. Location of rests
C. Orientation of guiding planes
D. Placement of porcelain on metal finish lines
E. All of the above.

14. An endodontically treated posterior tooth has 3 mm of circumferential clinical crown remaining. How many millimeters in length are necessary to forego a post, using an amalgam core build up in prepared post spaces?

A. Greater than 3 mm
B. Less than 3 mm
C. 5 to 6 mm
D. 2 mm
E. Greater than 2 mm

15. A patient with a complete upper denture and a bilateral lower partial denture presents in your office for the first time in 5 years. What can you expect to find after 5 years without RPD maintenance?

    A. Loss of vertical dimension of occlusion (VDO) and retrognathic facial appearance
    B. Decrease in VDO and prognathic facial appearance
    C. Premature posterior contacts and retrognathic facial appearance
    D. Increase in VDO and premature posterior contacts
    E. Decrease in VDO and prognathic facial appearance

16. Mechanical consideration in crown preparation design is an important factor that could dictate longevity of the fixed prosthesis. All of the following are categories for mechanical consideration, *except*:

    A. Providing retention form
    B. Providing resistance form
    C. Preventing deformation of the restoration
    D. Geometry of tooth preparation

17. Recognition of wall convergence angles in crown preparation will determine if undercuts are produced when taper is too small and if retention is undermined when taper is too large. What degree of wall convergence during crown preparation will give the prosthesis optimal retention?

    A. 1 to 3 degrees
    B. 3 to 6 degrees
    C. 4 to 8 degrees
    D. 6 to 9 degrees

18. Certain restorations (inlay, crowns, fixed partials, removable partials) require alloys intended for their use according to physical strength. In turn, this affects our selection of casting alloy. Which of the following correctly pairs the casting alloy with its intended restoration?

    A. Type III: Complex inlays
    B. Type IV: Simple inlays
    C. Type III: Crowns and FPDs

D. Type II: Crowns and FPDs
E. Type II: RPDs

19. A 56-year-old patient presents with moderate decay on tooth #30. After observing the bitewing and periapical radiograph of this tooth, you determine that a PFM is indicated. Since the restoration is in an area where the margin is of low esthetic concern, you decide to prepare the tooth with a supragingival margin. All of the following are advantages of a supragingival margin, *except*:

    A. Easily finished margins
    B. Cleansable of margins
    C. Less impingement of gingival tissue during impressions
    D. Improved clinical access for evaluation of margins at recall
    E. Increased retention

20. A 25-year-old patient presents in your office to restore a fractured maxillary central incisor. After evaluation, you determine that the tooth has insufficient structure for an operative restoration and that an all-ceramic crown is indicated. What type of finish line will you prepare?

    A. Feather edge
    B. Chamfer
    C. Shoulder
    D. Knife edge
    E. Bevel

21. In March 2003, the Journal of the American Dental Association revised the classification system of dental alloys. What are the requirements for a high noble alloy?

    A. Noble metal content $\geq$ 40% (gold + platinum group) and gold $\geq$ 60%
    B. Noble metal content $\geq$ 60% (gold + platinum group) and gold $\geq$ 40%
    C. Noble metal content $\geq$ 25% (gold + platinum group) and gold $\geq$ 40%
    D. Noble metal content $\geq$ 40% (gold + platinum group)
    E. Noble metal content $\geq$ 60% (gold + platinum group)

22. The pontic design selection with the most esthetic advantage for a 39-year-old female with an anterior bridge, teeth #7–#9, is:

A. Saddle-ridge-lap
B. Conical
C. Sanitary/hygienic
D. Modified ridge-lap
E. Modified sanitary
F. Ridge lap

23. Retraction cord is often used with a hemostatic agent to capture an accurate impression. Which hemostatic agents minimize tissue damage?

A. $Fe_2(SO_4)_3$ and $AlCl_3$
B. $ZnCl_2$ and $AlCl_3$
C. $Fe_2(SO_4)_3$ and $ZnCl_2$
D. $(SO_4)_2$ and $ZnCl_2$
E. Epinephrine and $Fe_2(SO_4)_3$

24. Ceramic shade matching is an important step in achieving natural esthetics in dental tooth restoration. What is the most important dimension of color for dental restorations?

A. Color
B. Hue
C. Value
D. Chroma
E. Metamerism

25. A 20-year-old female presents for her initial dental examination and prophylaxis. During the examination, you observe wear on the occlusal surfaces of many posterior and anterior teeth. The wear on the posterior teeth are cup like and smooth, and on the anterior, it has smoothed out the lingual anatomy of the incisors. This is most typical of which type of wear?

A. Attrition
B. Erosion
C. Abrasion
D. Abfraction
E. Bruxism

26. Addition silicone (aka polyvinylsiloxane) is one of many impression materials used for crown and bridge final impressions. Addition silicone has greater dimensional stability than polyethers

(e.g., impregum), but they also come with some disadvantages. Which of the following is *not* a disadvantage?

A. Hydrophobicity
B. Temperature sensitivity
C. Latex can interfere with setting
D. Surface detail
E. Wettability

27. Gypsum-bonded and phosphate-bonded investments each have their requirements to be selected as an ideal investment material. Phosphate-bonded investments are more stable at high temperatures and therefore better suited for casting metal–ceramic alloys. What is the correct order (first step, second step, . . . last step) of the "lost-wax casting" technique?

I.   Casting
II. Investing
III. Wax pattern
IV. Material selection (e.g., gypsum-bonded, phosphate-bonded)
V.   Spruing

A. I, V, IV, III, and II
B. III, IV, II, and I
C. III, II, I, V, and IV
D. V, III, IV, II, and I
E. IV, V, III, II, and I
F. V, III, II, and I

28. The addition of resin to glass ionomer cement in the 1990s was introduced to combine desirable properties of both luting agents. Which of following is not an advantage of a resin-modified glass ionomer-luting agent?

A. Low microleakage
B. Luting ceramic restorations
C. Fluoride release
D. Low solubility
E. Reduce postoperative sensitivity

Operative Dentistry and Prosthodontics

29. Alginate (irreversible hydrocolloid) is a hydrocolloid consisting of a solution of alginic acid and has a physical state that is changed by an irreversible chemical reaction forming insoluble calcium alginate. The setting reaction is represented by the following formula:

$$H_2O + Na\ alginate + Ca_2SO_4 \rightarrow Ca\ alginate$$
$$gel\ (insoluble) + NaSO_4$$

What are the methods for decreasing setting time of the alginate?

A. Increase water temperature, mix more rapidly, decrease water:powder ratio
B. Decrease water temperature, mix less rapidly, decrease water:powder ratio
C. Increase water temperature, mix less rapidly, decrease water:powder ratio
D. Decrease water temperature, mix more rapidly, increase water:powder ratio

30. A 51-year-old female patient presents to your office requiring full mouth extractions. You explain the treatment options to her, and she elects upper and lower complete dentures. You explain to the patient that fabricating an immediate denture (I/D) to insert after the full mouth extractions is a great option to control bleeding and inflammation. What is the time frame an immediate denture can be used?

A. An I/D can continue to be used as a prosthesis for the rest of the patients life
B. An I/D should only be used for about 1 to 2 days post oral surgery
C. An I/D can be used up to 1 full year post oral surgery
D. An I/D can be used up to 6 months post oral surgery
E. An I/D is not a viable option for full mouth extractions

31. Fabricating a complete denture requires many important steps from impression taking to tooth shape and shade selection. What are the three factors for successful fit of a complete denture once it has been fabricated?

A. Stability, resiliency, and temperature
B. Stability, support, and retention
C. Retention, resiliency, and temperature
D. Support, temperature, and retention
E. Retention, flexibility, and support

32. It is important to select an esthetic tooth shape and to consider alignment features when fabricating any type of prosthesis. Considered in treatment planning and evaluation of patients smile analysis, what is the acceptable midline deviation?

A. 1 mm
B. 2 mm
C. 3 mm
D. 4 mm
E. 5 mm

33. An articulator is a mechanical instrument used to represent the temporomandibular joint and mandible. A classification system was developed to determine the variable movements an articulator can produce. Which of the following is the most commonly used type of articulator?

A. Class I
B. Class II
C. Class III
D. Class IV
E. Class V

34. Articulators are further distinguished by design. What is the advantage an ARCON (ARticulator, CONdyle) design has over a non-ARCON design?

A. The ARCON design has condylar elements in the upper member
B. The ARCON design has condylar elements in the lower member
C. The non-ARCON design has the condylar inclination of the mechanical fossae at a fixed angle to the maxillary occlusal plane
D. The ARCON design has the condylar inclination of the mechanical fossae at a variable angle to the maxillary occlusal plane as the articulator opens
E. None of the above

35. A 68-year-old male presents to your office for complete upper and lower denture try-in. At insertion and after some adjustments, the patient continually complains of an uncomfortable clicking when he talks. Which of the following could be contributing to the clicking described by the patient?

I. Cheek biting
II. Excess VDO
III. Habit
IV. Lack of tissue adaptation at posterior palatal seal

A. I and IV
B. I
C. II and III
D. II
E. I, II, and III
F. All of the above

36. A 54-year-old female presents for an initial examination. She admits to periodontal issues in the past and you observe this in the panoramic examination upon evaluation. You recommend the extraction of her remaining teeth and fabrication of complete upper and lower dentures. You discuss the physiologic nature of the maxillary and mandibular bone because of the possibility of a reline or even a fabrication of new dentures in the future. Which statement below best describes the reaction of maxillary and mandibular bone to edentulism?

A. The maxillary ridge resorbs superiorly and anteriorly, while the mandibular ridge resorbs inferiorly and posteriorly
B. The maxillary ridge resorbs inferiorly and posteriorly, while the mandibular ridge resorbs superiorly and anteriorly
C. The maxillary ridge resorbs superiorly and posteriorly, while the mandibular ridge resorbs inferiorly and posteriorly
D. The maxillary ridge resorbs superiorly and posteriorly, while the mandibular ridge resorbs inferiorly and anteriorly
E. The maxillary ridge resorbs superiorly and anteriorly, while the mandibular ridge resorbs inferiorly and anteriorly

37. A 70-year-old patient presents for her recall appoint. She has been wearing her complete dentures for over 15 years and is ready for a new set of complete dentures. As you evaluate her oral mucosa during your routine cancer screening, you observe that her oral mucosal tissue is erythematous likely from overuse of her denture. Which of the following are issues should you address with the patient?

I. Removal of unacceptable dentures from the mouth for an extended period of time before impressions
II. Reline the dentures with a tissue conditioner
III. Educate the patient
IV. Massage of the tissues and warm saline rinses

A. I and IV
B. I and II
C. II and III
D. I and III
E. III and IV
F. All of the above

38. During the denture border molding and final impression appointment, it is important to observe which support and relief areas are for primary support in both maxilla and mandible. What are the primary denture support areas on the maxilla and mandible?

A. Rugae, residual ridge
B. Residual ridge, buccal shelf
C. Residual ridge, residual ridge
D. Rugae, buccal shelf
E. Incisive papilla, residual ridge
F. Incisive papilla, buccal shelf

39. A 51-year-old male patient presents for the final impression appointment for the fabrication of a complete upper denture. As you remove the final impression from the patient's mouth in the custom tray, which of the following structures are you attempting to accurately capture?

I. Residual ridge
II. Labial and buccal frenum
III. Labial and buccal vestibules
IV. Tuberosities
V. Hamular notches
VI. Posterior palatal seal
VII. Fovea
VIII. Hard palate
IX. Rugae
X. Incisive papilla

A. I, II, III, IV, and V
B. II, IV, VI, VIII, and X
C. I, III, V, VII, and XI
D. VI, VII, VIII, IX, and X
E. All of the above

40. Border molding is the shaping of the denture border areas with impression materials typically compound. The shape and size of the vestibule is duplicated by either functional and/or manual manipulation of the soft tissue adjacent to the borders. Rubber base (polysulfide) is an elastomeric impression material for taking impressions after border molding has been completed on the custom tray. What are the advantages of using rubber base for this purpose?

    I.   Long setting time
    II.   Long working time
    III. Flexible and tear resistant
    IV.   Very unpleasant odor and taste
    V.   Highest permanent deformation

    A. I, III, and IV
    B. I, II, and III
    C. III, IV, and V
    D. II and III
    E. II and V

41. While anterior tooth selection is based on shape, size, and shade, the posterior tooth selection is based on cusp angle. Which one of the follow occlusal schemes is correctly paired with its cusp angle?

    A. Anatomic: 0 degrees
    B. Semi-anatomic: 33 to 45 degrees
    C. Nonanatomic/flat: 10 to 20 degrees
    D. Semi-anatomic: 10 to 20 degrees
    E. Anatomic: 33 to 45 degrees

42. You are at the tooth try-in appointment where you will evaluate if you have captured the correct VDO for your patient's dentures. Which of the following are VDO guidelines that you can follow to aid in your evaluation?

    I.   Parallelism of residual ridges
    II.   Phonetics
    III. Patient's proprioception
    IV.   Appearance
    V.   Comparison to old dentures

    A. I, III, and V
    B. II, III, and IV
    C. II, III, IV, and V
    D. I, III, IV, and V
    E. All of the above

43. In 1 hour, you will see your first complete denture patient as a "real dentist." In your excitement and just to keep on the safe side, you review the proper steps for each appointment from beginning to end for the fabrication of a complete upper and lower denture. Which of the following complete denture appointments is the longest appointment?

    A. Diagnosis and preliminary impressions
    B. Border molding and final impressions
    C. Wax rim try-in, VDO, CR
    D. Tooth setup try-in
    E. Delivery/insertion
    F. 24-hour follow-up

44. During the delivery appointment of your patient's complete dentures, you are always sure to give proper instructions for oral tissue and denture care. You remind your patient that the denture should be kept off oral tissue for at least 6 to 8 hours each day, preferably when sleeping. Which of the following are the benefits of resting the oral tissue?

    I.   Blood and lymph flow is improved
    II.   Cheek and tongue function will massage the mucosa
    III. The constant film of stagnant saliva between the dentures and the mucosa is removed
    IV.   Bruxing will not impinge on denture supporting tissue

    A. I and II
    B. I, II, and III
    C. II, III, and IV
    D. III and IV
    E. I and IV
    F. All of the above

45. A 62-year-old male presents to your office for the first time in several years. He has complete dentures that have been feeling loose for the last few months. Upon examination, you observe that the denture borders do not extend to cover all the supporting soft tissue. The patient is not ready for the fabrication of a new complete denture because he is comfortable with the way the teeth come together. What is the best treatment for this patient?

A. Stress that fabricating new dentures is the only treatment option
B. Reline the denture
C. Instruct the patient on how to use denture adhesive
D. Rebase the denture
E. Tell the patient that he will adjust to his existing dentures with time

46. A 35-year-old female presents for a comprehensive oral examination. She admits that this is her first dental visit in 15 years when they extracted all four third molars. Upon examination, you observe decay in several maxillary anterior teeth, and #4, #5, #12, and #13 require root canal therapy. The mandibular anterior teeth have heavy calculus. After explaining all of her treatment options, the patient elects to extract all the teeth requiring endodontic treatment and restoring them with an upper partial denture. What is the Kennedy classification for the partial denture you will design for this patient's final dentition after extractions?

A. Kennedy Class I, Mod 1
B. Kennedy Class II, Mod 2
C. Kennedy Class III, Mod 1
D. Kennedy Class IV, Mod 2
E. Kennedy Class III, Mod 2
F. Kennedy Class I, Mod 2

47. Which of the following is false concerning Applegate's rules governing the application of Kennedy Classification?

A. If a third molar is missing and is not to be replaced, it is not considered in the classification
B. If a second molar is missing and is not to be replaced, it is not considered in the classification
C. The most posterior edentulous area always determines the classification
D. Edentulous areas other than those determining the classification are referred to as modifications and are designated by their number
E. There can be only one modification area in Class IV arches
F. All of the above are true

48. A patient presents to your office for a framework try-in this afternoon. You are evaluating the removable prosthesis prior to the appointment and are concerned with the factors that a major connector requires to be stable in the patient's mouth. Which of the following are requirements for a functional major connector?

I.   Be rigid
II.   Join clasps, rests, and indirect retainers
III.   Provide vertical support and protect the soft tissue
IV.   Reciprocating stabilization
V.   Provide means of obtaining indirect retention where indicated
VI.   Provide an opportunity of positioning denture bases where needed
VII.   Maintain patient comfort
VIII. Connect parts of the prosthesis from one side of the arch to the other

A. I, II, III, IV, V, and VI
B. II, III, V, VI, and VII
C. I, III, IV, V, VII, and VIII
D. I, III, V, VI, VII, and VIII
E. III, IV, VI, VII, and VIII
F. All of the above

49. A 43-year-old male presents to your office for a comprehensive dental examination. In your review of the panoramic radiograph, you observe periodontal disease in the lower anterior dentition. During your clinical examination, you are surprised to only observe +1 mobility on teeth #22, #23, #25, and # 26. In addition, your patient will require the extraction of his last remaining molar #19. Following a gross debridement and the extraction of tooth #19, your patient will have teeth #20 to #28 remaining. Which of the following major connectors will be the most likely indicated for your mandibular partial denture design?

I.   Lingual bar
II.   Lingual plate
III. Double lingual bar or Kennedy bar
IV.   Labial bar

A. I
B. I and II
C. II and III
D. I, II, and III
E. II, III, and IV
F. All of the above

50. A combination clasp is a circumferential clasp that has a retentive arm made of wrought metal, thus making it more flexible than a similar arm constructed from cast alloy. The reciprocating arm, made of cast metal, must be rigid to counteract the forces generated by the flexible wrought metal. What part of the retentive is the most flexible?

   A. The terminal half
   B. The middle third
   C. The terminal third
   D. The shoulder half
   E. The proximal third

51. Which of the following are not basic requirements for clasp design?

   I.   Retention
   II.   Support
   III.   Rigidity
   IV.   Stability
   V.   Reciprocation
   VI.   Durability
   VII.   Encirclement
   VIII.   Esthetic
   IX.   Passivity
   X.   Restorability

   A. III, VI, VIII, and X
   B. II, IV, V, VI, and IX
   C. I, III, IV, V, and VI
   D. I, III, VI, and VII
   E. V, VI, and 1X
   F. None of the above are basic requirements for a clasp design

52. A 30-year-old female patient presents to your practice with no upper molars. You present all her treatment options, and she chooses the option of upper partial dentures. There are many factors to consider when designing a removable prosthesis. At this time, you are most concerned about indirect retention. Which of the following statements is not true of an indirect retainer?

   A. It prevents the distal extension from moving away from the underlying tissue during function
   B. The ideal location is determined by an imaginary line drawn perpendicular to the fulcrum line and as anterior as possible
   C. Must be flexible

   D. Must be placed in the rest seats that transmit applied forces through the long axis of the abutment tooth
   E. A distal extension partial denture uses the mechanical advantage of leverage by moving the fulcrum line further from the force
   F. Cingulum rests designed on maxillary canines are of great advantage

53. During a recall appointment, your patient states that he has finally decided to take your recommendation of extraction of his upper posterior teeth. You discuss with him the sequence of his treatment plan that includes partial upper and lower dentures. After extractions, root canal therapy, and periodontal therapy, you must survey and contour natural teeth and crowns. What is the modification sequence one should follow to complete tooth preparations for final impressions?

   A. Heights of contour, parallel guiding planes, retentive contours, rests
   B. Rests, retentive contours, heights of contour, parallel guiding planes
   C. Retentive contours, rests, parallel guiding planes, heights of contour
   D. Heights of contour, retentive contours, rest, parallel guiding planes
   E. Parallel guiding planes, heights of contour, retentive contours, rests
   F. Parallel guiding planes, heights of contour, rests, retentive contours

54. A 33-year-old male presents with pain. Upon examination, you see severely decayed teeth #6 to #11 with edematous exudate from the buccal mucosa of several teeth. You recommend the extraction of all upper anterior teeth #6 to #11 as they are unrestorable. What Kennedy classification is this partially edentulous arch?

   A. Kennedy Class IV, Mod 2
   B. Kennedy Class I, Mod 1
   C. Kennedy Class IV
   D. Kennedy Class II, Mod 2
   E. Kennedy Class I, Mod 2
   F. Kennedy Class II

55. The design for a lower partial denture will require wrought metal clasps on the direct

retainers. You evaluate the patient's mounted cast with an undercut gauge. What is the undercut required for the retentive arm of a c-clasp direct retainer?

A. 0.005 inch
B. 0.010 inch
C. 0.015 inch
D. 0.020 inch
E. 0.030 inch

56. All of the following are true for Class II amalgam preparations, except one. Which one is the EXCEPTION?

A. Proximal retention locks if placed, should be entirely in dentin, and are deeper gingivally than occlusally
B. The axiopulpal line angle is beveled or rounded to reduce stress
C. The uninvolved proximal wall should converge slightly toward the occlusal
D. The pulpal depth aids in the resistance form of the preparation
E. The buccal and lingual walls should converge to provide mechanical retention to the restorative material

57. All of the following are advantages of glass ionomer cements except one. Which one is the EXCEPTION?

A. Anticariogenic
B. Biocompatibility
C. Bond chemically to tooth structure
D. Set via an acid–base reaction
E. More soluble in the conditions of the oral cavity than zinc phosphate cements

58. All of the following techniques can decrease the setting time for Gypsum except one. Which one of the following is the EXCEPTION?

A. Increasing the powder to liquid ratio
B. Decreasing the rate and time of spatulation
C. Contamination of the mixture
D. Decreasing the mixing temperature
E. Increasing the rate and time of spatulation

59. What is the ideal amount of remaining dentin thickness that is required for an amalgam preparation?

A. 0.5 mm
B. 1.0 mm
C. 1.5 mm
D. 2.0 mm
E. 2.5 mm

60. All of the following are characteristics of a Class V (five) composite preparation except one. Which one is the EXCEPTION?

A. All internal line angles should be rounded
B. Retention provided by undercuts made into the axial walls
C. Cavosurface margins when placed on enamel should be beveled
D. Outline form of the prep is determined by the extent of the carious lesion
E. A butt joint is not indicated when finishing the preparation on root surfaces

61. Which of the following marginal designs is the best for cast gold restorations?

A. Shoulder
B. Shoulder bevel
C. Chamfer
D. Shoulder with retention groves

62. What are the requirements of a good provisional restoration?

A. Provide pulpal protection
B. Be able to be easily cleaned
C. Have nonimpinging margins
D. All of the above

63. What is the recommended prosthodontic treatment of a patient missing four maxillary incisors with severe ridge resorption and limited finances?

A. No treatment
B. Fixed bridgework
C. Maxillary removable partial denture
D. Maryland bridge

64. The most rigid palatal connector is:

A. Anterior–posterior palatal bar connector
B. Palatal palate
C. Palatal horseshoe-shaped connector
D. Single palatal bar

65. "T" and "D" sounds are formed by:

    A. The tongue protruding slightly between the maxillary and mandibular anterior teeth
    B. Contact of the tip of the tongue with the anterior palate and lingual surfaces of the maxillary teeth
    C. The lips only
    D. None of the above

66. Which of components of zinc oxide eugenol impression paste functions as an accelerator of the setting time?

    A. Rosin
    B. Resinous balsam
    C. Oil of cloves
    D. Calcium chloride

67. When fabricating dentures, posterior teeth that are set edge to edge may cause:

    A. Lip biting
    B. Tongue biting
    C. Cheek biting
    D. Gagging

68. Change in dentinal structure as a response to slowly progressive or mild irritations such as mechanical abrasion or chemical erosion is known as:

    A. Physiologic dentinal sclerosis
    B. Reactive sclerosis
    C. Reparative dentin
    D. Smear layer

69. All of the following describe the compositional and structural aspects of dentin EXCEPT:

    A. Contains 70% inorganic hydroxyapatite
    B. Contains 18% organic type I collagen and 12% water
    C. Organic and inorganic constituents of dentin are homogenous in structure
    D. Dentin is a vital and dynamic tissue due to the odontoblastic processes serving as a direct connection to the vital pulp

70. Primers serve as the adhesion-promoting agents and contain both hydrophobic and hydrophilic monomers dissolved in organic solvents such as acetone or ethanol.

    A. Both statements are TRUE
    B. Both statements are FALSE
    C. The first statement is TRUE, the second statement is FALSE
    D. The first statement is FALSE, the second statement is TRUE

71. A stimulus on a tooth such as cold or air drying can cause fluid movement to become rapid, which is then interpreted as pain to the nerve endings in the pulp. This theory is known as the:

    A. Pulpal inflammation theory
    B. Hydrodynamic theory
    C. Thermal sensitivity theory
    D. Thermal expansion theory

72. Which of the following teeth retain sealants the best?

    A. Permanent first molars
    B. Primary second molars
    C. Permanent second premolars
    D. Permanent second molars
    E. Primary first molars

73. Which of the following teeth retain sealants the worst?

    A. Permanent first molars
    B. Primary second molars
    C. Permanent second premolars
    D. Permanent second molars
    E. Primary first molars

74. All of the following can cause damage to the pulp during cavity preparation except for:

    A. Heat during cutting
    B. Pressure applied
    C. Size of bur
    D. Amount of time of cutting
    E. Amount of tooth reduction

75. All of the following cavity classifications can involve any teeth except for:

    A. Class I
    B. Class II
    C. Class V
    D. Class VI

76. Conservative tooth preparation is a fundamental principle of sound restorative dentistry. Which of the following strategies regarding tooth preparation will result in an unsatisfactory result?

A. Preparing the occlusal surface anatomically to create uniform thickness in the restoration
B. Axial wall preparation should be minimal at approximately 6-degree taper
C. Crown preparations should utilize partial ceramic coverage rather than full ceramic coverage in nonesthetic areas
D. Use of a shoulder margin on all full metal crown restorations

77. A patient presents to your office with tooth #14 with a large restoration and recurrent decay. You make the determination that the tooth will require a full metal crown. Which of the following statements would be incorrect regarding your treatment plan for the preparation of this tooth?

A. The functional cusp should be reduced to provide 1.5-mm clearance
B. The nonfunctional cusp should be reduced to provide 1.5-mm clearance
C. The axial reduction should allow 0.5 mm of metal thickness at the margin
D. The functional cusp bevel should be placed at 45 degrees to the long axis

78. You are treatment planning a patient who has selected a PFM (Porcelain Fused to Metal) crown restoration for tooth #8. The patient would like to know how much tooth structure will be removed during your PFM preparation. Which one of the following statements about your reduction for tooth preparation would be incorrect?

A. The desired incisal reduction for a PFM crown is 2.0 mm in intercuspal position and in excursive movements
B. A labial reduction of 1.2 to 1.5 mm (one plane) is mandatory for PMF preparations
C. The lingual concavity is prepared to allow 1-mm clearance if the contacts are to be located on metal
D. Shoulder must extend at least 1-mm lingual to proximal contact area

79. A patient from your practice is a singer with a high esthetic requirement and is requesting a full coverage porcelain crown. Which of the following statements about crown preparation of an all ceramic crown is incorrect?

A. The recommended facial surface reduction for an all ceramic crown is 1 mm of reduction in two planes anatomically following contour surface of tooth
B. Incisal reduction of 1.5 mm including lateral and protrusive excursions
C. A lingual chamfer preparation of 1-mm depth
D. Axial wall taper of 6 degrees is ideal to help preserve tooth structure and provide retention form for the restoration

80. An insurance company has asked you to consult on a claim for an implant supported fixed prostheses. The insurance company is seeking to determine if an implant is appropriate in a patient and has asked you which if any of the following patients are candidates for implant placement followed by a fixed prosthesis:

A. A patient with uncontrolled diabetes
B. A patient with a history of nasopharyngeal cancer that required head and neck radiation to include the maxilla and mandible
C. A patient who is 7-months pregnant
D. An 80-year-old female with no medical problems
E. None of the above

81. When preparing a tooth for a composite restoration, the dimension of the preparation is solely determined by the access and:

A. Removing sound tooth structure to obtain the most optimal preparation
B. The extent of the caries
C. Removing sound tooth structure to obtain mechanical retention
D. The shade of the tooth.

82. What are the structural components of composite?

A. Polymer matrix and filler particles
B. A coupling agent and initiator
C. Polymer matrix and coupling agents
D. All of the above

Operative Dentistry and Prosthodontics

83. When preparing an anterior tooth for a metal–ceramic crown, the ideal preparation requires that approximately_____of tooth structure reduction is needed.

    A. 1.0 mm
    B. 0.8 mm
    C. 2.5 mm
    D. 1.5 mm

84. What is an advantage of using a cast-gold restoration?

    A. Gold is a strong material and rarely fractures
    B. A cast-gold restoration has esthetics superior to other restorations
    C. The impression material that is used for cast-gold restorations is less expensive
    D. Gold has a wear rate that is similar to porcelain

85. When restoring an endodontically treated tooth, what are the first two things that must be considered?

    A. The canal configuration and if a post will be necessary
    B. Which restoration is indicated and if a post will be necessary
    C. The canal configuration and which restoration is indicated
    D. Which restoration is indicated and the function of the restored tooth

86. The following are true of dental caries *except*:

    A. The critical pH is 5.5
    B. Incipient caries are able to remineralize
    C. Frank caries describe caries that have progressed into dentin
    D. Dentin caries progress faster than enamel caries
    E. Saliva is carioprotective

87. The most common cariogenic bacteria responsible for coronal caries are:

    A. *Streptococcus mutans* and *Lactobacilli*
    B. *Actinomyces viscosus*
    C. *Streptococcus sanguis*
    D. *Veillonella*
    E. *Actinomyces naeslundii*

88. There are four zones of carious enamel, the zones of incipient lesions. Which of the four zones is the largest?

    A. Translucent zone
    B. Dark zone
    C. Body zone
    D. Surface zone
    E. Alfi zone

89. All of the following are associated with Rampant caries *except*:

    A. Acute onset
    B. Rapid progression
    C. Children
    D. Deep and wide
    E. Associated with pain

90. Which of the following are known as high-risk factors for caries?

    A. Visible cavitation
    B. Restoration in past 3 years
    C. Exposed roots
    D. Deep pit and fissures
    E. A and B
    F. A, B, and C
    G. All of the above

91. Which of the following bone graft materials area osteoconductive, osteoinductive, and osteogenic?

    A. Xenograft
    B. Alloplast
    C. Allograft
    D. Autogenous graft
    E. Both D and C

92. All of the following are considered to be drugs used for oral conscious sedation *except*:

    A. Triazolam (Halcion®)
    B. Fentanyl (Duragesic®)
    C. Lorazepam (Ativan®)
    D. Diazepam (Valium®)
    E. All of the above can be used

93. Single-tooth implants show a decreased risk of caries to the adjacent teeth BECAUSE of the patients improved ability to clean the proximal surfaces of these teeth.

A. Both the statement and the reason are correct and related
B. Both the statement and the reason are correct but NOT related
C. The statement is correct, but the reason is NOT
D. The statement is NOT correct, but the reason is correct
E. NEITHER the statement NOR the reason is correct

94. Defects in color vision primarily affect 8% to 10% of the female population. Types of defects in color vision include achromatism, dichromatism, and anomalous trichromatism.

A. Both statements are TRUE
B. Both statements are FALSE
C. The first statement is TRUE, and the second statement is FALSE
D. The first statement is FALSE, and the second statement is TRUE

95. In a Provisional Fixed Partial Denture that is seated immediately after the extraction of a tooth, which of the following pontic forms will result in tissue blanching and provide the best support to the surrounding papillae while also providing for the best esthetic outcome following healing of the extraction site?

A. Sanitary (hygienic) pontic
B. Conical pontic
C. Ovate pontic
D. Modified ridge lap pontic
E. None of the above

Operative Dentistry and Prosthodontics

1. **The correct answer is C.** The patient has amelogenesis imperfecta, a rare hereditary condition that results in a reduced amount of enamel, which is softer than normal enamel and is yellow in color and pitted. Both primary and permanent teeth are affected. The dentin and pulps are normal, and there is no increase in rate of caries. The only necessary treatment is cosmetic treatment, which is best accomplished by full coverage crowns. Answer choice D refers the patient to an eating disorders clinic. This would be inappropriate in this case, but if the patient exhibits enamel erosion on the lingual surfaces of the teeth, referral to a therapist who specializes in treatment of eating disorders may be appropriate.

2. **The correct answer is D.** The patient has a congenitally missing permanent right mandibular second premolar and an over-retained primary second molar in that space. Primary teeth are likely to exhibit furcation canals, and if infection is present radiographically in the furcation, the most appropriate treatment is to extract the tooth. Ideal replacement of the missing tooth in a healthy patient would be to place a single-unit implant. However, this patient is HIV positive and smokes two packs per day. Both are likely to impede healing, so placement of an implant is not the most desirable treatment option. A three-unit fixed partial denture would be the most appropriate treatment.

3. **The correct answer is B.** Incipient caries and enamel hypocalcification appear similar clinically. To properly diagnose, wet the surface of the tooth. If the lesion fully or partially disappears, and drying it again causes it to reappear, the diagnosis is smooth surface incipient caries. Neither radiograph nor transillumination will show facial incipient lesions. Caries detector will appear similar with both lesions. Both lesions will appear hard and smooth, so a sharp explorer will not diagnose.

4. **The correct answer is A.** In interproximal or smooth surface caries, demineralization starts wide at the enamel surface and converges with the apex toward the DEJ. Then in dentin, caries progresses faster because of less mineral content. V-shaped caries has a broad base at the DEJ and converges to the apex toward the pulp.

5. **The correct answer is D.** Turbid dentin is the only zone listed, which is infected dentin. Bacterial invasion has occurred in dentinal tubules of turbid dentin. Normal, subtransparent, and transparent dentin are all affected dentin and are capable of remineralization. The dentin in an arrested or remineralized lesion is eburnated or sclerotic dentin.

6. **The correct answer is A.** Swallowing, mastication, and speech are considered functional movements of the mandible. Parafunctional movements are sustained activities that occur beyond the normal functions of those mentioned above. Bruxism is initiated at a subconscious level diurnal, nocturnal, or both. It is the sustained grinding, rubbing together, or gnashing of the teeth with greater than normal chewing force. Nail biting is an example of parafunctional activity. Parafunctional activity can cause excessive wear, widening of the PDL, and mobility, migration, or fracture of the teeth. Clenching is the pressure and clamping of the jaws and teeth together, frequently associated with acute nervous tension or physical effort.

7. **The correct answer is C.** It is recommended to restore the patient to a functional status by eliminating caries and controlling periodontal disease prior to treatment planning with fixed prosthodontics. Veneers, crowns, fixed partial dentures, and partial coverage restorations are contraindicated with both active caries and active periodontal disease. Extraction is a final treatment option but may not be required at this point. Caries control and treatment planning prior to restoration of edentulous space(s) is recommended. Endodontically treated tooth often require cast post and core fabrication prior to fixed restorations.

8. **The correct answer is A.** The working condyle is rotational, while the nonworking condyle demonstrates translational movement.

9. **The correct answer is A.** Vertical dimension is a combination of relaxed muscles, lips at rest, varying freeway space, harmony between lower and middle one-third of the face, ability to speak without bite rims contacting, tongue room for making the "th" sound, satisfaction of the patient's tactile sense, and a consistent rest position measurement.

Since the maxillary plane "appears" close, and there is light contact near centric relation, face bow is not the error. Remember the problem is the straining lips to contact each other.

Answer choice C would be true if lips were contacting "too much," and there was a lack of harmony with lower and middle one-third of the face.

Freeway space is the space between the occluding surfaces of the maxillary and mandibular teeth when the mandible is in physiologic position.

10. **The correct answer is C.**

11. **The correct answer is C.** The best anterior esthetic will be achieved by using the adjacent tooth to a space for path of withdrawal because the contour of the artificial tooth can be manipulated to fit existing natural tooth. Extraction of the remaining anterior teeth may be an option if these remaining teeth are compromised. Although occlusion with the lower mandibular teeth is a consideration for esthetics, it is not because of its path of draw. All treatment options should be considered and presented to the patient.

12. **The correct answer is D.** Most endodontic texts advocate maintaining a 5-mm apical seal. Ideally, the post should be as long as possible without jeopardizing the apical seal or the strength or integrity of the remaining root structure.

If the post is shorter than the coronal height of the clinical crown of the tooth, the prognosis is unfavorable. Stress is distributed over a smaller surface area and more likely to cause radicular fracture. If the root is short, a 3-mm apical seal may be considered acceptable.

As post length increases, retention increases. However, the relationship is not linear. A post that is too short will fail, whereas one that is too long may damage the seal of the root canal fill or risk root perforation if the apical third is curved or tapered. Posts less than 3 mm in length are unacceptable.

13. **The correct answer is E.** All are considerations for fabrication of a crown under an existing RPD. Path of draw or withdrawal is planning both guide planes and reciprocal planes surfaces, as well as areas that require survey lines in the gingival third. Location of rests (at least 1mm deep) will help you determine RPD design and evaluate where rest seat will be in new crown. Orientation of guide planes is important because of path of draw. Finally, it would be unesthetic if porcelain were to chip because of the stress from retentive metal arms of RPD design.

14. **The correct answer is A.** If more than 3 to 4 mm of coronal tooth structure remains, use of a post in the root for retention is not necessary, and this avoids the chance of perforation. Answer choices B, D, and E are incorrect because more tooth structure is required for a secured core without a post.

15. **The correct answer is B.** All patients using removable prosthodontics should visit his or her dentist no less than one time a year, preferably every 3 months.

16. **The correct answer is D.** Geometry of tooth preparation is a subcategory of retention and resistance form. It is not considered a category of mechanical consideration. Providing retention form can be further divided to include (1) magnitude of the dislodging forces, (2) geometry of the tooth preparation, (3) roughness of the fitting surface of the restoration, (4) materials being cemented, and (5) film thickness of the luting agent. Providing resistance form can be further divided to include (1) magnitude and direction of the dislodging forces, (2) geometry of the tooth preparation, and (3) physical properties of the luting agent. Preventing deformation of

Operative Dentistry and Prosthodontics

the restoration can be further divided to include (1) alloy selection, (2) adequate tooth reduction, and (3) margin design.

17. **The correct answer is B.** Three to six degrees has been shown to have the optimal retention in crown preparation. One to three degrees is too small a degree of convergence; therefore, a possibility of undercuts exists. Four to eight degrees is incorrect because any angle greater than 6 will undermine retention. Likewise, 6 to 9 degrees will undermine retention.

18. **The correct answer is C.** Crowns and FPDs are best fabricated with Type III alloys. Complex inlays are best fabricated with Type II alloys. RPDs and pinledges are fabricated with Type IV alloys. Nickel-chromium alloys are stronger than Type IV alloys. Some patients may present with an allergic reaction to nickel-chromium. Simple inlays are best fabricated with Type I alloys. Type III alloys are used to fabricate Crowns and FPDs.

19. **The correct answer is E.** When the margin preparation is taken subgingivally, there is an increase in surface area; this in turn increases retention. Keeping the margin above the gingival tissue decreases the complications of tooth preparation. Patients are able to keep the restoration clean with daily oral hygiene if the margin in maintained above the gingival tissue. Impression material will have better access to margins if maintained supragingivally. The clinician will have direct visual access for evaluation of the PFM during recall if the margin in maintained supragingivally.

20. **The correct answer is C.** All-ceramic crowns, such as those often used in areas of high esthetic consideration, are best prepared with a shoulder finish line. The shoulder finish line is used to minimize risk of porcelain fracture. Featheredge is usually contraindicated when preparing for ceramic crowns because of over-contouring of the crown near the margin. It typically does not provide sufficient bulk on the restoration, although it is the most conservative type of finish line. Chamfer finish lines are best suited for margins prepared for metal restorations. This type of finish line can cause a lip on the margin if the tooth is overprepared. Bevels are rarely indicated except for full-gold crowns, inlay and onlay preparations. Often this type of finish line is used to relieve a lip when overprepared with a chamfer finish line.

21. **The correct answer is B.**

Revised Classification System for Alloys for Fixed Prosthodontics

Classification	Requirement
High noble alloys	Noble metal content $\geq$ 60% (gold + platinum group*) and gold $\geq$ 40%
Titanium and titanium alloys	Titanium $\geq$ 85%
Noble alloys	Noble metal content $\geq$ 25% (gold + platinum group*)
Predominantly base alloys	Noble metal content < 25% (gold + platinum group*)

*Metals of the platinum group are platinum, palladium, rhodium, iridium, osmium, and ruthenium.

22. **The correct answer is D.** A modified ridge lap is recommended in areas of high esthetic concern (i.e., anterior teeth). This design is moderately easy to clean. Pontic design is classified into two categories, mucosal contact and no mucosal contact. A modified ridge lap is categorized by mucosal contact.

Saddle-ridge lap is not recommended pontic design because its concave fitting surface overlaps the residual ridge of missing tooth. This tight fit with the tissue does not allow for adequate hygiene and will accumulate plaque causing tissue inflammation.

A conical pontic is easy for the patient to keep clean. It has only one point of contact with the gingival tissue as the design is convex, heart shaped. This type of design would be recommended in the posterior region where esthetics is not a high concern.

The sanitary/hygienic design is categorized by no mucosal contact; therefore it is most hygienic. However, with poor esthetics, it is typically considered for posterior areas with increased bone loss. It is the least "toothlike."

The modified sanitary is a modification of the sanitary design, but its archway design between the abutment teeth allows this design to increase connector size while decreasing the stress to the pontic.

23. **The correct answer is A.** Ferric sulfate and aluminum chloride are good hemostatic agents that minimize tissue damage. Zinc chloride causes tissue necrosis and is no longer used. Potassium aluminum sulfate is less effective than epinephrine. Epinephrine causes vasoconstriction and should be used with caution especially in lacerated tissue. It may cause tachycardia, so it is contraindicated in cardiac patients.

24. **The correct answer is C.** Value is the relative lightness/whiteness or darkness/blackness, and brightness of a color. Hue, value, and chroma are the three dimensions of color. Hue is the actual color. Chroma is the amount of saturation of the hue. Metamerism is when two objects appear to color match under one light source but not another.

25. **The correct answer is B.** Erosion (acid erosion) is wear because of chemical means (e.g., bulimia, GERD). It does not involve bacterial action-producing defects (deep facial and cervical wedge-shaped depressions). Attrition is normal wear of occlusal and/or incisal surfaces of opposing teeth during mastication but can turn excessive with parafunction. Abrasion is abnormal wear because of mechanical process other than mastication (e.g., toothbrush). Biomechanical loading forces that lead to flexure fatigue degradation at a distant location on the tooth cause abfraction. Bruxism is not a type of wear but is rather the parafunctional habit of grinding teeth.

26. **The correct answer is D.** PVS has excellent surface detail. Along with dimensional stability, these are the advantages of using a PVS material for final impressions. Hydrophobicity is a disadvantage of PVS. Polyether's advantages are low permanent deformation, dimensional stability second only to PVS, and hydrophilicity. Temperature sensitivity is a disadvantage of PVS. Polyether's main disadvantage is rigidity during removal of impression. Latex gloves will retard PVS setting. Wettability is a disadvantage of PVS.

It is also a disadvantage of polyethers, causing expansion when contacted with moisture.

27. **The correct answer is B.** A wax pattern is made on the die. A sprue is attached to the wax pattern. There is no such spruing step. A sprue is a cast metal or plastic acting as a channel, connecting the casting to a sprue button. Investment material selected once the choice of alloy is selected. Once the investment of material is inserted, reaching the wax pattern and has time to set, the wax pattern is eliminated by burn out. Finally, the casting send melted alloy into investment space, producing a replica of the wax pattern.

28. **The correct answer is B.** All ceramic restorations are contraindicated from using R-MGI luting agents because of associated risk of fracture. Low microleakage is an advantage of R-MGIs. Fluoride release is an advantage of R-MGIs. Low solubility is an advantage of R-MGIs. Reduced sensitivity is an advantage of R-MGIs. Luting agents containing phosphoric acid have a history of postoperative sensitivity such as with zinc phosphate.

29. **The correct answer is A.** Since set irreversible hydrocolloid is largely water, it will absorb (imbibition) and give off (syneresis) liquid causing a distortion in the impression. Therefore, the alginate impression should be poured immediately. Be sure to always follow manufacturer's instructions.

30. **The correct answer is D.** As inflammation decreases, mucosal tissue heals, and bone resorbs and remodels. As a result, the I/D may not support or retain itself on the ridge. This may lead to pain or fracture of the denture. The denture will need to be relined or be remade after 6 months.

An immediate denture should never used as a complete denture. Once time has allowed the tissue to heal properly, a better impression can be taken to fabricate a complete denture meant for a use over a longer term. Complete dentures also will not last forever but are fabricated for multi-year use.

An immediate denture is used to control inflammation and protect the surgical site from further trauma that may occur within 1 to 2 days post oral surgery. In addition, an I/D will aid to maintain VDO and a more natural esthetic while tissue heals.

Depending on the patients healing process, a year may be too long. Six months is typically enough time for bone remodeling to occur in the maxilla and the mandible.

31. **The correct answer is C.** Stability is the resistance of the denture base against lateral forces. Support is the resistance to the forces directed against the tissues. Retention is the resistance to the dislodgement of the denture base away from the tissues.

Temperature should not affect a denture once it has been fabricated. Resiliency and flexibility are more important fit factors for partial dentures.

32. **The correct answer is B.** Studies show that midlines up to 2 mm off center are not noticeable unless they become canted obliquely.

33. **The correct answer is C.** The semiadjustable (Class III) articulator provides diagnostic information while minimizing clinical adjustment at the try-in appointment. It simulates condylar pathways by using averages or mechanical equivalents for all or part of the motion. Class I articulators are nonadjustable and only accept a single registration. Class II articulators are also nonadjustable; however, they accept a horizontal and vertical registration. Movements are not oriented to the TMJ. Class IV articulators are fully adjustable. They accept a three-dimensional dynamic registration. These instruments allow for orientation of casts to the TMJ and simulation of mandibular movements. Class V articulators do not exist.

34. **The correct answer is B.** The ARCON is anatomically correct, which makes the understanding of mandibular movements easier. The condylar element is in the lower member, and its condylar inclination to maxillary occlusal plane angle is fixed. The non-ARCON design has its condylar elements in its upper member, and its condylar inclination to maxillary occlusal plane angle changes as the articulator opens.

35. **The correct answer is C.** Excess VDO is usually the primary problem that can be corrected by resetting the tooth setup to decrease the VDO to a more comfortable and stable height. Clicking is also commonly the result of habit. If the problem is habit, this is more difficult to correct. The dentist should refrain from using porcelain teeth.

Check biting is caused by insufficient VDO and horizontal overlap of posterior teeth. This can be corrected by resetting tooth setup prior to processing. The lack of posterior palatal seal adaptation may lead to gagging. A reline will be required to achieve a proper seal. You may also consider the posterior length of the denture if gagging is a problem and reduce to a comfortable length.

36. **The correct answer is D.** The direction of ridge resorption for the maxilla is superior and posterior, while the mandible is inferior and anterior. This discussion with the patient is important so the patient understands that the denture does not last forever.

37. **The correct answer is F.** All of the answer choices are reasonable actions to be taken with this patient. Patient education regarding denture care and use is particularly important because without it, the patient will recreate the same mistakes in denture care and use.

38. **The correct answer is B.** The residual ridge is the primary maxillary area for denture support and the buccal shelf is the primary mandibular area for denture support.

The secondary area for denture support in maxilla is rugae. Relief areas are the incisive papilla, prominent midline suture, and areas of the residual ridges that are highly displaceable.

The secondary area for denture support in the mandible is the residual ridge. Relief areas are the sharp spiny ridges with overlying displaceable tissue, mental foramen if exposed by severe resorption, sharp mylohyoid ridges, tori, and prominent genial tubercles.

39. **The correct answer is E.** Landmarks of the mandible that should be accurately captured are the residual ridge, labial and lingual frenum,

buccal frenae, buccal shelf areas, external oblique lines, retromolar pads, lingual sulci, and retromylohyoid spaces.

40. **The correct answer is D.** The advantages of using polysulfide are the long working time, its flexibility, and its tear-resistant properties. Long setting time, unpleasant odor, and highest permanent deformation are disadvantages of polysulfides.

Final impressions are beaded with rope wax and boxed with boxing wax to create master casts with proper land areas along the borders of the impression and an adequate base.

An interim denture base is fabricated on the master cast to support the occlusal rim. The occlusal rim is made of wax to help with jaw relation records and the setting of the teeth. The rim is contoured and adjusted in the mouth.

41. **The correct answer is E.** Thirty-three to 45 degrees is the correct angle for an anatomical posterior tooth setup. There are six factors relevant to selection of posterior teeth: (1) occluso-gingival length, (2) mesiodistal width, (3) buccolingual width, (4) shade, (5) type of occlusal surface, and (6) material.

The semi-anatomical posterior setup is 10 to 20 degrees, while the nonanatomical setup is 0 degree. Anatomical setup is used for easier penetration of food, better esthetics, interdigitating cusps offer a guide for jaw closure, and can be ground to harmonize with the TMJ and jaw closure. The nonanatomical set-up is used as a simpler technique requiring less instrumentation. It is also used when closure is in more than one position and adapts more easily to Class II and III jaw relationships.

42. **The correct answer is E.** Parallelism of the residual ridges is an excellent guide if the ridges have not experienced excessive bone resorption. Once casts have been mounted, the maxillary and mandibular casts can be evaluated for parallelism, which will aid in VDO approximation.

The closest speaking space, or 1 mm, is considered when the patient speaks. Special consideration should be given to "ch," "s," and "j" sounds. Teeth should not touch during normal conversation.

The patient should feel comfortable with the denture. Teeth should not prematurely contact each other and should not interfere with the patient's proprioception.

Check the patient's profile. An increased VDO would cause strained facial expression. A decreased VDO would cause a drooping at the corners of the mouth and a prognathic appearance.

Evaluating and measuring an old denture can be one of the most important tools to determining a patient's VDO.

43. **The correct answer is E.** The delivery/insertion appointment is typically the longest because all discrepancies in tissue adaptation, border extension, VDO, occlusal harmony, and esthetic value must be addressed. When the corrections are accompanied by patient education and instructions, the adaptation should be a pleasant learning experience for the patient. It is very important to have a 24-hour follow-up to adjust undetected errors. Delivery should not be schedule on Friday unless your office is open on Saturdays.

44. **The correct answer is F.** These are all benefits of resting the oral tissue from the constant contact of the denture on it.

45. **The correct answer is D.** Rebasing is the replacement of the entire denture base while keeping the same denture teeth in their current occlusal relationship. This option can also be utilized when the denture base has been fractured or has become stained or discolored.

Although the fabrication of new dentures would be the best option, especially if dentures have been used over a long period, personal and economical issues may make this option unreasonable.

Relining is the replacement of the intact surface of the denture base with a new layer of material to make up for loss of supporting tissue. It is important to understand that a visual reference of the loss of supporting tissue is important before recommending this treatment option.

The use of denture adhesive should never be the solution to an ill-fitting denture.

The maxilla and mandible will continue to resorb, thus causing the denture to become even more unstable over time.

46. The correct answer is C.

Kennedy Class I—Bilateral distal extension

Kennedy Class II—Unilateral distal extension

Kennedy Class III—All tooth supported

Kennedy Class IV—Single anterior area crossing the midline. This classification (IV) cannot have a modification. An easy method to determine modification is to count the number of missing spaces (spans not teeth) in a single arch and subtract that number by 1.

47. The correct answer is E. Applegate's rule 8 states that there can be no modification areas in Class IV arches. The following are Applegate's rules:

Rule 1—Classifications should always follow rather than precede any extractions of teeth that might alter the original classification.

Rule 2—If a third molar is missing and is not to be replaced, it is not considered in the classification. Answer B is Rule 4, Answer C is Rule 5, and Answer D is Rule 6. All are true statements and therefore the incorrect answers.

Rule 3—If a third molar is present and is to be used as an abutment, it is considered in the classification.

Rule 4—If a second molar is missing and is not to be replaced, it is not considered in the classification.

Rule 5—The most posterior edentulous area always determines the classification.

Rule 6—Edentulous areas other than those determining the classification are referred to as modifications and are designated by their number.

Rule 7—The extent of the modification is not considered, only the number of additional edentulous areas.

48. The correct answer is D. Answer choices II and IV describe minor connector functions. Minor connectors connect all the remaining components of the RPD to the major connector and provide stress distribution. These remaining components include clasp assemblies, direct retainers, indirect retainers, auxiliary rests, and denture bases.

The types of maxillary major connectors include:
1. Single posterior palatal bar
2. Palatal strap
3. Anterior posterior or double, palatal bar
4. Horseshoe or U-shaped connector
5. Closed horseshoe or anterior posterior palatal strap
6. Complete palatal coverage

49. The correct answer is C. A lingual plate and Kennedy bar will both provide support, such as with a splint, to anterior teeth that have lost support of the bone. They also provide additional indirect retention when most, if not all, posterior teeth are being replaced with the partial denture. Remember that the major connector itself is not an indirect retainer; however, the support given by the rests on the anterior teeth supply indirect retention. Since the bar is contacting all anterior teeth, the force is distributed along the bar to all teeth contacted, thus reducing total force on a single tooth. The lingual plate should be considered before the Kennedy bar because of food entrapment between the double bar and tongue annoyance with the Kennedy bar.

The lingual bar is the most commonly used major connector. Its advantage is its simplicity and its minimal contact of oral tissue.

The labial bar is indicated for patients with severe lingually inclined lower anterior teeth and/or premolars where a traditional lingualized bar cannot be fabricated. This major connector should only be used when absolutely necessary and all other options have been exhausted.

50. The correct answer is C. A retentive clasp is divided into three parts: the proximal, middle, and terminal. The terminal third is placed beneath the height of contour, allowing it to engage at the undercut.

Although there is a variable amount of flexibility in the middle part, as the wrought wire transforms from rigid (proximal) to flexible (terminal), the terminal end is still more flexible. The proximal part is the most rigid and is positioned above the height of contour.

51. The correct answer is A. Rigidity, durability, esthetic, and restorability are not requirements for clasp design. The six basic requirements for clasp design are as follows:

1. Retention—provide retention against dislodgement
2. Support—property of clasp to resist displacement in a gingival direction
3. Stability—resistance to horizontal displacement
4. Reciprocation—to resist horizontal forces exerted on the tooth by the retentive arm
5. Encirclement—each clasp must encircle more than 180 degrees of the abutment tooth
6. Passivity—for insertion and removal of partial denture

52. The correct answer is C. An indirect retainer must be rigid. If the retainer were to flex, forces would be multiplied instead of dissipated. The remaining statements are true regarding indirect retainers. Indirect retainers are most often incorporated when there is a unilateral or bilateral distal extension.

53. The correct answer is E. After examination, diagnosis, and the treatment planning phases, the sequence of mouth preparation appointments must be planned with the goal of conserving as much time as possible.

54. The correct answer is C. Kennedy Class IV is a single, but bilateral (crossing the midline), edentulous area located anterior to the remaining teeth.

  Kennedy Class I—Bilateral distal extension
  Kennedy Class II—Unilateral distal extension
  Kennedy Class III—All tooth supported
  Kennedy Class IV—Single anterior area crossing the midline. This classification (IV) does not have a modification.

55. The correct answer is D. Wrought alloy clasps are placed in an undercut of 0.020 inch. Chrome metal cast clasps are placed in an undercut of 0.010 inch. Golf cast clasps are placed in an undercut of 0.015 inch.

56. The correct answer is C. Retention form of the preparation prevents dislodging of the amalgam restoration. By having the buccal and lingual walls converge occlusally will lock the restoration in place. Proximal retention locks should be placed 0.2 mm into the DEJ. Entirely in dentin maintaining enamel support, regardless of the axial depth. If the retention locks are placed entirely into the axial wall, there is no effective retention obtained, and there is the increased risk of pulpal exposure.

Beveling or rounding the axiopulpal line angle increases the bulk of and decreases the stress concentration within the restorative material. This aids in the resistance form of the preparation.

The uninvolved proximal wall should be slightly obtuse (6 degrees) and diverge toward the occlusal. This will provide adequate support and prevent undermining of the uninvolved marginal ridge and fracture of the restoration.

The resistance form aids in the resistance of the restoration and the tooth to fracture as a result of occlusal forces. The pulpal depth of the restoration is preferred to be a minimum of 2.0 mm as measured from the central fossa and entirely into an even layer of hard dentin.

57. The correct answer is E. Glass ionomer cements are made of a polyacrylic acid liquid and an acid-soluble calcium fluoroaluminosilicate glass powder. Glass ionomer releases fluoride over a sustained period of time, which aids in the remineralization of tooth structure and has been shown in studies to inhibit the progression of secondary caries. Glass ionomer bonds chemically to tooth structure by having the carboxyl groups of the polyacids chelated by the calcium, which is in the apatite of the enamel and dentin. Enamel has a higher inorganic composition than dentin, and thus the bond strength to enamel is higher. Calcium hydroxide liners should only be used if the remaining dentin thickness is less than 0.5 mm. This is done to protect these deep areas from direct contact with unset glass ionomer. Glass ionomer shows mild pulpal effects that tend to subside within a month's time. When glass ionomer cements are compared with zinc phosphate cements, glass ionomer cements have shown a lower solubility in the environment of the oral cavity. Mechanical properties with the exception of a lower elastic modulus are similar in comparison as well.

58. **The correct answer is B.** The setting time is the time needed from the start of mixing to the time for a material to reach a state of hardness. The penetration test is used to determine the end point of the reaction. The setting time of Gypsum can be manipulated as to increase or decrease. The following chart below shows ways to decrease the setting time of Gypsum:

Variable	Decrease setting time
P:L ratio	By ⇑ P:L ratio, have less liquid per unit volume at start of mixing
Rate and time of spatulation	Longer and more rapid the plaster is mixed, the shorter setting time that can be achieved
Contamination of P:L	If impurities are added to mixture, it will decrease the set time; this can be done by the addition of slurry water/terra alba. This is the addition of small amounts of set Gypsum in watery mixture
Temperature	Temperature has shown to have minimal effect; it, however, slightly shortens the set time of the reaction

59. **The correct answer is D.** The pulpal depth of an amalgam preparation should extend to a minimum of 0.5 mm into sound dentin. This will aid in the resistance form of the cavity preparation. The ideal remaining amount of dentin to provide thermal insulation to the pulp is 2.0 mm. If the remaining dentin thickness is less than 2.0 mm, a base or liner should be used to replace the destroyed dentin.

ZOE (zinc oxide and eugenol) cannot be used on restorations where bonding to enamel or dentin is needed since the eugenol will interfere with the curing phase (polymerization) of resin-based composites. Picking a desirable base for a deep restoration is required to replace the amount of dentin that has been destroyed. A base is needed when the restoration to be placed is very deep and they will provide thermal insulation, thus protecting the pulp. With composite restorations, a base is not needed for thermal insulation; however, with small pulpal exposures, calcium hydroxide is still used for its ability to aid in the formation of secondary dentin bridges. A small amount of calcium hydroxide can be placed on a pinpoint exposure and covered with a liner (usually, a zinc phosphate) to provide pulpal protection. This is a direct pulp cap procedure. An indirect pulp cap is when a small amount of carious dentin is left behind and then covered with calcium hydroxide. This procedure utilizes the antimicrobial properties of calcium hydroxide.

60. **The correct answer is E.** Composite restorations should have all internal line angles rounded; this allows for better banking of the composite material. It is easier to place composite into rounded line angles than sharp ones. Remember, sharp internal line angles are needed for retention in gold restorations. Micromechanical bonding through acid etching provides primary retention for composite restorations when needed additional retention can be obtained. Undercuts can be made into the gingivo-axial and inciso-axial lines angles with a small round bur; this will provide a form of mechanical retention. This is usually done for larger carious lesions. The cavosurface margins when placed on enamel should be beveled. This is true as beveling will allow the acid-etch attack to occur at the ends of enamel rods, allowing for better adhesion and retention of the restorative resin material. Beveling also aids in preventing microleakage. Outline form of the prep is determined by the extent of the carious lesion; this holds true for all restorative materials. A butt joint is indicated when the preparation does not end on enamel. This allows for increased retention and a better seal when bonding to cementum or root dentin.

61. **The correct answer is C.** A chamfer margin provides the best support of a cast gold restoration. A shoulder is used for porcelain jacket and all ceramic crowns. A shoulder bevel is used for proximal boxes of inlays and occlusal shoulders of mandibular three-fourth crowns.

62. **The correct answer is D.** All of the statements are requirements of a good provisional restoration. The restoration must be fabricated of material that prevents the conduction of temperature extremes. The temporary restoration must be made of material and possess contours that the patient will be able to clean easily. It is of great importance that gingival margins of the temporary not impinge upon the gingival tissues.

63. **The correct answer is C.** This patient needs to function and needs a replacement for esthetics; therefore, no treatment would be appropriate. In this case, a fixed bridge prosthesis would be a very long span over this edentulous gap, which requires sufficient abutments to adequately place force and support. In addition, the severe bone resorption would compromise result of both an FPD and a Maryland bridge. Because of all of the above, a removable partial denture would be the best choice in this instance.

64. **The correct answer is A.** An anterior posterior palatal bar connector can be used in almost any maxillary partial denture to attain symmetry. A palatal palate is a thin broad connector that may be used for simple edentulous area and full palatal coverage. A palatal horseshoe-shaped connector should only be used when a large non-operable torus exists. The use of a single palatal bar is limited to tooth borne restorations for bilateral short-span edentulous areas.

65. **The correct answer is B.** Contact of the tip of the tongue with the anterior palate and lingual surfaces of the maxillary teeth produce "T" and "D" sounds. "P" and "B" sounds are produced by the lips only. "Th" sounds are produced by the tongue protruding slightly between the maxillary and mandibular anterior teeth.

66. **The correct answer is D.** Calcium chloride accelerates the setting time. Rosin facilitates the speed of the reaction and results in a smoother, more homogenous product. Resinous balsam is used to increase flow and improve mixing properties. Oil of cloves is used in preference to eugenol because it reduces burning sensation of the soft tissues of the mouth.

67. **The correct answer is C.** Posterior denture teeth that are set edge to edge can cause cheek biting. Lip biting after denture fabrication can be caused by reduced muscle tone or a large anterior horizontal overlap. Tongue biting may be caused by having the denture teeth set too far lingually. Gagging may be caused by a denture's posterior palatal seal extended too far posteriorly.

68. **The correct answer is D.** Physiologic dentinal sclerosis is the natural aging process of dentin. Reparative dentin is produced in the pulp chamber at the lesion site in response to insults such as caries, dental procedures, or attrition.

   The smear layer is any debris, calcific in nature, produced by reduction or instrumentation of dentin, enamel, or cementum.

69. **The correct answer is C.** Dentin has unevenly distributed intertubular and peritubular dentin and is therefore heterogeneous in nature. Enamel, however, is almost entirely homogenous in nature.

70. **The correct answer is A.** Primers contain hydrophilic monomers that have an affinity for the exposed collagen fibril arrangement and hydrophobic properties for the copolymerization with adhesive resins.

71. **The correct answer is B.** The hydrodynamic theory proposes that when a stimulus causes the slow fluid movement to become more rapid, nerve endings in the pulp are deformed, and this is interpreted as pain. Stimuli such as tooth preparation, air drying, and application of cold have been suggested as causes of sudden, rapid movement.

72. **The correct answer is C.** Premolars retain sealants best because the patient is older and it is easier to get better isolation for moisture control to place the sealant. It is harder to achieve adequate isolation on primary teeth and in younger patients. Permanent second molars are also noted for difficulty of isolation and moisture control.

73. **The correct answer is A.** Permanent first molars erupt when the patient is young. It is more difficult to get optimal isolation for restoration placement at this young age. Sealants are rarely placed on primary first molars and primary second molars.

74. **The correct answer is C.** The size of the bur does not matter in this situation. Heat and pressure are the most common causes of pulp damage during cavity preparation. The longer the cutting time, the more heat is generated, and the more damage can be caused. Greater tooth reduction would lead a cavity preparation to be closer in proximity to the pulp. Proximity to the pulp chamber increases the potential for pulpal damage.

75. **The correct answer is B.** Class II classification is for interproximal lesions on posterior teeth only. Cavity Classes I, V, and VI can involve both anterior and posterior teeth.

76. **The correct answer is D.** A shoulder margin is unnecessary for a full metal crown; a chamfer margin is sufficient. The use of depth cuts along anatomical planes of the occlusal surface will ensure adequate reduction and prevent over-reduction. The final preparation of the occlusal surface should follow a similar anatomical contour of the crown prior to reduction. Axial reduction should be approximately 6 degrees and should be slightly convergent to provide the maximum retention for the restoration. Increased taper results in excessive reduction of tooth structure. The use of PFM or partial ceramic coverage in nonesthetic areas will preserve tooth structure.

77. **The correct answer is B.** The recommended dimensions for a complete cast crown are a minimum of 1-mm clearance on nonfunctional cusps and 1.5 mm on functional cusps. The functional cusp bevel must be at a flatter angle than the cuspal plane to provide adequate reduction, which should be placed at about 45 degrees to the long axis of the tooth. A chamfer margin on a full metal crown allows for a 0.5-mm metal thickness, which provides adequate strength for the restoration.

78. **The correct answer is B.** The labial reduction should be in two planes (cervical and facial planes). A minimum of 1.2 mm in required to create a satisfactory appearance, but 1.5 is preferred. The incisal reduction for a PMF crown is 1.5 to 2.0 mm. The lingual reduction is 1 mm in excursion if contacts are in metal, but 1.5 mm of reduction is necessary if contact is in porcelain.

79. **The correct answer is C.** A lingual chamfer is insufficient in this situation. A full porcelain restoration will require a shoulder margin. Adequate reduction is imperative for an all-ceramic restoration. The facial surface requires a two-plane anatomical reduction of 1-mm depth. The incisal edge requires 1.5-mm reduction in intercuspation and excursive movements. The lingual surface of the tooth must be reduced 1.0 mm to provide adequate relief for porcelain coverage

80. **The correct answer is D.** Age is not an absolute contraindication for implant placement or restoration. Patients with acute or terminal illness are not candidates for implant placement. Patients with unrealistic expectations, poor motivation, or poor oral hygiene are not sound candidates for implants placement. Elective dental work on pregnant patients is not indicated. Implant placement in patients who have received IV bisphosphonates or head and neck radiation is relatively contraindicated because of the risks of bisphosphonate-related necrosis and osteoradionecrosis, respectively.

81. **The correct answer is B.** The extent of caries is important because that is all that needs to be removed without removing sound tooth structure. Removing sound tooth structure is unnecessary when performing a composite restoration, and doing so would not produce the most optimal preparation. A composite restoration does not require mechanical retention. The preparation does not correspond with the tooth shade.

82. **The correct answer is D.** The *polymer matrix* is the phase to which the other ingredients get added. The *filler particles* are silicon dioxide or glass that improves the physical properties of the

matrix. The *coupling agent* assists in the adhesion of the matrix to the filler particles. The *initiator* is what allows the polymerization of the composite to be activated.

83. **The correct answer is D.** 1.5 mm is the proper amount of reduction because 0.3 to 0.5 tooth structure reduction is needed to accommodate the metal and an additional 1.0 mm is needed for the porcelain. 0.8 and 1.0 mm are not enough reduction to accommodate both metal and porcelain. 2.5 mm is too much reduction.

84. **The correct answer is A.** Gold is a strong material. As opposed to other materials, gold rarely fractures. When used in restorations, it has the greatest functional longevity. Gold esthetics are inferior to other materials as gold does not look like natural teeth. The impression material used is dictated by the operator, not the restoration. Gold has a wear rate that is actually similar to enamel. Gold, unlike porcelain, will not cause wear on the opposing teeth to be accelerated

85. **The correct answer is B.** It is important to know which restoration is going to be the best for the specific tooth, and depending on the amount of remaining tooth structure, if a post will be necessary. The canal configuration is not going to affect the final outcome of how the tooth is restored. The function of the restored tooth is not one of the first things to be considered.

86. **The correct answer is C.** Frank Caries describe caries that have progressed just into the dentinoenamel junction (DEJ). Carious lesions occur when a mass of bacteria adhere to the tooth surface forming a dental plaque. The plaque bacteria feast on refined carbohydrates, metabolize the sugars, and produce acidic byproducts. The acid lowers the pH of the plaque adherent to the tooth; when the pH drops to 5.5, demineralization begins to take place; this is known as the critical pH (answer A). Early lesions are capable of remineralization or arrest if the pH is in favor of building and mineral content like fluoride is abundant. Incipient caries describe caries that have not progressed farther than enamel; these are reversible and capable of remineralization (answer B). Caries in enamel have different

properties than those in dentin; the mineral content in dentin is relatively sparse and arranged in a more tubular structure, allowing for more rapid progression of caries (answer D).

87. **The correct answer is A.** *Actinomyces viscosus* is the most common cariogenic bacteria in root surface or smooth surface caries (answer B). *Streptococcus sanguis* is the earliest organism found in dental plaque (answer C). A good way to remember common cariogenic bacteria: SALIVA: *S. mutans, sanguis. A. viscosus. Lactobacilli. Veillonella. A. naeslundii.*

88. **The correct answer is C.** The four zones of incipient lesions are listed above in correct order A to D. These characterize separate zones seen in a sectioned enamel lesion. The translucent zone is the deepest zone and is named for its absent or composition-less appearance seen under polarized light. The dark zone represents remineralization and is named after its characteristic inability to transit polarized light. The body zone is the largest zone and represents a demineralization phase. The surface zone is the outermost zone and seems to be unaffected by the caries.

89. **The correct answer is D.** Rampant caries are rapidly progressing and widespread caries. They are often the result of histological disadvantages, poor hygiene, drug abuse, radiation, high sugar diets, or disadvantaged saliva. They present acutely (A), are most often associated with pain (E), are seen in children (C), and result in large cavitation because of its deep and **narrow** presentation.

90. **The correct answer is E.** While all of the above are known risk factors for caries, A and B are high-risk factors, B and C are moderate-risk factors. Other high-risk factors for caries include visible plaque, frequent between meals snacks, inadequate saliva, and dental appliances.

Moderate-risk factors include: interproximal enamel lesions, other white spots or discolorations, and recreational drug use.

91. **The correct answers is D.** Autogenous graft.

Xenograft and alloplastic grafts are only osteoconductive and will not grow new bone without the presence of surrounding cells, such as osteoblasts, that will form bone. They only act as a scaffold to which new bone can be added onto.

Allografts can be osteoconductive and osteoinductive, meaning that they act as a scaffold onto which new bone forms and their bone matrix contains inducing agents that cause new bone to form.

Only autogenous bone is osteoconductive, osteoinductive, and osteogenic, meaning in addition to acting as a scaffold for new bone to adhere to and having a matrix with inducing agents to stimulate new bone, it also has the capability of forming new bone on its own, without the aid of surrounding growth factors.

92. **The correct answer is B.** Fentanyl.

Triazolam, lorazepam, and diazepam are all benzodiazepines that can be delivered by an oral route and are routinely used for oral conscious sedation.

Fentanyl is considered to be an IV drug used in IV sedation

93. **The correct answer is A.** Both the statement and the reason are correct and related.

Taken straight from advantages of single tooth implants section of the "Contemporary Implant Dentistry" textbook by Dr. Carl Misch, 3rd edition.

94. **The correct answer is D.** The first statement is FALSE and the second statement is TRUE.

Defects in color vision primarily affect 8% to 10% of the MALE population, for example, about 10% of all males are color blind.

The second statement is TRUE. Achromatism is the complete lack of hue sensitivity. Dichromatism is sensitivity to two of the primary hues. Anomalous trichromatism is sensitivity to all three primary hues with a deficiency or abnormality of one of the three primary pigments in the retinal cones.

95. **The correct answer is C.** Ovate pontic.

Sanitary (hygienic) pontics have the best access for oral hygiene but usually provide you with the worst esthetic outcomes once the gingival tissues have healed.

Conical pontics typically provide for good access for oral hygiene but again tend to have poor esthetic outcomes with the final prosthesis

Modified ridge lap pontics are moderately easy to clean and can provide good esthetics.

Ovate pontics: generally accepted to provide the best esthetics for the final prosthesis because of its support of the gingival architecture around the extraction site following healing.

CHAPTER 3

Oral and Maxillofacial Surgery and Pain Control

QUESTIONS

1. Which of the following statements about the temporomandibular joint (TMJ) is/are true?
   I.   It is a synovial joint
   II. It is a ginglymoarthrodial joint
   III. It allows for translational (gliding) movement
   IV. Posterior TMJ dislocations are more common than anterior dislocations

   A. I, II, and III
   B. II and IV
   C. IV only
   D. All the above
   E. None of the above

2. Trigeminal neuralgia presents with:
   I.   Generally presents bilaterally
   II. Common complaints include stabbing, burning, shocking pain
   III. It is uncommon for the pain to be triggered by benign events
   IV. Carbamazepine is more effective than amitriptyline

   A. I, II, and III
   B. II and IV
   C. IV only
   D. All the above
   E. None of the above

3. An elderly patient with a history of atrial fibrillation and recent cardiac stent placement presents to your clinic for mandibular lingual bony exostosis removal. The procedure occurs without incident, but you are concerned because of the potential immediate postoperative complications that can occur in this situation.
   I.   You are worried about infection
   II. You are worried about a pathologic fracture.
   III. You are worried that the patient will have difficulty eating
   IV. You are worried about postoperative bleeding

   A. I, II, and III
   B. II and IV
   C. IV only

   D. All the above
   E. None of the above

4. Regarding common bacteria found in oral infections, the following statements are true *except*:
   I.   Aerobic bacteria compose roughly 75% of oral infections
   II. Anaerobic bacteria involved in oral infections include *Neisseria* spp. and the *Bacteroides* spp.
   III. Odontogenic infections involve the predominance of one bacterium
   IV. Alpha hemolytic *Streptococcus* spp. are Gram-positive cocci in pairs

   A. I, II, and III
   B. II and IV
   C. IV only
   D. All the above
   E. None of the above

5. A patient presents to your clinic with a diagnosis of an *abscess*. Which characteristics support your diagnosis?
   I.   History of pain and swelling for 3 days
   II. History of pain and swelling for 1 week
   III. Predominance of anaerobic bacteria with a well-circumscribed border
   IV. Predominance of aerobic bacteria with a diffuse border

   A. I, II, and III
   B. II and IV
   C. IV only
   D. All the above
   E. None of the above

6. Necrotizing fasciitis:
   I.   Is a slowly progressing infection of the skin and fascia
   II. Is a rapidly progressing infection of the skin and muscle
   III. Has a low mortality rate with administration of antibiotics
   IV. Is a rapidly progressing infection of the skin and fascia

A. I, II, and III
B. II and IV
C. IV only
D. All the above
E. None of the above

7. A patient presents for dental implant evaluation. You do an oral examination and notice that he is completely edentulous and has minimal alveolar bone. You consider bone augmentation surgery. The following are true, *except*:

   I. An allograft is composed of tissue obtained from an animal such as a cow or pigs
   II. Augmentation of an atrophic mandible prior to implant placement is indicated in a patient with less than 10 mm of bone height
   III. Smokers, alcoholics, and uncontrolled diabetics are an absolute contraindication to dental implants
   IV. An autograft is an excellent choice for bone augmentation. Donor sites include the mandibular ramus, tibial plateau, anterior, and/or posterior hip

   A. I, II, and III
   B. II and IV
   C. IV only
   D. All the above
   E. None of the above

8. Clark's rule of pediatric dosing of local anesthetics is:

   A. Used to calculate the therapeutic dose
   B. Defined by (weight of child in kg/150) (maximum adult therapeutic dose)
   C. Not applicable to local anesthetics that have epinephrine
   D. Only calculated by a complex algorithm
   E. None of the above

9. Which of the following relate to the esters group local anesthetics?

   I. The esters local anesthetics include novocaine, procaine, and bupivacaine
   II. All are metabolized by the microsomal P450 enzymes of the liver
   III. Esters are metabolized by the liver
   IV. Esters are metabolized by pseudocholinesterase in the plasma

A. I, II, and III
B. II and IV
C. IV only
D. All the above
E. None of the above

10. What is the correct sequence for Guedel's stages of anesthesia?

    A. Amnesia and analgesia; delirium and excitement; surgical anesthesia; medullary paralysis
    B. Delirium and excitement; amnesia and analgesia; surgical anesthesia; medullary paralysis
    C. Amnesia and analgesia; surgical anesthesia; delirium and excitement; medullary paralysis
    D. Amnesia and analgesia; delirium and excitement; medullary paralysis; surgical anesthesia

11. You are performing full-mouth extractions for a patient when he starts to complain of tinnitus, circumoral numbness, and appear drowsy. What do you do next?

    A. You continue with the procedure because the patient is likely anxious
    B. Discontinue the procedure and send the patient home
    C. The patient is probably feeling some pain and is anxious. The patient needs more local anesthetic
    D. Discontinue the procedure; monitor the patient for local anesthetic toxicity

12. Regarding the mechanism of action for local anesthetics, the following are true, *except*:

    A. An inactive nerve cell has a resting membrane potential of -50 to -70 mV
    B. During the repolarization of the peripheral nerve, potassium ions pass out of the cell to restore the resting cell to resting membrane potential
    C. During depolarization, there is an influx of Ca^{2+}
    D. Nonionized molecules enter through nerve cell membranes more readily than ionized molecules

13. Infection causes tissue to be more resistant to the anesthetic effect of local anesthetics because:

    A. This results in a decrease in the ionized form of the local anesthetic; in turn, the local anesthetic has difficulty penetrating the cell membrane of the neuron
    B. Infected tissue has many bacteria that create buffers that hinder the diffusion of local anesthetic toward the nerve cell
    C. This results in an increase of the nonionized form of the local anesthetic; in turn, the local anesthetic effect is diminished because of an increased refractory period because of the abundance of local anesthetic in the neuron
    D. This results in an increase in the ionized form of the local anesthetic at the expense of the unionized form of the local anesthetic

14. What is the amount of local anesthetic in a cartridge with 3% local anesthetic and a volume of 2 mL?

    A. 60 mg/mL
    B. 20 mg /mL
    C. 30 mg
    D. 60 mg

15. What is the amount of epinephrine (mg) in a 5-mL vial labeled with 1:100,000 epinephrine?

    A. 0.01
    B. 0.05
    C. 0.1
    D. 0.5

16. In methemoglobinemia, all of the following are true except:

    A. Hemoglobin is oxidized to methemoglobin
    B. Methemoglobin cannot bind and carry oxygen
    C. Methemoglobin levels can only be detected by arterial blood draws
    D. Patients who have glucose-6-phosphate dehydrogenase (G6PD) are more sensitive to excessive doses of local anesthetics and antibiotics such as prilocaine and dapsone

17. The proper treatment for an avulsed tooth that occurred less than 25 minutes ago would include which of the following?

    A. Minimize contact with root and replant primary teeth
    B. Placement of a rigid splint for 4 to 6 weeks
    C. Replant and splint for 7 to 10 days
    D. Immediate pulpectomy and reimplantation

18. Nonrigid splints are recommended for all of the following situations except:

    A. Subluxation of a tooth or a group of teeth
    B. Avulsion. Tooth outside of socket less than 30 minutes
    C. Nonrigid splints should be made with thinner, 28 gauge, rather than thicker, 20 gauge, stainless steel wire
    D. Mid-root fracture

19. In decreasing order of frequency, what is the correct sequence for mandible fractures?

    A. Symphyseal/parasymphyseal>body> angle>ramus>coronoid>alveolar
    B. Symphyseal/parasymphyseal>condyle> alveolar>coronoid
    C. Symphyseal/parasymphyseal>angle> body>condyle
    D. Symphyseal/parasymphyseal>ramus> angle>coronoid

20. Signs and symptoms of alveolar osteitis include all of the following except:

    A. Pain commencing 2 to 5 days following the extraction
    B. Accompanied by a foul taste or smell
    C. It is a self-limiting condition that will improve and resolve with time
    D. Treat with antibiotics and pain medications

21. A dentist removes a maxillary premolar and notices that she has created an oroantral communication, which is 4 mm in diameter. Which of the following is an appropriate treatment?

    A. No surgical treatment
    B. Figure-of-eight sutures to maintain integrity of the blood clot within the socket
    C. Requires a buccal fat pad flap advancement
    D. Tongue flap advancement

22. The following drugs act as an agonist on mu (μ) receptors in the central nervous system (CNS) for analgesia, *except*:

    A. Fentanyl
    B. Ibuprofen
    C. Meperidine
    D. Tramadol

23. Benzodiazepines have all the following effects *except*:

    A. Anxiolytic
    B. Amnestic
    C. Analgesic
    D. Anticonvulsant

24. You are a first responder to a man found unresponsive, lying supine with a pulse at the scene of an unwitnessed motor vehicle accident. He is an unrestrained driver and was recovered 40 yards from his car. His leg appears broken, and there are no obvious open wounds. You initiate cardiopulmonary resuscitation (CPR). How do you establish an airway?

    A. Head tilt
    B. Placement of an oropharyngeal airway
    C. Perform a cricothyroidomy
    D. Jaw thrust

25. You are observing an orthognathic surgery in the operating room, when the healthy patient, who is under general anesthesia, begins to develop hypercarbia, rigidity, elevated temperature, and tachycardia. The anesthetist has his hands full and asks you to get the medication that is used to treat this condition.

    A. This condition is benzodiazepine overdose and should be treated with flumenazil
    B. This condition is an opioid overdose and should be treated with naloxone
    C. This condition is neuroleptic malignant syndrome and should be treated with dantrolene
    D. This condition is malignant hyperthermia and should be treated with dantrolene

26. A 60-year-old female comes to the emergency department with significant left periorbital edema, ptosis, mydriasis, and a history consis-tent with a dental infection of an upper left molar for the past 7 days. Her signs and symptoms suggest cavernous sinus thrombosis. This complication involves which of the following cranial nerves?

    A. IV, V, VII, IX
    B. II, III, IV, X
    C. IV, VI, VII, VIII
    D. III, IV, V, VI

27. A 24-year-old male presents to the emergency department very toxic and ill appearing. He is having difficulty breathing, is febrile, and is notably swollen below the jaw line. He complains of pain and difficulty swallowing and is also noted to be drooling. His mother mentions that he has had a toothache for the past 2 weeks. Initial management would include:

    A. Administration of antibiotics
    B. Administration of intravenous fluids and pain medications
    C. Establishment and maintenance of an adequate airway
    D. Incise and drain the most fluctuant area of the swelling
    E. Extract offending tooth

28. A 43-year-old male presents with trismus and pain localized to the right preauricular region. On examination, he has limited range in jaw movements, and it is noted that he has a right posterior open bite. CT maxillofacial shows a calcified growth of his right condyle, which you suspect to be an osteochondroma. You plan to resect the right condyle and condylar neck. What muscle would be required to be stripped, according to your plan, to remove the condylar segment successfully?

    A. Temporalis
    B. Masseter
    C. Lateral pterygoid
    D. Medial pterygoid

29. You are a member of the craniofacial team at the local hospital. As the team dentist, you are approached by the mother of an 8-day-old baby girl. She is curious about the timing of cleft palate repair. What is the appropriate timing of treatment?

    A. Rule of tens. When the patient is at least 10 lbs, has 10 mg /dL of hemoglobin, and is at least 10 weeks of age
    B. The palate repair is usually performed between 9 and 18 months of age
    C. As soon as possible. Usually between the first week of life and 6 months
    D. It only has to be repaired if the baby develops problems with speech

30. A 35-year-old male presents to the emergency department after an incident with his girlfriend. He was stabbed in the face with a box cutter, and upon your arrival, his vitals are stable and the bleeding is controlled with direct pressure. You assess the patient and note that portions of the parotid gland are herniating out of the wound. Your examination would include which of the following?

    I.   Facial nerve function
    II.   Mandibular nerve function
    III. Maxillary nerve function
    IV.   Vitality of his teeth
    V.   Patency of Stensen's duct
    VI.   Patency of Wharton's duct
    VII. Patency of nasolacrimal gland

    A. I, II, IV
    B. VI, VII
    C. I, II, III, IV, V, VI
    D. I, V
    E. III, VII

31. A 10-year-old generally healthy male presents for endodontic treatment of #30, he is extremely anxious and in acute pain. Because of the acute nature of the disease process, it has taken numerous carpules of local anesthesia to obtain any relief. Not soon after anesthesia is achieved, the patient begins to become confused and systolic blood pressure increases by 50 torr from baseline. What other signs would you also see the patient exhibit?

A. Relaxation
B. Increase in visual acuity
C. Decreased blood pressure over time
D. Increased respiratory rate over time

32. Which local anesthesia is associated with causing methemoglobinemia?

    A. Lidocaine
    B. Bupivicaine
    C. Prilocaine
    D. Procaine

33. After giving two cartridges of 2% lidocaine to anesthetize the inferior alveolar nerve, the patient develops facial drooping on the side of the injection. This complication occurred because the needle was directed:

    A. Too far lateral
    B. Too far inferior
    C. Too deep
    D. Too far superior

34. Which factor determines local anesthetic onset time?

    A. Lipid solubility of the anesthetic
    B. The percentage of protein binding
    C. The presence of a vasoconstrictor
    D. The degree of ionization

35. A 5-month-old mentally retarded patient presents to your office and on clinical examination, you note brachycephaly, midface hypoplasia, hypertelorism, and syndactyly of hands and feet. These findings are consistent with the diagnosis of what syndrome?

    A. Apert syndrome
    B. Treacher–Collins syndrome
    C. Eagle syndrome
    D. Beckwith–Wiedemann syndrome

36. What is the initial force direction with forceps placed on a tooth for a successful extraction?

    A. Apical
    B. Buccal
    C. Palatal
    D. Occlusally

37. A 24-year-old male with history of 1-ppd smoking and occasional alcohol use presents to your office 4 days after a routine extraction of #30 with complaints of severe throbbing pain and a foul taste, but on examination, there is no drainage or erythema of the area. What is the most likely diagnosis?

   A. Inferior alveolar nerve injury
   B. Alveolar osteitis
   C. Infection
   D. Osteomyelitis

38. A 64-year-old female with history of atrial fibrillation controlled medically with labetalol and taking coumadin presents for extraction of remaining lower teeth. Her current INR is 1.5. What is the most appropriate method of treating this patient?

   A. Remove the teeth and use local hemostatic materials and sutures
   B. Remove teeth and start saline rinses day of procedure
   C. Stop coumadin for 1 day and then remove teeth
   D. Stop coumadin for 3 days and then remove teeth

39. To remove maxillary tori, the necessary nerve blocks include which of the following?

   A. Incisive
   B. Incisive and posterior superior alveolar
   C. Greater palatine and incisive
   D. Greater palatine and posterior superior alveolar

40. The most difficult mandibular third molar impaction position is classified as:

   A. Mesioangular
   B. Soft tissue
   C. Distoangular
   D. Erupted

41. A 75-kg male presents for extraction of several teeth. He has a noncontributory medical history. What is the maximum amount of 2% lidocaine with 1:100 K epi patient can safely be administered (in mg)?

   A. 225
   B. 375
   C. 525
   D. 750

42. Which of the following suture materials is classified as nonresorbable?

   A. Vicryl
   B. Chromic gut
   C. Plain gut
   D. Nylon

43. What is the minimal safe distance for implant placement from the mental foramen?

   A. 2 mm
   B. 0.5 mm
   C. 2 cm
   D. 1 mm
   E. 3 mm

44. A 64-year-old female presents for removal of #2 and #3 under local anesthesia. Her past medical history is significant for type II diabetes and a history of rheumatic heart disease as a child. Medications: none, Allergies: Pen VK. What is the appropriate method of proceeding?

   A. Administer adequate local anesthesia and proceed with the removal of #2 and #3
   B. Give 2-g amoxicillin PO 1 hour prior to the procedure and remove #2 and #3
   C. Give 1-g ampicillin IV 30 minutes prior to the procedure and remove #2 and #3
   D. Give 600-mg clindamycin PO 1 hour prior to the removal of #2 and #3

45. What are the most common teeth that may cause referred pain to the ear?

   A. Maxillary central incisors
   B. Mandibular central incisors
   C. Mandibular molars
   D. Maxillary premolars
   E. Maxillary molars

Oral and Maxillofacial Surgery and Pain Control

46. A 54-year-old male presents with a 4-day history of tooth pain and swelling of his right mandible. Trismus of 10 mm, odynophagia, and dysphagia findings are noted. PMH: HTN, DM II Meds: HCTZ All: Pen VK. What is the necessary treatment for this patient?

    A. Incision and drainage
    B. Antibiotic therapy with pen VK
    C. Antibiotic therapy with clindamycin
    D. Incision and drainage followed by IV antibiotics

47. A 63-year-old male presents with pain and swelling in the floor of mouth and superior neck. PMH: Hyperlipidemia Meds: Lipitor All: NKDA. He notes that the pain is more evident prior to eating. What is the most likely diagnosis based on this history and radiograph?

    A. Sialolith
    B. Lingual artery atherosclerosis
    C. Normal findings on occlusal radiograph of mandible
    D. Supernumerary tooth

48. A 30-year-old male presents for routine examination, when a lesion is noted in the left mandible. PMH: none, Meds: none, All: NKDA. What is the most likely diagnosis?

    A. Odontogenic keratocyst
    B. Pindborg tumor
    C. Calcifying odontogenic cyst
    D. Squamous cell carcinoma

49. What medication reverses the effects of benzodiazepines?

    A. Narcan
    B. Naloxone
    C. Flumazenil
    D. Neostigmine
    E. Decadron

50. Which is the first muscle incised in a floor of mouth lowering procedure?

    A. Geniohyoid
    B. Genioglossus
    C. Buccinator
    D. Mylohyoid

51. Fentanyl, a synthetic derivative of morphine, has the relative potency:

    A. 10 times that of morphine
    B. Equal to morphine
    C. Half of that of morphine
    D. 100 times that of morphine

52. Which of the following describes a graft material derived from genetically unrelated members of the same species?

    A. Autogenous
    B. Allogeneic
    C. Xenogeneic
    D. Synthetic

53. A 34-year-old female presents with a non-painful 0.5 × 0.5 cm lesion on the underside of her tongue that was noted on routine examination (see photo). She states that it has been present for approximately 1 year. She has no past medical history and takes no medications. What is the treatment for this lesion?

    A. Incisional biopsy
    B. Excisional biopsy
    C. Nothing
    D. Resection

54. The panoramic radiograph depicts what type of fracture in the left mandible?

    A. Pathologic fracture
    B. Comminuted fracture
    C. Closed fracture
    D. No fracture present

55. Bell's palsy is caused by injury to what cranial nerve?

    A. CN V
    B. CN VII
    C. CN XII
    D. CN XI

56. Which peripheral nerve fibers are the thickest?

    A. Motor fibers
    B. Pain fibers
    C. Autonomic fibers
    D. Proprioception fibers
    E. Touch fibers

57. What is the primary effect of local anesthetics on the heart?

    A. Decreases the maximum rate of depolarization of Purkinje fibers and myocardium
    B. They have dose-dependent negative inotropic effect on myocardium
    C. Depress spontaneous pacemaker activity in the sinus node
    D. Blocks the intracellular release of calcium

58. Which of the following would be most likely encountered in the preoperative examination of a patient with Treacher–Collins syndrome?

    A. Mental retardation
    B. Pulmonary hypertension
    C. Cleft palate
    D. Glossoptosis

59. Extraction wounds heal by which method?

    A. Primary intention
    B. Secondary intention
    C. Tertiary intention
    D. None of the above

60. A 25-year-old female presents with past history of biting her lower lip for several weeks and now presents with a lesion that increases and decreases in size (Photo 30). PMH: asthma, Meds: Albuterol, All: NKDA. On the basis of the symptoms and clinical presentation, what is the treatment of choice?

    A. NS rinses four times daily
    B. Pen VK 500 mg every 6 hours for 7 days
    C. Excisional biopsy
    D. Incisional biopsy

61. A 16-year-old male presents with an unerupted maxillary upper left canine (Figure). He has no past medical history. What is the diagnosis?

    A. Mucous retention cyst
    B. Antrolith
    C. Condensing osteitis
    D. Odontoma

62. A 12-year-old girl sustains a traumatic right subcondylar fracture and a left parasymphyseal fracture. Radiographs show that the right condylar head is displaced laterally out of the glenoid fossa, with medial rotation of the condylar neck; the left parasymphyseal fracture is nondisplaced. Which of the following is the most appropriate management?

    A. Intermaxillary fixation for 4 weeks followed by passive/active physical therapy
    B. Closed reduction and intermaxillary fixation for 2 weeks and passive/active physical therapy
    C. Open reduction and internal fixation of the right subcondylar fracture followed by intermaxillary fixation for 6 weeks and passive/active physical therapy thereafter
    D. Open reduction and internal fixation of both the right subcondylar fracture and the left parasymphyseal fracture followed by intermaxillary fixation for 2 weeks and passive/active physical therapy thereafter

63. A 40-year-old African-American female with a chief complaint of needing "a cleaning."

    PMH: type II diabetes (diet controlled)
    Meds: none
    All: IV contrast

    Multiple areas of radiolucent lesions are seen in the panoramic radiograph, but the patient does have any symptoms of pain and on examination has no bony expansion or lesions associated with the overlying mucosa. Next step in treatment includes:

    A. Resection of the mandible
    B. Aspiration biopsy alone
    C. Aspiration and excisional biopsy
    D. No treatment indicated

64. A 50-year-old male presents to your office for evaluation and is noted to have a radiolucency in his left posterior mandible underneath the inferior alveolar nerve and is asymptomatic. The appropriate next step in treatment includes which of the following?

    A. Resection of the mandibular angle
    B. Aspiration biopsy
    C. Excisional biopsy
    D. No treatment needed

Oral and Maxillofacial Surgery and Pain Control

65. On removal of #14, you have broken off a root tip. The tooth is missing a portion of its palatal root. Unable to visualize the root tip, you take a radiograph and note its position to be:

    A. In the infratemporal fossa
    B. In the nerve canal
    C. In the maxillary sinus
    D. In the nasal floor

66. The nerve injury classified as neurotmesis is described as?

    A. A contusion of the nerve
    B. Complete loss of nerve continuity
    C. Loss of epineural sheath but intact axon
    D. A stretching of the nerve

67. Dental elevators are used for which of the following purposes?

    A. To retract the gingival crest tissue
    B. To reflect a full mucoperiosteal flap
    C. To engage the tooth apical to the cementoenamel junction
    D. To engage the tooth coronal to the cementoenamel junction

68. The levator veli palatini muscle is primarily innervated by the:

    A. V2 branch of the trigeminal (V) nerve
    B. V3 branch of the trigeminal (V) nerve
    C. Facial (VII) nerve
    D. Vagus (X) nerve
    E. Hypoglossal (XII) nerve

69. A right unilateral cleft lip is most likely to result from incomplete union between which of the following prominences?

    A. The frontonasal prominence to the lateral nasal prominence
    B. The frontonasal prominence to the medial nasal prominence
    C. The lateral nasal prominence to the maxillary prominence
    D. The lateral nasal prominence to the medial nasal prominence
    E. The medial nasal prominence to the maxillary nasal prominence

70. The mental nerve exits the mental foramen at which of the following sites?

    A. Below the canine halfway down the mandible
    B. Below the first premolar halfway down the mandible
    C. Below the first premolar, directed posteriorly
    D. Below the second premolar halfway down the mandible
    E. Below the lateral incisor

71. During a LeFort I maxillary osteotomy, the tooth most likely to be injured by a low osteotomy line is the:

    A. Central incisor
    B. Cuspid
    C. First bicuspid
    D. Lateral incisor
    E. Second bicuspid

72. The cervical branch of the facial nerve is transected during parotidectomy. Which of the following functions is most likely to be affected?

    A. Forward flexion of the neck
    B. Lateral flexion of the neck
    C. Pursing the lips
    D. Retraction and depression of the angle of the mouth
    E. Upward and downward movement of the hyoid bone

73. Which of the following glandular structures receives innervation from the auriculotemporal nerve?

    A. Lacrimal
    B. Meibomian
    C. Parotid
    D. Sublingual
    E. Submandibular

74. A 40-year-old woman develops Frey syndrome after undergoing parotidectomy. The most likely cause is injury to branches of which of the following nerves?

    A. Auriculotemporal
    B. Facial
    C. Great auricular

D. Posterior auricular

E. Vagus

75. Which tooth cannot be removed by only rotation motion?

A. Maxillary central incisor
B. Maxillary lateral incisor
C. Maxillary canine
D. Maxillary first premolar

76. Which of the following is the most common site of squamous cell carcinoma of the oral cavity?

A. Buccal mucosa
B. Floor of the mouth
C. Mandibular gingivae
D. Palate
E. Tongue

77. In adults, the normal range of vertical mandibular opening is from:

A. 20 to 30 mm
B. 30 to 40 mm
C. 40 to 50 mm
D. 50 to 60 mm

78. Each of the following is a muscle of mastication *except* the:

A. Buccinators
B. Lateral pterygoid
C. Masseter
D. Medial pterygoid
E. Temporalis

79. Which of the following structures is a branch of the mandibular division of the trigeminal nerve?

A. Infraorbital nerve
B. Lingual nerve
C. Nasopalatine nerve
D. Posterosuperior alveolar nerve
E. Posterosuperior nasal nerve

80. Stensen's duct can be found at which of the following anatomic sites?

A. Mandibular angle
B. Preauricular border
C. At the zygomatic arch

D. Between the superficial and deep lobes of the parotid gland

E. Within the buccal space

81. A 62-year-old man is 6 years status post right hemimaxillectomy for the treatment of a benign tumor. He is otherwise in good physical shape, with a noncontributory medical history. He complains that when he speaks and eats, his maxillary obturator becomes loose. He has had a new obturator fabricated less than 4 months ago, and the new one is just as ill fitting as his previous ones. He asks if there is anything that can be done to improve the retention of his obturator. Physical and radiographic examinations (including computerized tomography (CT) dentascan and panorex radiographs) show absence of the right hemimaxilla and complete maxillary edentulism with inadequate maxillary bone for placement of standard endosseous implants. Which of the following is the best possible treatment plan to improve retention of this patient's obturator?

A. Placement of bilateral zygomaticus implants
B. Soft reline of the existing obturator
C. Nothing can be done to improve this patient's condition
D. Take new impressions to fabricate a new obturator
E. Placement of standard endosseous implants and a prescription for long-term prophylactic oral antibiotics

82. A 15-year-old boy presents to your office with his mother 2 days after sustaining facial trauma after falling while riding his bicycle. He was referred to you from the local hospital emergency department, where he had a full workup. He suffered no bony injury; however, his permanent maxillary right central incisor (#8) has a small fracture of the crown (enamel only). The maxillary left central incisor (#9) was completely avulsed and accidentally discarded by the emergency department team. The maxillary right central incisor is treated with good cosmetic result by smoothing down of the sharp edges. The mother asks you if placement of an endosseous implant is a possible treatment of her child's missing tooth. Which of the following statements best answers the mother's question?

A. Because this patient is under 18, he is not a candidate for endosseous implant replacement of his missing tooth. He should wait at least 3 years prior to implant placement

B. This patient is currently a candidate for endosseous implant replacement of his missing tooth

C. Placement of endosseous implants in children will cause increased and faster erosion of alveolar ridge height

D. Placement of endosseous implants in children is inherently unstable and will not prevent supraeruption of opposing teeth or help maintain a stable occlusion

E. Endosseous implants have not been reported to migrate when placed in children. The patient should wait until he is 21 to have implants placed

83. A 21-year-old female patient with a right-side unilateral cleft lip and palate is referred by an orthodontist to an oral surgeon for an alveolar cleft bone grafting procedure. Clinical examination reveals a missing permanent right maxillary lateral incisor. All other permanent teeth have erupted. Orthodontic appliances are aligning the arches, and space has been maintained for the replacement of the lateral incisor. A panorex radiograph confirms that all permanent teeth have erupted, no supernumerary or impacted teeth are evident, and the alveolar cleft site is deficient in bone. A decision is made to graft the alveolar cleft site with autogenous iliac marrow. How long should the consolidation period be for the alveolar cleft bone graft before the placement of an endosseous implant to replace the missing lateral incisor?

A. 4 weeks
B. 8 months
C. 4 months
D. 1 year
E. 2 years

84. A 45-year-old female patient has three implant supported crowns in her right posterior mandible with three individual, nonconnected implants replacing missing teeth #28, #29, and #30. On clinical evaluation, the patient reports pain in her jaw during percussion of the crown on the most mesial implant. Periapical radiographs show a generalized radiolucency surrounding the implant in the #28 position, and just less than one-half of the surrounding bone has resorbed around the implant in the #29 position. No radiographic abnormalities are associated with the implant in the #30 position. There is no discharge, pus, erythema, or discoloration of the peri-implant gingiva. Which of the following implants meet the criteria for failure?

A. #28
B. #29
C. #30
D. #28 and #29
E. #28 and #30
F. #29 and #30

85. A 45-year-old female patient has presented for restoration of a previously placed endosseous implant in the right maxillary canine tooth #6 position. She has a full maxillary and mandibular dentition, with the exception of tooth #6, which was extracted secondary to a failed root canal treatment. The patient has a slight distocclusion relationship between her maxillary and mandibular dental arches, and the canine classification directly correlates to the Angle molar relationship. Bilaterally, the mesiobuccal cusp of her maxillary first permanent molars articulates mesial to the mesiobuccal groove of the

mandibular first permanent molar. Currently, her occlusion is balanced, stable, and reproducible. She is without TMJ pain or symptoms. How would you restore the canine tooth implant to preserve a functional and balanced occlusion?

A. The maxillary canine tip should oppose the embrasure between the mandibular canine and first premolar
B. The maxillary canine tip should occlude distal to the embrasure between the mandibular canine and first premolar
C. The maxillary canine tip should be flattened and taken out of occlusion
D. The maxillary canine tip should occlude mesial to the embrasure between the mandibular canine and first premolar
E. It does not matter where the maxillary canine tip ends up. Normal wear of the restoration will result in a functional and stable occlusion

86. A 27-year-old female patient presents for a cosmetic restoration of a previously placed endosseous implant in the left maxillary central incisor position. Which of the following descriptive terms describes relationship in which the incisal edges of the maxillary teeth follow the curvature of the border of the lower lip in a posed, social smile?

A. Smile arc
B. Dental display
C. Esthetic line of the dentition
D. Curve of Spee
E. Centric occlusion

87. A 65-year-old Caucasian female patient presents to your office because she is interested in replacing her missing mandibular teeth with endosseous implants. Her medical history is significant for osteoporosis, for which she has taken alendronate 10 mg/d for the past 2 years. She does not report any other comorbidities and has never taken any other medications. Which of the follow statements is the most appropriate treatment philosophy for this patient?

A. This patient's history of bisphosphonate use disqualifies her as a potential endosseous implant recipient

B. This patient may undergo surgical placement of endosseous implants using standard implant surgery techniques without modification
C. This patient should undergo a 2-month "drug holiday" prior to endosseous implant placement
D. This patient should undergo a 2-month "drug holiday" immediately after endosseous implant placement
E. This patient should undergo a 1-year "drug holiday" prior to endosseous implant placement and is restricted from ever taking bisphosphonate medications again in her lifetime

88. An 18-year-old male patient with anhidrotic ectodermal dysplasia presents to your office for evaluation and treatment planning. He displays hypodontia, hypohidrosis, and hypotrichosis. The patient's existing dentition consists of bilateral maxillary canines, bilateral maxillary first molars, bilateral maxillary primary molars, bilateral mandibular primary molars, bilateral mandibular first molars, and bilateral mandibular second molars. All other permanent maxillary and mandibular teeth are missing. His alveolar ridges are extremely narrow and are concave lingually. Which of the following will provide the most accurate information regarding the patient's alveolar height and width for implant treatment planning?

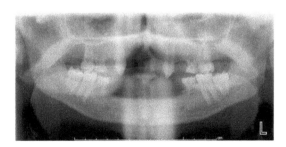

A. Computed tomography with dental CT software (i.e., dentascan)
B. Orthopantogram
C. Full-mouth periapical radiographs
D. Occlusal radiographs
E. Bitewing radiographs

89. A 43-year-old female patient is scheduled for placement of endosseous implants to replace her missing maxillary central incisor teeth #8 and #9. Her medical history is significant for mitral valve prolapse with mild regurgitation. She tells you that she is allergic to penicillin. Which antimicrobial prophylaxis regimen should be followed for this patient?

    A. The patient should be administered clindamycin 600 mg PO 1 hour prior to the dental procedure
    B. The patient should be administered clindamycin 600 mg PO 1 hour prior to the dental procedure, and clindamycin 300 mg 1 hour after the dental procedure
    C. The patient should be administered amoxicillin 2 g PO 1 hour prior to the dental procedure
    D. The patient should be administered vancomycin 2 g PO 1 hour prior to the dental procedure
    E. Antimicrobial prophylaxis is not indicated at this time

90. According to the original two-stage Branemark method of endosseous implant placement, which of the following describes the recommended healing time for maxillary and mandibular bone in patients without bone grafts, soft bone, or oral parafunctional habits?

    A. Maxilla: 5- to 6-month healing period. Mandible: 3- to 4-month healing period
    B. Maxilla: 1- to 2-month healing period. Mandible: 1- to 2-month healing period
    C. Maxilla: 1- to 2-month healing period. Mandible: 3- to 4-month healing period
    D. Maxilla: 3- to 4-month healing period. Mandible: 1- to 2-month healing period
    E. Maxilla: 5- to 6-month healing period. Mandible: 1- to 2-month healing period

91. A 57-year-old male patient is scheduled for surgical endosseous implant placement. He has a history of right prosthetic hip total joint replacement 4 months ago. He reports that he has a penicillin allergy. Which of the following antibiotic prophylaxis regimens is most appropriate for this patient?

    A. The patient should be administered clindamycin 600 mg PO 1 hour prior to the dental procedure, and clindamycin 300 mg 1 hour after the dental procedure
    B. The patient should be administered amoxicillin 2 g PO 1 hour prior to the dental procedure
    C. The patient should be administered cephradine 2 g PO 1 hour prior to the dental procedure
    D. The patient should be administered clindamycin 600 mg PO 1 hour prior to the dental procedure
    E. No antimicrobial prophylaxis is indicated at this time

92. Large postablative palatomaxillary defects are often treated prosthodontically with the fabrication of a maxillary obturator. Which of the following forces are properly matched with the destabilizing effect most likely encountered with prosthetic obturation of the defect?

    A. Cantilever forces causing the obturator to tip toward the defect
    B. Rotational forces causing the obturator to spin uncontrollably with function
    C. Tensile forces causing the obturator to stretch
    D. Compressive forces causing compaction of the obturator

93. Which of the following definitions describes the process by which new bone formation occurs from osteoprogenitor cells that are present in the graft, survive the transplant, and proliferate and differentiate to osteoblasts?

    A. Osteoinduction
    B. Osteogenesis
    C. Osteoconduction
    D. Osseointegration
    E. Angiogenesis

94. Which of the following is considered the "gold standard" in bone grafting?

    A. Autologous bone
    B. Allograft
    C. Xenograft
    D. Alloplast
    E. Bone morphogenetic protein (BMP)

95. A 30-year-old female patient presents to your office for reevaluation 1 week after surgical placement of a single endosseous implant in her posterior right mandible. The implant was placed in a long-standing edentulous region to replace her missing second molar tooth (#31). The patient complains of total "numbness" in her right lip and chin that has persisted since the surgery.

A complete sensory evaluation is performed including testing of the patient's responses to light touch, pain, temperature, directional movements, and two-point discrimination. Vitality testing of all mandibular teeth is also performed. Comparisons are made with the normal, contralateral side.

Upon examination and mapping of the distribution of her right mandibular nerve, an area of right-side mental region skin and oral mucosa displayed marked decreased perception of stimulation. Which of the following nerve injury terminologies best describes the sensations experienced by the patient?

A. Hypoesthesia
B. Dysesthesia
C. Hyperesthesia
D. Allodynia
E. Hyperalgesia
F. Hyperpathia
G. Anesthesia

96. A 33-year-old male patient is diagnosed with a closed nerve injury 1 week after endosseous implant placement in his posterior right mandible. Upon examination and mapping of the distribution of his right mandibular nerve, the following areas of hypoesthesia are noted.

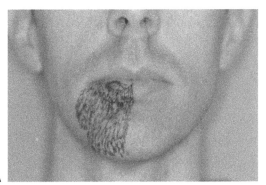

A

Panoramic and periapical radiographic examinations of the posterior right mandible fail to show any abnormality or disruption of the inferior alveolar canal.

He is followed closely with serial sensory examinations. During a repeat examination 4 weeks later, he reports improvement of symptoms and returning sensation to his right mental region. Sensory mapping at this examination shows a decreased size of the area of altered sensation.

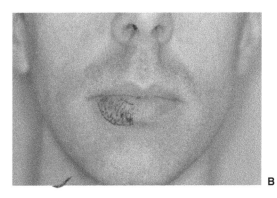

B

Which of the following of nerve injury classifications best describes the sensations experienced by the patient?

A. Neurapraxia
B. Axonotmesis
C. Neurotmesis
D. Hyperpathia
E. Allodynia

97. A 60-year-old male patient with chronic renal failure secondary to long-standing type I diabetes mellitus presents requesting dental implant replacement of his missing mandibular molar teeth. He reports that he undergoes hemodialysis three times weekly. What special considerations must be taken in the care of this patient?

    A. Consult with the patient's physician regarding his current medical status. No antibiotic prophylaxis is currently recommended for end-stage renal disease patients undergoing hemodialysis. Oral surgery procedures should be done on the same day as dialysis
    B. There is no need to consult with the patient's physician. He can undergo surgical dental implant placement without special considerations
    C. Consult with the patient's physician regarding his current medical status, antibiotic prophylaxis recommendations, and dialysis schedule. It is recommended that oral surgery procedures be performed the day after dialysis. The patient will require antibiotic prophylaxis
    D. This patient is not a candidate for surgical implant therapy

98. A 31-year-old female patient is 9 weeks into her first pregnancy. She reports that while biting into an apple, her retained left primary molar tooth "fell out." There are no clinical signs of infection. She is interested in dental implant replacement of her missing maxillary left first premolar tooth. A review of a panorex radiograph taken 1 year ago shows an impacted left maxillary first premolar tooth apical to a retained deciduous molar. The patient would like to know when she will undergo dental implant replacement of her missing tooth. You tell the patient:

    A. Elective surgical procedures such as implantology should be delayed until after delivery
    B. This patient can undergo dental implant treatment immediately as there is no risk to the fetus at this time
    C. It is best to wait until the third trimester to undergo surgical dental implant treatment

as there is less risk to the mother during this time
    D. Because of the presence of an impacted, ankylosed tooth, this patient is not a candidate for dental implant treatment in that region

99. A 29-year-old female patient presents to your office 1-week status postsurgical dental implant placement in her posterior right maxilla. She reports that since her last visit she has found out that she is pregnant. She informs you that she is still in mild-to-moderate pain from the surgical procedure. The patient asks you what she can use for the pain. She has no known allergies to medications. Which of the following pain medications is best suited for this pregnant patient?

    A. None
    B. Acetaminophen
    C. Aspirin
    D. Codeine
    E. Hydromorphone

100. Which of the following diseases would contraindicate the placement of dental implants in an elderly patient?

    A. None
    B. Dementia
    C. Hypertension
    D. Hypercholesterolemia
    E. Atrial fibrillation

101. When treatment planning the placement of osseointegrated endosseous implants, which of the following is true?

    A. As a general rule, always use the smallest possible implant diameter
    B. As a general rule, the diameter of the implant does not affect stability
    C. As a general rule, always use the longest length implant available, even if there is potential impingement of vital structures such as the inferior alveolar nerve
    D. As a general rule, always use the largest possible implant diameter

102. When treatment planning implant placement, what is the minimal mesiodistal distance from

the implant shoulder to the adjacent tooth at bone level?

A. A minimal distance of 1.5 mm is recommended between the implant shoulder and the adjacent tooth at bone level
B. A minimal distance of 1.0 mm is recommended between the implant shoulder and the adjacent tooth at bone level
C. A minimal distance of 0.5 mm is recommended between the implant shoulder and the adjacent tooth at bone level
D. A minimal distance of 3.0 mm is recommended between the implant shoulder and the adjacent tooth at bone level

103. How much bone is recommended at a minimum on the facial and palatal surfaces of the implant to support the ideal orofacial implant position?

A. 0.25 mm
B. 0.5 mm
C. 1.0 mm
D. 2.0 mm

104. What is the maximum torque that should not be exceeded when inserting the implant fixture?

A. 25 Ncm
B. 35 Ncm
C. 45 Ncm
D. 50 Ncm

105. Traditionally, what comprises the "Second Stage" implant surgical procedure?

A. Placement of the healing abutment
B. Torque testing of the implant cover screw
C. Placement of the closure screw
D. Placement of the implant fixture

106. You are about to provide supplemental oxygen to a patient in your dental chair scheduled for implant placement under IV sedation. The regulator gauge on the portable E-cylinder of oxygen reads 1,000 psi. You plan to use a flow of 10 L/min. Using this flow rate, approximately how much time is remaining in this oxygen E-cylinder?

A. 30 minutes
B. 45 minutes

C. 60 minutes
D. 120 minutes

107. You are about to provide supplemental oxygen via nasal cannula to a patient sitting in your dental chair with chronic obstructive pulmonary disease (COPD). Although the patient is not in any significant distress, the patient's pulse oximeter reading is 80%, which is lower than her usual value. Which of the following statements is correct?

A. Oxygen supplementation is never indicated in patients with COPD
B. One can provide whatever concentration of supplemental oxygen is required to maintain oxygen saturation above 90%, as measured by pulse oximeter
C. One should administer 100% oxygen by non-rebreather mask to all COPD patients exhibiting even the slightest signs of dyspnea.
D. A nasal cannula is not an appropriate method for administration of supplemental oxygen in this case

108. A man is diagnosed as having extremely inflamed retrodiscal tissue as a result of functional loading of an internally deranged TMJ. All conservative treatment has failed to resolve the problem. What is the next course of action?

A. Arthrocentesis
B. Arthroscopic surgery
C. Prosthetic restoration
D. Occlusal adjustment
E. Orthognathic surgery

109. A patient presents to your office with symptoms that include stabbing, shocking pain lasting a few seconds to minutes. He says that the pain is provoked by cold and only occurs on the left side. What is the most likely diagnosis for this patient?

A. Myofascial pain dysfunction syndrome
B. Trigeminal neuralgia
C. Osteoarthritis
D. TMJ ankylosis
E. Disk displacement

110. A 150-lb man presents for extraction of #30. The patient has an abscess and severe swelling in the area around the tooth to be extracted. You have already administered six carpules of 2% Lidocaine with 1:100,000 epinephrine to the patient. How many more carpules can you give without putting the patient at risk?

    A. 6
    B. 8
    C. 10
    D. 14

111. A patient presents with tooth pain after being punched in the mouth. Upon examination, the tooth causing the pain is fractured at the coronal portion of the root. There is no mobility or displacement. What is the proper treatment for this patient?

    A. Removal of coronal segment and pulpectomy
    B. Rigid splint

C. Occlusal adjustment
D. Extraction

112. A 55-year-old woman presents for extraction of #28. She intends to have an implant placed in the extraction site. The woman has a medical history of controlled type II diabetes. She is currently taking oral bisphosphonates for mild osteoporosis. #28 has a small abscess and +1 mobility. There is 9 mm of vertical bone height in the area. The abscess is drained and the patient notes immediate relief upon extraction. What, if any, is a contraindication for immediate placement of an implant at the extraction site?

    A. Not enough bone height
    B. Bisphosphonate therapy
    C. Active infection
    D. Osteoporosis
    E. type II diabetes

1. **The correct answer is A.** The temporomandibular joint is classified as a ginglymoarthrodial joint that consists of a translational (gliding) movement and a rotational (hinging) movement. It is also a synovial joint. There are superior and inferior synovial cavities that provide an articular surface for the movement of the articular disk and the mandibular fossa, of the temporal bone, and also against the mandibular condyle.

Anterior dislocations are more common than posterior TMJ dislocations because of the posterior boundary that is the posterior glenoid process. The articular tubercle is relatively less prominent than the posterior glenoid process; in turn, less energy is required to cause the mandibular condyle to be dislocated and entrapped by the articular tubercle. Anterior dislocations are more common than posterior dislocations. Posterior TMJ dislocations are not as common as anterior dislocations.

2. **The correct answer is B.** Trigeminal neuralgia is commonly described as stabbing, burning, shocking pain that lasts for seconds to minutes. It generally presents unilaterally. Medications that are used to treat trigeminal neuralgia include: antiepileptics, tricyclic antidepressants, muscle relaxants, and benzodiazepines. Carbamazepine, tegretol, is a preferred treatment for trigeminal neuralgia. Amitriptyline can be tried, but the success rate is lower. Other antiepileptics that can be used include: lamotrigine, gabapentin, and phenytoin. Amitriptyline is a tricyclic antidepressant that is also used for neuropathic pain.

Carbamazepine is an antiepileptic drug that has a mechanism of sodium channel blockade. It is a versatile drug that has multiple indications such as for seizures disorders, mood disorders, and also for neuropathic pain.

Trigeminal neuralgia is generally unilateral and is commonly reported by patients to be triggered by relatively benign events such as light touch, thermal stimulation, and wind.

3. **The correct answer is C.** An elderly patient with a history of atrial fibrillation and recent cardiac stent placement should alert you to the likely use of anticoagulants such as coumadin. International normalized ratio (INR) between the ranges of 2 to 3 is therapeutic for patients diagnosed with atrial fibrillation. Recent cardiac stent placements also require anticoagulation to prevent clot formation on newly placed stents. The removal of mandibular lingual bony exostosis can lead to the development of postoperative bleeding, hematoma formation, and airway compromise. A temporary acrylic stent could be fabricated to assist in hemostasis at the surgical site to prevent the development of a sublingual/submandibular hematoma.

Infection should be a concern; however, it would not be suspected in the immediate postoperative course. Although the removal of extensive bony tori may predispose one to a pathologic fracture, the potential for postoperative bleeding is more likely in this case presentation. Difficulty eating would not be suspected in the immediate postoperative course.

4. **The correct answer is C.** Alpha hemolytic *Streptococcus* spp. are aerobic Gram-positive cocci in pairs. Aerobic bacteria roughly compose 25% of oral infections. *Neisseria* spp. are anaerobic Gram-negative cocci. *Bacteroides* is an anaerobic Gram-negative rod. Odontogenic infections are from indigenous bacteria and polymicrobial in nature, composed of both aerobic and anaerobic bacteria.

5. **The correct answer is A.** An abscess is characterized by a disease process of chronic duration. Abscesses generally develop from cellulitic processes and form 2 to 3 days after the onset of symptoms of pain and swelling. They may persist for long periods of time since purulence that is not drained will remain until the body removes the necrotic tissue, which can be a lengthy process dependent on the extent of the abscess formation. As the infection progresses into a mature abscess, the purulence produced

will compress the surrounding tissue to create granulation tissue, which helps to contain the infection from spreading. This containment of the infection produces a well-circumscribed border.

Abscesses are composed of predominantly anaerobic bacteria with a well-circumscribed border. Cellulitic processes are composed of a predominance of aerobic bacteria with a diffuse border. There is a lack of a well-circumscribed border in cellulitis because of the lack of purulence. Abscesses are predominantly anaerobic bacteria with a well-circumscribed border. They have a chronic duration, pain is generally localized, and the borders are well circumscribed. On palpation, they are fluctuant because of the presence of purulence.

6. **The correct answer is C.** Necrotizing fasciitis is a rapidly progressing infection of the skin and fascia. It has a high mortality rate (30%–50%) even with antibiotic administration. In many cases, surgical debridement is required for adequate treatment and can lead to disfiguring results.

Necrotizing fasciitis is a rapidly progressing infection of the skin and fascia. Etiology is attributed to Group A strep, mixed aerobic–anaerobic bacteria or *Clostridium perfringens*. It has a high mortality rate (30%–50%) and without prompt surgical debridement of necrotic/infected tissue can lead to death and significant disfigurement. The muscle that is affected by necrotizing fasciitis occurs secondary to the progression via the skin and fascia.

7. **The correct answer is C.** An autograft is the transplantation of tissue from one region to another within the same individual. Donor sites include the mandible (chin, ramus, maxillary tuberosity), iliac crest (anterior/posterior hip), tibia, and even the cranium. An allograft is the transplantation of tissue from one individual to another genetically nonidentical individual of the same species. Xenograft is the transplantation of tissue from one species to another. Augmentation of an atrophic mandible prior to implant placement is indicated in a patient with less than 8 mm of bone height. The edentulous maxilla can be classified depending on

the deficiency of alveolar bone and can be defined by Parel's classification system.

8. **The correct answer is E.** Clark's rule is (weight of child in lb/150) (maximum adult dose in mg). This rule helps define the maximum pediatric dose and is not affected by the presence of epinephrine. It is a simple formula that should be calculated prior to pediatric procedures.

9. **The correct answer is C.** Esters are metabolized by pseudocholinesterase in the plasma. Amides are metabolized by the microsomal P450 enzymes of the liver via N-dealkylation and hydroxylation. Ester local anesthetics include procaine, benzocaine, and tetracaine. Amide local anesthetics generally have the letter "I" plus "-caine" in their drug names (lidocaine, mepivacaine, bupivacaine). All local anesthetics comprised a lipophilic aromatic ring linked to a hydrophilic amino group. The link is either an ester or an amide bond, and this determines its classification. Children and the elderly are at greatest risk for local anesthetic toxicity.

10. **The correct answer is A.** Amnesia and analgesia; delirium and excitement; surgical anesthesia; medullary paralysis.

Amnesia and analgesia is the stage in which induction occurs; preservation of protective reflexes, and this ends with loss of consciousness. Delirium and excitement is the second stage and consists of the presentation of involuntary movements, obtunded reflexes, and ends with the onset of total anesthesia. Nausea and vomiting are common in this stage. Surgical anesthesia is the third stage and is composed of three planes—light, medium (ideal for surgical procedures), and deep. Medullary paralysis is very deep anesthesia with loss of cardiovascular function and imminent death.

11. **The correct answer is D.** The patient is demonstrating initial signs of local anesthetic toxicity. These include circumoral numbness, tachycardia, hypertension, drowsiness, confusion, tinnitus, and metallic taste.

Full-mouth extractions generally require a lot of local anesthetic, and at times if one is not careful, the threshold for toxicity may be exceeded. The assumption of local anesthetic toxicity should be ruled out before considering a diagnosis of anxiety. Drowsiness is unlikely with anxious patients.

Although it is correct to discontinue the procedure, one should monitor the patient for progression of symptoms. Treatment for the initial signs of toxicity are supportive measures; however, if later signs of CNS compromise (e.g., tremor, hallucinations) appear, in conjunction with cardiovascular collapse, immediate referral to the hospital is required.

Patients who are in pain are unlikely to appear drowsy. Most will wince or complain of inadequate anesthesia. The presentation with CNS and cardiovascular signs/symptoms suggest local anesthetic toxicity.

12. **The correct answer is C.** During the depolarization of the neuron, there is an influx of sodium. Local anesthetics act by increasing the threshold for the opening of sodium channels.

An inactive nerve cell has a resting membrane potential of -50 to -70 mV. The cytoplasm of a resting nerve cell has a high concentration of potassium ions and a low concentration of sodium ions. This gradient is maintained by a Na/K ion pump.

During the repolarization of the peripheral nerve, potassium ions pass out of the cell to restore the resting cell to resting membrane potential.

Non-ionized molecules enter through nerve cell membranes more readily than ionized molecules. The local anesthetics lipophilic aromatic ring facilitates passage through the nerve sheath and membrane.

13. **The correct answer is D.** The acidic environment of infected tissue has a tendency to shift the balance regarding a local anesthetic's equilibrium toward more of the ionized form of the local anesthetic. In turn, there is a decrease in the non-ionized form of local anesthetic and less penetration of local anesthetic through the cell membrane of the neuron. Non-ionized molecules readily diffuse across cell membranes. Infected tissue is acidic; thereby, readily ionizing local anesthetic to an ionized form,

which is not effective at traversing a neuron's cell membrane. There is a decrease in the non-ionized form of the local anesthetic. A shift toward more ionized local anesthetic molecules prevents the local anesthetic from exerting their effect on the sodium channels.

14. **The correct answer is D.** The percentage of local anesthetic is measured in grams per 100 mL (i.e., 1% is 1 g/100 mL or 1,000 mg/100 mL or 10 mg/mL). Therefore, the concentration in a 3% solution is 30 mg/mL. In 2 ml of this solution, there would be 60 mg of local anesthetic. Answer choice A is incorrect because 60 mg/mL is the concentration, and not the amount, in a cartridge with 6% local anesthetic. In answer choice B, there is 30 mg/mL in a 3% local anesthetic. Since there is a volume of 2 mL, the total amount of local anesthetic is 60 mg. Answer choice C is incorrect because this is the amount of local anesthetic in 1 mL of a 3% local anesthetic.

15. **The correct answer is B.** 1:100,000 means 1 g/100,000 mL. Converting into milligrams, a 1:100,000 solution contains 1,000 mg/100,000 mL or 0.01 mg/mL. The concentration 0.01 mg/mL in the vial is then multiplied by 5 mL (the volume in the vial) for a total of 0.05-mg epinephrine. If the vial had a volume of 1 mL, 0.01 mg would be correct.

16. **The correct answer is C.** Methemoglobin levels may be obtained by both arterial and venous blood draws. Hemoglobin is oxidized to methemoglobin. Elevated levels of methemoglobin in the blood are caused when the mechanisms that defend against _oxidative stress_ within the red blood cell are overwhelmed and the oxygen carrying _ferrous ion_ (Fe^{2+}) of the _heme_ group of the hemoglobin molecule is oxidized to the _ferric state_ (Fe^{3+}). This converts hemoglobin to methemoglobin, which is a non-oxygen binding form of hemoglobin that binds a water molecule instead of oxygen. Patients with G6PD deficiency lack the production of sufficient amounts of NADPH, an oxidizing agent. Normally, the production of methemoglobin is reduced back to a normal state by protective enzymes such as

cytochrome b5 reductase (major pathway), and to a lesser extent NADPH methemoglobin reductase, glutathione, and ascorbic acid.

17. **The correct answer is C.** Replant and splint the avulsed tooth for 7 to 10 days (3–4 weeks for a tooth with an immature/open apex). Primary teeth are not reimplanted because this action could jeopardize the underlying adult dentition. A space maintainer may be required if loss of dental arch space is an issue. Avulsed teeth should not be splinted for greater than 7 to 10 days, except in the case of an avulsed tooth with an immature apex (3–4 weeks). Rigid splint placement is recommended for alveolar process fractures, but not isolated tooth avulsions. Minimal contact with a tooth, especially the root, should be practiced to limit any loss of PDL. Immediate pulpectomy is generally reserved for root fractures where less than one-third of the root is involved.

18. **The correct answer is D.** With dental root fractures of the apical or mid-root, the tooth should be reimplanted and a rigid splint placed for 2 to 3 months. Subluxation is trauma to a tooth that causes mobility without displacement from the tooth socket. Avulsion of a tooth from a socket less than 30 minutes should be placed in a nonrigid splint after reimplantation. Compared with rigid splints, this will have less chance of causing ankylosis. Thinner wire will allow for physiologic dental movement, whereas thicker wire will act more like a rigid splint and predispose tooth to ankylosis.

19. **The correct answer is B.** The quoted frequencies of mandible fractures are: Symphyseal/parasymphyseal 22%; condyle 24.5%; alveolar 3.1%; coronoid 1.3%; body 16%; angle 24.5%; ramus 1.7%. Fractures of the condyle will result in deviation on opening to the fractured side because of unopposed muscle action of the contralateral medial pterygoid muscle. Therefore, fracture of the right condyle will cause deviation of the mandible to the right upon mouth opening. When considering the entire facial complex, nasal bone fractures are the most common facial fracture.

20. **The correct answer is D.** Alveolar osteitis (dry socket) is a self-limiting condition that will improve and resolve with time. Antibiotics are not indicated without the signs of infection. It generally presents after extraction of teeth. Alveolar osteitis is a painful phenomenon that most commonly occurs a few days following the removal of mandibular (lower) *wisdom teeth*. It occurs when the *blood clot* within the healing *tooth* extraction site is disrupted. In rare cases, the removal of the upper *wisdom teeth* can also result in possible alveolar osteitis.

Signs of alveolar osteitis include worsening, throbbing pain 2 to 5 days after extraction of a tooth. Radiation of pain from the socket up and down the head and neck. Fetid odor and bad taste are common complaints.

Management is palliative with interventions that decrease pain during an episode of dry socket. These treatments consists of a gentle rinsing of the inflamed socket followed by the direct placement within the socket of a sedative dressing, which soothes the inflamed bone for a period of time and promotes tissue growth. This is usually done without anesthesia. The active ingredients in these sedative dressings usually include natural substances like *zinc oxide*, *eugenol*, and *oil of cloves*. Additional *analgesics* are sometimes prescribed.

21. **The correct answer is B.** Oroantral communications 2 to 6 mm in size can be repaired with a figure-of-eight suture to maintain the integrity of the blood clot within the socket. Additional measures such as the placement of gelfoam can further assist in blood clot stability and formation. Oroantral communications less than 2 mm can be monitored. No acute surgical treatment required. Oroantral communications greater than 7 mm should be repaired with flap closure such as a buccal fat pad flap advancement. A tongue advancement flap should be reserved for situations where failure of localized advancement flaps.

22. **The correct answer is D.** Ibuprofen is a nonsteroidal anti-inflammatory drug. It is believed to work through inhibition of *cyclooxygenase* (COX), thus inhibiting *prostaglandin* synthesis. Fentanyl is a synthetic primary μ agonist

opioid, currently the most widely used synthetic opioid analgesic worldwide, with a primary potency approximately 81 times that of *morphine*. Tramadol is a *monoamine* uptake inhibitor and centrally acting *analgesic*, used for treating moderate-to-severe *pain*. It is a synthetic agent, and it appears to have actions at the μ-*opioid receptor* as well as the *noradrenergic* and *serotonergic* systems. Meperidine acts as an *agonist* at the μ-*opioid receptor*. In addition to its strong opioidergic and anticholinergic effects, it has *local anesthetic* activity related to its interactions with *sodium ion channels*.

23. **The correct answer is C.** Benzodiazepines do not act as an analgesic. Additional medication is required locally or systemically to produce an analgesic effect. Benzodiazepines enhance the binding of GABA to the GABA receptor complex; in turn, binding increases the frequency of chloride channel opening to cause less neuronal stimulation. They can cause anterograde amnesia and are recommended as an anticonvulsant for the treatment of status epilepticus.

24. **The correct answer is D.** A jaw thrust is the least traumatic manipulation of the head and neck to establish an airway when no adjunctive measures are readily available. One should be concerned of a cervical spine fracture and minimal manipulation of the neck should be practiced. A head tilt would not be advised since the fact this man was found ejected from his vehicle, unresponsive, and with a fractured leg, it is very likely that he may have a fractured neck as well. Placement of an oropharyngeal airway may be conducted; however, the first attempt to establish an airway should be a jaw thrust. If an airway cannot be obtained with a jaw thrust, one should use an oropharyngeal airway to assist in establishing an airway. A cervical collar should be placed to limit unnecessary manipulation while placing the oropharyngeal airway. A cricothyrotomy should be reserved for cases in which more conservative measures are unsuccessful.

25. **The correct answer is D.** This patient has malignant hyperthermia. It is believed to be triggered by halogenated general anesthetics and/or succinylcholine. Susceptibility to malignant hyperthermia is often inherited as an *autosomal dominant* disorder. The potential for malignant hyperthermia is caused in a large proportion (50%–70%) of cases by a *mutation* of the *ryanodine receptor* (type 1), located on the *sarcoplasmic reticulum* (SR), the *organelle* within *skeletal muscle cells* that store *calcium*. It results from the massive release of calcium from the sarcoplasmic reticulum into the skeletal muscle cell to cause persistent muscle contraction. Signs and symptoms include rigidity, fever, tachycardia, metabolic acidosis, hypercarbia, and hypoxia. Considering that the patient is ventilated and monitored by anesthesia, overdose is generally not a concern and can be controlled symptomatically.

Neuroleptic malignant syndrome (NMS) is a life-threatening neurological disorder most often caused by an adverse reaction to *neuroleptic or antipsychotic drugs*. It generally presents with muscle rigidity, *fever*, autonomic instability, and cognitive changes such as *delirium* and is associated with elevated *creatine phosphokinase* (CPK). The setting and history of this presentation is unlikely to be caused by NMS.

26. **The correct answer is D.** The cavernous sinus exists in the middle cranial fossa and receives tributaries from the surrounding dural sinuses and venous plexuses from the face. These veins are valveless and are susceptible to retrograde flow; in turn, this can be a pathway for septic emboli from facial infectious to travel into the cavernous sinus. Patients generally have sinusitis or a midface infection for 5 to 10 days. The cavernous sinus contains cranial nerves III, IV, V (V1, V2), and VI, in addition to the internal carotid artery and associated sympathetic nerve branches. Lateral gaze palsy (isolated cranial nerve VI) is usually seen first since CN VI lies freely within the sinus in contrast to CN III and IV that lie within the lateral walls of the sinus. Without effective therapy, signs appear in the contralateral eye by spreading through the communicating veins to the contralateral cavernous sinus. Eye swelling begins as a unilateral process and spreads to the other eye within 24 to 48 hours via the

intercavernous sinuses. This is pathognomonic for cavernous sinus thrombosis.

27. **The correct answer is C.** Initial management should be the establishment and maintenance of an adequate airway is the sine qua non of therapy. Death is most likely from the acute phase of cellulitis by airway obstruction. Ludwig's angina results from the involvement of infection/cellulitis of the bilateral submandibular, sublingual, and submental spaces. In light of signs and symptoms of an impending loss of the patient's airway (difficulty breathing, pain on swallow, uncontrolled secretions, edema noted in the submandibular region), the acute problems need to be addressed first; in turn, establishment of a secure airway is required as the initial management. Following the establishment of a secure airway, intravenous antibiotics, and incision and drainage with the removal of the offending tooth/teeth is generally curative. Without an airway, the patient cannot ventilate. Antibiotics should be started upon establishment of an airway to treat the underlying infection. Generally, an empiric broad spectrum antibiotic is used to cover for Gram-positive and anaerobic bacteria. Administration of intravenous fluids and pain medications are indicated since the patient is likely dehydrated from his difficulty in swallowing and general malaise and discomfort. Caution is used with regard to pain control prior to a secure airway since it could further depress the patient's respiratory drive. Incision and drainage is an effective treatment if the patient did not show signs of respiratory distress (difficulty breathing, pain on swallow, uncontrolled secretions). This procedure will likely follow the establishment of an airway to irrigate and debride the areas of infection. Drains are usually left in the drainage site to prevent reaccumulation of purulence. The extraction of the source of infection is generally curative; however, with the extension of the infection into multiple fascial spaces, further treatment with incision and drainage is required.

28. **The correct answer is C.** The lateral pterygoid is composed of a superior head that originates from the infratemporal surface of the greater wing of the sphenoid and an inferior head that originates from the lateral surface of the lateral pterygoid plate. These will insert into the anterior portion of the condylar neck and TMJ capsule. The other muscles are not specifically located around the condyle or condylar neck.

Temporalis:
   Origin: floor of temporal fossa, deep surface of temporal fascia;
   Insertion: coronoid process, anterior border of mandibular ramus.

Masseter:
   Origin: superficial portion—anterior two-thirds of lower border of zygomatic arch; deep portion—medial surface of zygomatic arch.
   Insertion: lateral surface of ramus, coronoid process, and angle of mandible.

Medial pterygoid:
   Origin: deep head—medial surface of lateral pterygoid plate; pyramidal process of palatine bone; superficial head—maxillary tuberosity.
   Insertion: medial surface of ramus inferior to mandibular foramen.

29. **The correct answer is B.** The palate repair is usually performed between 9 and 18 months of age to promote proper speech development. The babies' first words are usually noted on average at 12 months of age. Cleft lip repair is recommended to occur when the infant is at least 10 pounds in weight, has 10 mg/dL of hemoglobin, and is at least 10 weeks of age. The recommended period of 9 to 18 months is suggested because any further delay could affect the patient's speech development. Cleft palate repair attempts to prevent delays in speech development.

30. **The correct answer is D.** The extra cranial segment of the facial nerve exits from the stylomastoid foramen to dive between the deep and superficial layers of the parotid gland to branch and form the five branches of the sensory segment of the facial nerve: temporal, zygomatic, buccal, marginal mandibular, and

cervical branches. Injury to these branches will manifest as paralysis of the muscles they innervate. Damage to the temporal branch will cause paralysis of the forehead and ptosis of the ipsilateral side.

Also traversing within the parotid gland is Stensen's duct that delivers salivary fluid to the oral cavity. The ampulla of the duct is generally located buccal to the second maxillary molar. Expression of saliva upon manipulation of the parotid gland demonstrates intact patency of Stensen's duct. Also, the duct may be cannulated with a lacrimal probe to assess for any perforations visible through the external wound.

With respect to trauma, the mandibular nerve is associated with injury to the mandible. Local injury to an area of dentition or injury to the ipsilateral mandibular nerve would lead to loss of vitality in teeth.

Damage to the floor of the mouth or submandibular gland/ducts would be associated with Wharton's duct. Injury to the medial aspect of the eye can damage the nasolacrimal duct. Damage to the maxillary nerve is associated with injuries to the midface and not the parotid area.

31. **The correct answer is C.** The patient is exhibiting signs of local anesthetic overdose. Toxicity occurs when too high levels enter the systemic blood stream because of either intravascular injection or a large dose. Answer choice A is wrong because the patient would become increasingly agitated. Answer choice B is incorrect because with LA toxicity visual and auditory disturbances can occur, not improve. Other neurologic signs and symptoms would include tremors, loss of consciousness, and seizures. Answer choice C is correct because after an initial chorionic villus sampling (CVS) stimulation, including increase in heart rate, blood pressure, and respiratory rate (answer D), there is rapid fall of all of these parameters.

32. **The correct answer is C.** Prilocaine is metabolized in the liver to O-toluidine, capable of oxidizing hemoglobin to methemoglobin. They will clinically appear cyanotic. It is reversed by the administration of methylene blue IV.

33. **The correct answer is C.** Having the needle directed to high (superior) can cause anesthetic to move through the sigmoid notch into the parotid gland, anesthetizing the facial nerve. An injection to inferior would cause lingual nerve anesthesia but will miss the main branch of the IAN. Too far lateral will place the needle into the buccinator. Too deep a needle placement may cause complications such as hematoma but will not likely cause CNVII nerve dysfunction.

34. **The correct answer is D.** Answer choice D is correct because the closer the pKa (the pH at which the ionized and unionized forms exist in equal concentrations) of the local anesthetic is to tissue pH, the more rapid the onset time. Answer choice A is incorrect; the lipid solubility affects the potency; the higher the solubility, the greater the potency. Answer choice B is incorrect because the protein binding influences the duration of action not the timing of onset. Answer choice C is incorrect because a vasoconstrictor influences length of anesthetic duration.

35. **The correct answer is A.** Apert syndrome is a rare autosomal dominant disorder in patients has the traits described above as well as relative mandibular prognathism and cleft soft palate or uvula. Answer choice B is incorrect because Treacher–Collins syndrome is characterized by narrow, depressed cheeks, downward slanting palpebral fissures, and hypoplastic condylar and coronoid processes. Answer choice C, Eagle syndrome, is incorrect because it is a calcification of the stylohyoid ligament and has no other craniofacial deformities associated with it. Beckwith–Wiedemann syndrome, answer D, is not correct because it is a syndrome associated with gigantism, macroglossia, and visceromegaly.

36. **The correct answer is A.** The initial force is apically directed to wedge the crestal bone and also moves the fulcrum toward the apex of the tooth reducing possibility of root fracture. Buccal and palatal movements are only secondary to the initial apical force. Occlusal force is never used in the extraction process.

37. **The correct answer is B.** Alveolar osteitis or dry socket is delayed healing but is not associated with infection (answer C) because of the lack of the usual signs and symptoms of infection including swelling, erythema, and fever. Most common site for a dry socket is the mandible and can be associated with smokers. Answer choice A is incorrect because IAN injury would present with neuropathic-type pain or paresthesia. Answer choice C is incorrect because of the symptoms and signs mentioned above. Answer choice D is incorrect because the presentation of this chronic bony infection process would not present within the 3-day time frame.

38. **The correct answer is A.** Minor surgical procedures can be performed with an INR less than 3 with control of bleeding achieved with hemostatic packing and suture placement. Answer choice B is incorrect. Removing the teeth without sutures and starting rinses will precipitate bleeding. Answer choices C and D are incorrect because the INR is in the low range; if greater than 3, consulting the PCP and withholding for 3 days would be appropriate.

39. **The correct answer is C.** Bilateral greater palatine and incisive nerve blocks to properly anesthetize a patient for length-wise incision with anterior and posterior releases and reflection of a full mucoperiosteal flap in the palate. Answer choice A is incorrect. This alone would not provide anesthesia for the posterior palate. Answer choices B and D are incorrect. The posterior superior alveolar nerves do not innervate the palate.

40. **The correct answer is C.** Impactions in the mandible have several classification systems; the most common is positional relation. Distoangular impactions in the mandible have more bony coverage.

41. **The correct answer is C.** The maximum dosage of 2% xylocaine with 1:100 K epi is 7 mg/kg; therefore, answers A and B would be acceptable dosages but not the max. Choice D is incorrect because it exceeds the 7 mg/kg limit.

42. **The correct answer is D.** Nylon is a monofilament nonresorbable suture material that will need to be removed within 5 to 7 days of placement. Choices A, B, and C are incorrect because they are each types of resorbable suture materials. Plain Gut resorbs quickly (approximately 3–5 days), chromic gut holds tensile strength for 7 to 14 days, and vicryl can hold for up to 3 to 4 weeks.

43. **The correct answer is A.** 2 mm is the recommended distance from the mental foramen to the inferior aspect of the implant.

44. **The correct answer is D.** 600 mg of clindamycin PO 1 hour prior to the procedure is the recommended dose and antibiotic for a patient who requires premedication and has an allergy to the class of penicillins.

45. **The correct answer is C.** Mandibular molars frequently refer pain to the ear because of cross innervation of the inferior alveolar nerve.

46. **The correct answer is D.** The most appropriate treatment for a patient with a deep fascial space infection is incision and drainage followed by antibiotics.

47. **The correct answer is A.** The radiograph and clinical correlation of increased pain prior to salivation are pathognomonic for the diagnosis of a sialolith (a calcification that is formed within a salivary duct, most common being found within the submandibular duct because of it being a primary mucous secretions gland and anatomic position of the duct). Answer choice B is incorrect, although calcifications of arteries can be noted on radiographic examination, this does not correlate with the pts presenting symptoms. Answer C is incorrect because these are not normal radiographic findings on an occlusal view of the anterior mandible. Answer D is incorrect because a supernumerary tooth would not be found outside of the bony confinements of the maxilla or mandible.

48. **The correct answer is A.** This radiograph depicts a radiolucent lesion in the left posterior mandible. The only pathology consistent with

this radiograph is an OKC; the others, a COC and Pindborg, have radio-opaque findings within the radiolucent lesion, and in SCC one would see bony destruction.

49. **The correct answer is C.** Flumazenil is a competitive benzodiazepine receptor antagonist at binding sites in the central nervous system. Answers A and B are the same medication and are used to reverse the effects of narcotics. Answer D is incorrect because neostigmine is an acetyl-cholinesterase inhibitor. Decadron, answer E, is incorrect because it is a steroid and has no effect on the mechanism of benzodiazepines.

50. **The correct answer is D.** The mylohyoid muscle is the most superficial muscle of the floor of the mouth followed by the genioglossus and finally by the geniohyoid. The buccinator is located on the lateral aspect of the mandible.

51. **The correct answer is D.** Fentanyl is 100 times stronger than morphine.

52. **The correct answer is B.** An allogeneic graft describes material derived from genetically unrelated members of the same species. Autogeneic is a material derived from the same person receiving the graft. A xenogeneic graft is the one derived from a different species than that into which it is placed. Synthetic grafts are chemically made.

53. **The correct answer is B.** An asymmetric raised white lesion that persists longer than 2 weeks should be biopsied since the lesion is less than 2 cm that appears clinically benign. Incisional biopsies are performed for lesions greater than 2 cm. Resection is not an applicable treatment option based on the history and clinical appearance of this lesion.

54. **The correct answer is A.** Pathology that evolves enough to involve the inferior border can cause weakness and eventual fracture, thus the term pathologic fracture. A comminuted fracture is one involving multiple fragmented segments. A closed fracture is a term used to describe a fracture that does not have exposure to the outside world; in the mandible, these are confined

to the subcondylar and condylar regions in a dentate patient.

55. **The correct answer is B.** Bell's palsy is weakness or severance of the seventh cranial nerve that controls motor function of the muscles of facial expression. CN V is involved in sensory innervation of the face and motor function of the muscles of mastication. CN XII controls motor function of the tongue. CN IX controls motor function of the trapezius and sternocleidomastoid.

56. **The correct answer is A.** Local anesthetics block nerve fibers at different rates. Thinner fibers are easier to block than thicker fibers. Accordingly, the blockade of peripheral nerves usually follows the following order: (1) peripheral vasodilation and skin temp, (2) pain and temperature, (3) proprioception, (4) touch and pressure sensation, and (5) motor paralysis.

57. **The correct answer is A.** All the answers are partially true. but the primary effect is decreasing the maximum rate of depolarization in the Purkinje fibers and myocardium.

58. **The correct answer is C.** Cleft palate is present in these patients approximately 30% of the time. Mental retardation is uncommon in patients with Treacher–Collins syndrome. Pulmonary hypertension usually occurs in those patients who have chronic airway obstruction.

59. **The correct answer is B.** Extraction sites heal by secondary intention, a healing process that entails clot formation, inflammatory phase and soft tissue coverage, and subsequent bone formation by osteoblasts surrounding the fibrin network. Primary intention is the process in wounds healing when adjacent structures are reapproximated. There is no healing process termed tertiary.

60. **The correct answer is C.** Excisional biopsy of a mucocele is the treatment of choice in this case on the basis of its size and location. NS rinses would not provide any beneficial component. Antibiotics are not indicated since there

is no infectious process involved. An incisional biopsy would only be indicated if the lesion was large and did not have the classic presentation of a mucocele noted by patient report.

61. **The correct answer is D.** The pathology noted around the permanent impacted canine is an odontoma. Odontomas are the most common types of odontogenic tumors. They can be further classified as compound and complex forms. The compound form is composed of multiple toothlike structures, whereas the complex subset consists of a conglomerate mass of enamel and dentin and bears no resemblance to a tooth. Answer A is incorrect because a mucous retention cyst is a dome-like structure on the floor of the maxillary sinus and would not prevent tooth eruption. Answer B is incorrect because an antrolith is a mass in the maxillary sinus that has undergone dystrophic calcification. Answer C is incorrect because it describes localized areas of bone sclerosis associated with teeth with pulpitis or large carious lesions not seen here.

62. **The correct response is D.** Open reduction of a fracture of the mandibular condyle is not commonly performed because the procedure may be complicated and closed reduction is usually sufficient. However, open reduction of the condyle is absolutely indicated in the following four situations: (1) displacement into the middle cranial fossa; (2) impossibility of obtaining adequate dental occlusion by closed reduction; (3) lateral extracapsular displacement of the condyle; and (4) invasion by a foreign body (e.g., a bullet from a gunshot wound). Because the condylar head is displaced in this patient, open reduction and internal fixation of the right subcondylar fracture and the left parasymphyseal fracture must be performed. Intermaxillary fixation should be applied before the procedure and should remain in place for 2 weeks after the surgery. Subsequently, active and passive physical therapy of the mandible should be performed to work the mandible and remold the subcondylar union. Closed reduction is contraindicated in this patient because of the displacement of the condylar head. Intermaxillary fixation applied for an extended time

period (>4 weeks) may result in postoperative ankylosis.

63. **Correct answer is D.** The radiographic and clinical findings are consistent with the diagnosis of florid cemento-osseous dysplasia. These lesions are commonly found in the African-American female population in their middle age, and the lesions showed marked areas of radiolucency and many times symmetric involvement. These lesions require no surgical intervention and can be watched unless areas become symptomatic.

64. **The correct answer is D.** The lesion seen and described is consistent with the diagnosis of a Stafne defect. This is an asymptomatic radiolucency below mandibular canal in the posterior mandible and no treatment is needed.

65. **The correct answer is C.** The most likely location to displace a root tip in a maxillary first molar is into the maxillary sinus.

66. **The correct answer is B.** Neurotmesis is the most severe nerve injury and involves loss of nerve continuity. Neurapraxia is the least severe and involves a contusion or stretching of the nerve, but there is no disruption of the epineural or axonal segments. In axonotmesis, the epineural sheath is disrupted, but there is an intact axon.

67. **The correct answer is C.** The single blade dental elevator is used to luxate a tooth apical to the cementoenamel junction prior to placement of forceps.

68. **The correct response is D.** The levator veli palatini muscle comprises a muscular sling in the posterior palate that is essential for effective palatal closure. It arises embryologically from the fourth pharyngeal arch and, therefore, is innervated by the pharyngeal plexus, a derivative of the vagus (X) nerve. This nerve also innervates several other muscles that figure prominently in speech development: the pharyngeal constrictors, the musculus uvulae, the palatoglossus, and palatopharyngeus. The trigeminal (V) nerve has three separate

divisions. The first branch, the ophthalmic division, is purely sensory as is the second division. The second, or maxillary, division is intermediate in size between the first and third divisions. The mandibular branch of the trigeminal nerve, the third division, is the largest branch and contains both sensory and motor nerves. Developmentally, the third division is a nerve of the first branchial (or mandibular) arch and provides motor innervation to the muscular derivatives of this arch, including the temporal, masseter, pterygoids, mylohyoid, tensor tympani, and the anterior belly of the digastric. The facial (VII) nerve provides motor innervation to the muscles of facial animation, including the buccinators. The hypoglossal (XII) nerve provides motor innervation to the tongue.

69. **The correct response is E.** Five facial prominences border the developing mouth. These include the bilateral mandibular prominences, the bilateral maxillary prominences, and the frontonasal prominence. The lateral nasal and medial nasal prominences are derived from the frontonasal prominence. A unilateral cleft lip results from incomplete union between the medial nasal prominence and the maxillary prominence on the affected side. The lateral and medial nasal prominences are derived from the frontonasal prominence. Clefting would not result from incomplete union of these structures. The lateral nasal prominence unites with the maxillary prominence. A patient with a unilateral cleft lip will have continuity between the lateral alar base and the lateral segment of the upper lip. The lateral nasal prominence does not normally unite with the medial nasal prominence. A lack of union between the lateral and medial nasal prominences will not result in a cleft lip.

70. **The correct answer D.** The mental nerve exits the mental foramen below the second premolar, halfway down the mandible. The mental nerve is the terminal branch of the inferior alveolar nerve, a major branch of the third division of the trigeminal (V) nerve. It provides sensation to the lower lip and skin overlying the chin. As such, its location must be known before using local anesthetic block techniques in this region. Moreover, knowing the mental nerve's exact location can be of use in avoiding inadvertent injury during osseous genioplasty.

71. **The correct answer is B.** The cuspids, or canine teeth, have the longest roots in both the maxilla and mandible. The average length of a cuspid tooth from the tip of the root to the tip of the crown is 27 mm. It is vital to know the length and position of the dental roots to avoid injuring the apices of the cuspid teeth during Le Fort I osteotomy and placement of internal fixation (interosseous miniplates or microplates and screws). The dentition may also be injured during stabilization of maxillary or mandibular fractures. The bicuspid, central and lateral incisor, and molar teeth all have roots that are shorter than the roots of the cuspid teeth; the average length of a molar tooth from the tip of the root to the tip of the crown, for example, is 24 mm. Consequently, these teeth are much less likely to be injured during LeFort I osteotomy.

72. **The correct answer is D.** Transection of the cervical branch of the facial nerve would result in loss of function of the platysma muscle, which acts to retract and depress the mandible. This muscle lies in a superficial position within the anterior neck and attaches to the superficial fascia of the pectoralis major and deltoid muscles as well as to the mandible and the skin and subcutaneous tissue of the lower face. With these multiple attachments, it acts in a synchronous motion with the other muscles of the lower lip to draw the oral commissure and lower lip downward. The marginal mandibular branch of the facial nerve innervates the lip depressor muscle. Because the lip depressor muscle compensates for the loss of function of the platysma muscle, weakened depression of the lower lip would only be a temporary finding. Forward flexion of the neck involves relaxation of the posterior muscles of the neck with the patient in the upright position or action of the sternocleidomastoid muscles bilaterally with the patient in the supine position. Muscles that contribute to lateral neck flexion include the sternocleidomastoid, splenius, and inferior obliquus capitis. Upward movement of

the hyoid bone is accomplished through the action of the digastric, stylohyoid, mylohyoid, and geniohyoid muscles; the sternohyoid, sternothyroid, thyrohyoid, and omohyoid muscles are used for downward movement. Pursing the lips is a function of the orbicularis oris muscle.

73. **The correct response is Option C.** The parotid gland receives its innervation from the auriculotemporal nerve, which is a branch of the glossopharyngeal nerve that communicates with the trigeminal and facial nerves. Because of its relationship with the parotid gland, the auriculotemporal nerve has been shown to be a cause of Frey syndrome (gustatory sweating) occurring after parotidectomy; division of the nerve has been recommended as a potential treatment option. The sympathetic plexus of the external carotid artery, the facial nerve, and the great auricular nerve also supply innervation to the parotid gland. The meibomian and lacrimal glands receive innervation from the lacrimal nerve, which is a branch of the ophthalmic division of the trigeminal nerve (V1). The sublingual gland is innervated by the lingual nerve, which is a branch of the mandibular division of the trigeminal nerve (V3). The submandibular gland is innervated by multiple sources, including the chorda tympani, which is a component of the facial nerve, the submandibular ganglion, which is a branch of the lingual nerve, and the mylohyoid branch of the inferior alveolar nerve. Each of these structures is derived from the trigeminal nerve.

74. **The correct answer is A.** This 40-year-old woman has Frey syndrome, which occurs as a result of peripheral autonomic dysfunction because of surgical injury. In patients who develop Frey syndrome following parotidectomy, the most likely cause is injury to branches of the auriculotemporal nerve, which is a branch of the mandibular division of the trigeminal nerve. The auriculotemporal nerve links the parasympathetic secretory fibers to the parotid gland. The preganglionic parasympathetic fibers course down the tympanic branch of the glossopharyngeal nerve and the lesser petrosal nerve to the otic ganglion; from there,

the postganglionic fibers travel via the auriculotemporal nerve to the parotid gland.

Following parotidectomy, the dermal sweat glands may be reinnervated abnormally by the parasympathetic fibers, resulting in innervation of the skin in the preauricular or temporal area. Patients with this abnormal innervation may have localized erythema and diaphoresis instead of saliva production from the parotid gland. Appropriate management for patients who develop this condition includes re-elevating the skin flap and using interposition grafts and flaps.

Frey syndrome does not develop following injury to motor nerves. Therefore, the facial (VII) nerve, which provides innervation for most of the facial muscles, cannot be injured in this patient.

The great auricular nerve arises from the second and third cervical nerves and emerges from the posterior border of the sternocleidomastoid muscle, then travels anterosuperiorly between the sternocleidomastoid and platysma muscles and divides into auricular, facial, and mastoid branches. The auricular branch provides sensation to the earlobe and posterior two-thirds of the ear and is prone to injury during surgery of the upper lateral neck.

The posterior auricular nerve arises from the facial nerve at the stylomastoid foramen, receives a contribution from the auricular branch of the vagus nerve, and supplies two nerve branches, one of which joins with the mastoid branch of the great auricular nerve and another that joins with the lesser occipital nerve. Both branches provide sensibility to the posterior side of the pinna and the concha. The posterior auricular nerve supplies motor innervation to the posterior auricular and occipitalis muscles.

The auricular branch of the vagus (X) nerve, also known as Arnold's nerve, arises from the superior ganglion, receives a contribution from the glossopharyngeal nerve, and travels along the temporal bone, emerging through the auricular fissure between the mastoid process and external auditory meatus. It supplies sensation to the posterior aspect of the ear and external auditory meatus.

75. **The correct answer is D.** A rotational movement of the forceps can only be used on teeth with a single root.

76. **The correct response is E.** The tongue is the most common site of squamous cell carcinoma of the oral cavity. Tongue carcinoma occurs most often in elderly persons but has been seen in adolescents and young adults. Excess alcohol and tobacco use are thought to be associated. Approximately 36% of all squamous cell carcinomas of the oral cavity affect the tongue.

In contrast, 30% of all oral squamous cell carcinomas involve the floor of the mouth, 16% involve the mandibular gingiva, and 10% involve the buccal mucosa, while only 3% involve the palate. Sites most likely to be affected by tongue carcinomas include the anterior two-thirds, lateral borders, and ventral surface of the tongue; lesions affecting the midline or dorsal surface are rare. Approximately 33% of these tumors arise behind the circumvallate papilla. Because tongue carcinomas are typically painless, affected persons often do not seek treatment until the tumor becomes advanced and begins to ulcerate and/or cause pain or difficulties with speech or swallowing. Tumor progression correlates directly with the size and extent of invasion of the tumor into the tongue muscles. Patients with extensive muscle infiltration typically have restricted tongue movement.

Approximately 30% of patients with tongue carcinomas have lymph node metastases at initial presentation. The midjugular, subdigastric, and submandibular lymph nodes are most likely to be affected, while the lower jugular, submental, and posterior cervical triangle nodes are rarely involved.

77. **The correct answer is C.** In adults, vertical mandibular opening measured from maxillary incisal edge to mandibular incisal edge (interincisal distance) typically ranges from 40 to 50 mm. In addition, normal range of motion of the mandible includes lateral jaw excursion (measured at the midline incisor) to 10 mm on each side. Decreased mandibular opening may indicate dysfunction of the temporomandibular joint (TMJ) or surrounding soft tissues.

Patients who may potentially have internal derangement of the TMJ may also experience painless clicking during attempted opening of the mandible.

78. **The correct answer is A.** The lateral and medial pterygoids, masseter, and temporalis muscles are muscles of mastication, capable of exerting force on the mandible. These muscles are innervated by the mandibular division of the trigeminal nerve (V3). The lateral pterygoid muscle has two heads that arise from the infratemporal surface and infratemporal crest of the greater wing of the sphenoid bone and the lateral surface of the lateral pterygoid plate, and insert on the mandibular neck and the articular capsule and disk of the temporomandibular joint. This muscle pulls the condylar process of the mandible and articular disk forward, opening the mouth. The medial pterygoid muscle arises from the medial surface of the lateral pterygoid plate and the pyramidal process of the palatine bone and inserts on the medial surface of the mandibular ramus and angle. It acts to elevate and protrude the mandible and produce side-to-side movements.

The masseter muscle arises from the zygomatic arch and inserts on the mandibular ramus and coronoid process; during mastication, it elevates the mandible to occlude the teeth.

The temporalis muscle arises from the temporal fossa, passes deep to the zygomatic arch, and inserts on the coronoid process and anterior border of the mandibular ramus. This muscle elevates the mandible and contributes to side-to-side grinding movements. The posterior fibers of the temporalis aid in retraction of the mandible once it has been protruded. The buccinator muscle arises from the alveolar process of the maxilla, from the mandible opposite the molars, and from the anterior border of the pterygoid mandibular raphe; it inserts into the submucosa of the cheeks and lips and is used to compress the cheeks against the teeth and gums. It is innervated by the facial (VII) nerve. Although it is not a muscle of mastication, it assists the tongue in directing food between the molars during mastication.

79. **The correct answer is B.** The lingual nerve, which supplies sensation to the anterior two thirds of the tongue, is a branch of the mandibular division of the trigeminal nerve (V3). Other structures that arise from this nerve include the inferior alveolar nerve, which supplies sensation to the mandibular teeth; the long buccal branch, which supplies sensation to the buccal mucosa; and the mental nerve, which supplies sensation to the skin of the chin and lower lip and the mucosa of the lip and adjacent gingiva. In addition, the auriculotemporal nerve divides from the posterior border of V3 immediately after exiting the foramen ovale, passes around the middle meningeal artery as two units, and then courses between the external auditory canal and temporomandibular joint (TMJ). This nerve supplies sensory innervation to the anterior auricle, a large portion of the temporal region, and part of the external auditory canal and gives off a branch to supply the TMJ.

The infraorbital nerve, nasopalatine nerve, posterosuperior alveolar nerve, and posterosuperior nasal nerve are branches of the maxillary division of the trigeminal nerve (V2).

80. **The correct answer is E.** Stensen's duct can be found within the buccal space, which is bordered anteriorly by the orbicularis oris muscle, posteriorly by the edge of the masseter muscle, superiorly by the zygomaticus major muscle, and inferiorly by the fascial attachment of the buccinator muscle to the mandible. The duct develops deep within the parotid gland and emerges from the superior third of the gland at its anterior border, then courses below the zygomatic arch and enters the buccal space, inserting into the buccinator and then entering the oral cavity opposite the upper second molar. The facial artery and vein, buccal branches of the facial nerve, and buccal fat pad can also be found within the buccal space. Although Stensen's duct and branches of the facial nerve are vulnerable to inadvertent dissection in the area of the parotid gland, there are no major arterial branches in this region. The external carotid artery can be found within the angle of the mandible, while the superficial temporal artery is located within the preauricular border.

The transverse facial artery is found at the zygomatic arch. These locations do not lie within the typical course of Stensen's duct.

81. **The correct answer is A.** Something, in fact, can be done for this patient as zygomaticus implants are a plausible option to enhance the retention of a maxillary obturator. Zygomaticus implants can be used to retain and support a maxillary obturator following extensive resection of the maxilla. Zygomaticus implants are placed in the zygomatic bone, engaging the junction of the temporal and frontal process. A soft reline of the patient's existing obturator would not offer long-term retention and stability. It is likely that the reline procedure would have to be repeated countless times, causing the patient and clinician much frustration. Zygomaticus implants are a more appropriate option in this otherwise healthy patient. Taking new impressions to fabricate a new obturator is not an acceptable treatment plan for this patient, who has had multiple obturators fabricated previously, all with poor retention. A better choice would be to place bilateral zygomaticus implants. Placement of standard endosseous implants and a prescription for long-term prophylactic oral antibiotics is not an appropriate treatment plan for this patient who has insufficient maxillary alveolar bone for placement of standard endosseous implants. A better option would be to place bilateral zygomaticus implants.

82. **The correct answer is B.** The ideal replacement of missing teeth in children is a fixed prosthesis restoration of osseointegrated implants. By age 12, vertical alveolar growth of the jaws is nearly complete. Implants placed after eruption of the permanent dentition have been shown to be successful in children. Vertical alveolar growth of the jaws is generally completed with the eruption of the 12-year molars. The patient is 15 years old and is a candidate for endosseous implant placement at this time. He does not have to wait until the age of 18 for surgical implant placement. Loaded endosseous implants help to maintain alveolar ridge height. Osseointegrated implants placed into alveolar bone do not cause excessive resorption of bone.

Placement of endosseous implants in children has been shown to be stable. As children are often noncompliant with removable appliances, endosseous implants offer a preferred method for the replacement of missing teeth in select children. Endosseous implants placed in a child's growing bone have been reported to migrate. Vertical growth of alveolar bone can cause submersion of endosseous implants. The patient in this vignette is 15 years old, and vertical growth of his alveolus should have neared completion by the age of 12. Implants would be a viable option in this 15-year-old child for replacement of his missing maxillary central incisor. He does not have to wait until he is 21 for surgical placement of implants.

83. **The correct answer is C.** Replacement of the missing lateral incisor with an osseointegrated implant depends on adequate volume and quality of bone. Studies have shown that the longer the interval beyond 4 months, the less likely there would be adequate bone volume to accept an implant in the bone grafted cleft site. Four weeks would be too short for a consolidation period in the alveolar cleft site. Placement of an endosseous implant in the grafted alveolar cleft should occur after a 4-month consolidation period. Eight months would be too long for a consolidation period in the alveolar cleft site. Placement of an endosseous implant in the grafted alveolar cleft should occur after a 4-month consolidation period. One year would be too long for a consolidation period in the alveolar cleft site. Placement of an endosseous implant in the grafted alveolar cleft should occur after a 4-month consolidation period. Two years would be too long for a consolidation period in the alveolar cleft site. Placement of an endosseous implant in the grafted alveolar cleft should occur after a 4-month consolidation period.

84. **The correct answer is A.** Failure of an implant is clinically and radiographically apparent by the following signs and symptoms:

- Horizontal mobility greater than 0.5 mm or any clinically observed vertical movement with less than 500 g applied force

- Rapid progressive bone loss refractory to stress reduction and peri-implant treatment
- Pain during function or percussion
- Continued uncontrolled exudate refractory to surgical attempts at correction
- Generalized radiolucency around the implant
- Greater than half of the surrounding bone is resorbed around the implant
- Implants placed in nonrestorable position
(Adapted from Misch, CE. *Contemporary Implant Dentistry, 2nd Edition.* Mosby, St. Louis; 1999.)

The implant-supported prosthesis causes the patient pain upon percussion. The implant in the position of missing tooth #28 has a generalized radiolucency surrounding it, satisfying the criteria for implant failure. Just less than one-half of the surrounding bone has resorbed around the implant in the position of missing tooth #29. This does not meet the criteria for implant failure, in which greater than one-half the bone has resorbed. As no radiographic abnormalities are associated with the implant in the position of tooth #30, it does not meet the criteria for implant failure. While implant #28 does meet the criteria for implant failure, implant #29 does not. While implant #28 does meet the criteria for implant failure, implant #30 does not. Neither implants #29 nor #30 meet the criteria for implant failure as described by Misch.

85. **The correct answer is D.** The patient has a preexisting Angle Class II malocclusion as evidence by her Class II molar relationship. The question stem explains that the canine relationship correlates to the molar relationship. To preserve the patient's existing, functional relationship, the right canine should be restored to a Class II canine relationship. The Class II canine relationship is best described as: the maxillary canine tip should occlude mesial to the embrasure between the mandibular canine and first premolar. If the maxillary canine tip opposes the embrasure between the mandibular canine and first premolar, the patient is in a Class I canine relationship. This patient has a Class II canine classification that should be

preserved with restoration of the maxillary right canine tooth in its characteristic position. If the maxillary canine tip occludes distal to the embrasure between the mandibular canine and first premolar, the patient is in a Class III canine relationship. This patient has a Class II canine classification that should be preserved with restoration of the maxillary right canine tooth in its characteristic position. Flattening the maxillary canine tooth and taking it out of occlusion would not result in an esthetic or functional outcome. The patient's right maxillary canine tooth should be restored to a Class II canine position. Restoring the maxillary canine without planning of the position of the tip would lead to a poor functional and esthetic result. It is likely that the restoration would cause the patient malocclusion, dysfunction, and pain. The best answer is to restore the patient's maxillary right canine into a Class II canine position.

86. **The correct answer is A.** Smile arc is the anterior arc of the esthetic line of the dentition. It is defined as the relationship of the curvature of the incisal edges of the maxillary teeth to the curvature of the lower lip in the posed social smile. It can be classified as consonant (parallel), reverse, or flat. Dental display is measured from the upper lip vermilion to the central incisal edge. The position of the upper lip in repose and smiling determines the amount of tooth show, which is also known as "dental display." The esthetic line of the dentition describes the facial surfaces of the maxillary teeth in relation to the smile. The curve of Spee is the curvature of the mandibular occlusal plane beginning at the tip of the mandibular canine and following the buccal cusps of the mandibular posterior teeth. Centric occlusion describes the relationship of the maxillary and mandibular jaws in which there is maximal contact of the inclined planes of the opposing cusps of the maxillary and mandibular teeth.

87. **The correct answer is B.** Estimated incidence of bisphosphonate-related osteonecrosis of the jaws (BRONJ) ranges from 0.8% to 12% for patients receiving intravenous formulations. For patients taking oral medications, the estimated incidence is 0.7 per 100,000 person years of exposure. This patient's 2-year history of oral bisphosphonate use makes her at risk for the development of BRONJ. Patients who have taken oral bisphosphonates for less than 3 years with no clinical risk factors require no alteration or delay in planned oral surgery. Therefore, this patient may undergo surgical placement of endosseous implants using standard implant surgery techniques without modification. The history of oral bisphosphonate use does not exclude this patient as a potential endosseous implant recipient. This patient has been taking an oral bisphosphonate (Alendronate) for 2 years. Patients taking oral bisphosphonates are at a considerable lower risk for BRONJ than patients taking IV bisphosphonates. Patients who have taken oral bisphosphonates for less than 3 years with no clinical risk factors require no alteration or delay in planned oral surgery.

Placement of dental implants should be avoided in patients with a history of taking the more potent IV bisphosphonate medications on a frequent dosing schedule.

The following bisphosphonates are available for use in the United States:

Generic Name	Brand Name	Route
Etidronate	Didronel	Oral
Tiludronate	Skelid	Oral
Alendronate	Fosamax	Oral
Risedronate	Actonel	Oral
Ibandronate	Boniva	Oral
Pamidronate	Areda	IV
Zoledronate	Zometa	IV
Clodronate	Bonefos	IV

The patient does not need to undergo a 2-month drug holiday prior to implant placement. A drug holiday is recommended for patients treated with oral bisphosphonates for 3 years or more, or patients that have taken concomitant steroid medication. The drug holiday should be arranged by the prescribing provider of the bisphosphonate and only be considered if systemic conditions permit it to be undertaken safely. Standard drug holidays are a discontinuation of bisphosphonate for at least 3 months prior to oral surgery.

The patient does not need to undergo a 2-month drug holiday following implant placement. A drug holiday is recommended for patients treated with oral bisphosphonates for 3 years or more, or patients that have taken concomitant steroid medication. The drug holiday should be arranged by the prescribing provider of the bisphosphonate, and only be considered if systemic conditions permit it to be undertaken safely. Standard drug holidays are a discontinuation of bisphosphonate for at least 3 months prior to oral surgery.

This asymptomatic patient does not require a 1-year drug holiday and is not restricted from taking bisphosphonates for life. This patient may resume bisphosphonate use after osseous healing has occurred. The patient should be placed on a regular recall schedule to monitor for the development of BRONJ, and the patient should be given appropriate informed consent regarding potential implant failure and possible osteonecrosis of the jaws if she continues to take oral bisphosphonates.

88. **The correct answer is A.** A CT Dentascan is a dental computed tomography (CT) imaging program that provides an image in true life-size format with vertical scale in millimeters. It provides for a cross-sectional view of the dental arch. The multiaxial reconstruction of the image allows for measurement of the alveolus, location of the inferior alveolar nerve, and accurate treatment planning for surgical implant placement. An orthopantogram or "panorex" is a scanning dental x-ray showing a two-dimensional view of the maxilla and mandible. Magnification of 15% to 30% is inherent in the panorex radiograph system. While an orthopantogram will provide important information for surgical implant treatment planning, a CT Dentascan will offer more accurate imaging. Periapical radiographs show the tip of the roots of the teeth. While periapical radiographs offer important information about the patient's dentition, the most accurate information about the patient's alveolar height and width would be provided by CT. The occlusal radiograph can provide information about the floor of the mouth or palate. The most accurate information regarding treatment planning for implant placement would be provided by CT. Bitewing radiographs show the crowns of posterior teeth and the alveolar bone height at the cementoenamel junction. Bitewing radiographs more accurately display bone levels than do periapical radiographs. However, the most accurate representation of alveolar bone height and width for implant treatment planning purposes would be provided by CT.

89. **The correct answer is E.** This patient does not require antibiotic prophylaxis. According to the 2007–2008 recommendations of the American Heart Association (AHA), only an extremely small number of cases of infective endocarditis might be prevented by antibiotic prophylaxis for dental procedures, even if such prophylactic therapy were 100% effective. Therefore, only those patients with underlying cardiac conditions associated with the highest risk warrant antibiotic prophylaxis.

Cardiac Conditions Associated with the Highest Risk of Adverse Outcome from Endocarditis for which Prophylaxis with Dental Procedures Is Reasonable

Prosthetic cardiac valve or prosthetic material used for cardiac valve repair

Previous infective endocarditis

Congenital heart disease (CHD)
- Unrepaired cyanotic CHD, including palliative shunts and conduits
- Completely repaired congenital heart defect with prosthetic material or device, whether placed by surgery or by catheter intervention, during the first 6 months after the procedure
- Repaired CHD with residual defects at the site or adjacent to the site of a prosthetic patch or prosthetic device (which inhibit endothelialization)

Cardiac transplantation recipients who develop cardiac valvulopathy

Modified with permission. *Circulation.* 2007;116: 1736–1754.

It is recommended that patients who meet these criteria receive antibiotic prophylaxis for all dental procedures that involve manipulation of gingival tissue or the periapical region of teeth or perforation of the oral mucosa.

Oral and Maxillofacial Surgery and Pain Control

The regimen of clindamycin 600 mg PO 30 minutes to 1 hour prior to the procedure would be appropriate in a patient requiring prophylaxis who is also allergic to penicillins. An antibiotic for prophylaxis should be administered as a single dose prior to the procedure. Administration of a post-procedure dose should only be considered when a patient has not received the preprocedure dose.

The regimen of 2 g of amoxicillin PO 1 hour prior to the procedure would be appropriate for an adult patient not allergic to penicillins. Vancomycin is not in the AHA recommended regimens for a dental procedure.

AHA Recommended Antibiotic Prophylaxis Regimens for Dental Procedures

Situation	Agent	Regimen: Single Dose 30–60 min Before Procedure	
		Adults	Children
Oral	Amoxicillin	2 g	50 mg/kg
Unable to Take Oral Medication	Ampicillin OR	2 g IM or IV	50 mg/kg IM or IV
	Cefazolin or Ceftriaxone	1 g IM or IV	50 mg/kg IM or IV
Allergic to Penicillins or Ampicillin Oral	Cephalexin OR	2 g	50 mg/kg
	Clindamycin OR	600 mg	20 mg/kg
	Azithromycin or clarithromycin	500 mg	15 mg/kg
Allergic to Penicillins or Ampicillin and Unable to Take Oral Medication	Cefazolin or ceftriaxone OR	1 g IM or IV	50 mg/kg IM or IV
	Clindamycin	600 mg IM or IV	20 mg/kg IM or IV

Modified with permission. *Circulation.* 2007;116:1736–1754.

90. **The correct answer is A.** According to Branemark's original two-stage technique, the recommended healing time was described as 3 to 4 months for mandibular bone and 5 to 6 months for the more cancellous bone of the maxilla. A healing period of 1 to 2 months for both the maxilla and mandible was not originally described by Branemark to ensure adequate osseointegration. A healing period of 1 to 2 months for the maxilla was not originally described by Branemark. However, a 3- to 4-month healing period in the mandible was described as appropriate time for osseointegration to occur. A healing period of 3 to 4 months for the maxilla and 1 to 2 months for the mandible was not originally described by Branemark. A healing period of 5 to 6 months for the maxilla is correct; however, a healing period of 1 to 2 months in the mandible was not originally described by Branemark to ensure adequate osseointegration.

91. **The correct answer is D.** This patient, who is allergic to penicillin, should be administered clindamycin 600 mg 1 hour prior to the dental procedure.

The following are the American Dental Association/American Academy of Orthopedic Surgeons suggested antibiotic prophylaxis regimens:

Clindamycin is a bacteriostatic antibiotic that acts to inhibit bacterial protein synthesis. It targets the 50S bacterial ribosomal subunit and is effective against anaerobes and

Patient Type	Recommended Drug	Single-Dose Regimen
Patients not penicillin allergic	Amoxicillin, cephalexin, or cephradine	2 g PO 1 hour prior to dental procedure
Patients not penicillin allergic, unable to take oral medications	Ampicillin or cefazolin	Ampicillin 2 g IM or IV or cefazolin 1 g 1 hour prior to dental procedure
Penicillin-allergic patients	Clindamycin	600 mg PO 1 hour prior to dental procedure
Penicillin-allergic patients, unable to take oral medications	Clindamycin	600 mg IV 1 hour prior to dental procedure

Modified with permission. *Stroke*. 1997;96:358–366.

Gram-positive bacteria. As it is highly effective against oral anaerobes, and it is not a β-lactam antibiotic, clindamycin is appropriate for use in patients who are allergic to penicillin.

The recommended antibiotic prophylaxis regimens are single-dose schedules administered 1 hour prior to the procedure. No second doses are currently recommended for any of the suggested regimens. This patient is allergic to penicillin, and therefore administering another β-lactam antibiotic such as amoxicillin at this time would be inappropriate. This patient has a documented penicillin allergy. Administration of cephalosporin would not be advisable as there is potential cross-hypersensitivity between penicillins and cephalosporins. The patient has undergone total joint replacement 4 months ago. The American Dental Association and the American Academy of Orthopedic Surgeons (AAOS) used to suggest that all patients during the first 2 years following total joint replacement are considered at potential increased risk of experiencing hematogenous total joint infection.

New guidelines proposed by the AAOS recommend that clinicians consider antibiotic prophylaxis in ALL total joint replacement patients prior to any invasive procedure that may cause bacteremia.

It is appropriate to consider antibiotic premedication for these patients. Therefore, the statement "No antimicrobial prophylaxis is indicated at this time" is incorrect.

92. **The correct answer is A.** Prosthetic obturation of postablative palatomaxillary defects can be associated with instability and poor retention. Prosthetic instability is characterized by a breakdown in the oronasal prosthetic-tissue seal, oro-nasal regurgitation, and compromised speech. Destabilizing cantilever forces in large palatomaxillary defects often lead the reconstructive team to consider reconstructive maxillofacial surgery including the utilization of free-flaps or bone grafts and later placement of osseointegrated implants. The most common destabilizing forces affecting obturators are cantilever forces causing the prosthesis to tip toward the defect. Rotational forces during function are not as common. A tensile force is a stretching force pulling at both ends of a structure along its length. Tensile forces are not the most common destabilizing forces affecting obturators. A compressive force applied to a material would result in its compaction or decrease in volume. Compressive forces are not the most common destabilizing forces affecting obturators.

93. **The correct answer is B.** Autologous bone, the gold standard in bone grafting, is the only graft material that contains all four qualities of osteogenesis, osteoinduction, osteoconduction, and osseointegration. Osteogenesis is the process of laying down new bone material by osteoblasts. Osteoinduction is the active process by which osteogenesis is induced. Osteoinduction involves the recruitment of immature cells, and the stimulation of these cells to develop into preosteoblasts through chemical signaling. Osteoconduction is the (passive) process by which bone grows on a scaffolding, matrix, or surface. Osseointegration, as originally described by Branemark, is the apparent direct

Oral and Maxillofacial Surgery and Pain Control

connection of osseous tissue to an inert alloplastic material without intervening connective tissue. Angiogenesis is the physiological process by which new blood vessels grow from preexisting blood vessels.

94. **The correct answer is A.** Autologous bone, the gold standard in bone grafting, is the only graft material that contains all four qualities of osteogenesis, osteoinduction, osteoconduction, and osseointegration. An autologous graft (autograft) is composed of cells or tissues that are reimplanted into the same individual from whom the graft was harvested. An allograft is composed of cells or tissues that are transplanted into a different individual from whom the graft was harvested. These grafts are also known as homologous grafts. A xenograft is composed of cells or tissues that are harvested from one species and transplanted into another. An alloplast is an inert material originating from a nonliving source that is surgically implanted. An alloplast may be a metal, polymer, (plastic, silicone, etc.), or other nonbiologic material. Recombinant human bone morphogenetic protein-2 (rhBMP-2) is a growth factor produced using recombinant DNA technology that has been used to promote bone growth. The osteoinductive agent (BMP) is combined with an osteoconductive matrix (collagen) to promote osteogenesis. This material is not considered to be the gold standard of bone grafting.

95. **The correct answer is A.** "Numbness" is an ill-defined, subjective lay term that can describe any altered or abnormal sensation after nerve injury. It is important for the clinician to investigate the patient's symptoms and interpret them into scientific terms. Hypoesthesia is the decreased perception of stimulation by a noxious or non-noxious stimulus in an area of skin or mucosa. Dysesthesia describes an unpleasant abnormal sensation, spontaneous or evoked. Hyperesthesia is increased sensitivity to any noxious or non-noxious stimulus. Allodynia, a subclass of hyperesthesia, describes pain because of a stimulus that normally does not provoke pain. Hyperalgesia, a subclass of hyperesthesia, is an increased response to a stimulus that is normally painful. Hyperpathia is char-

acterized by an exaggerated subjective painful response to any stimulus. Anesthesia is the absence of perception of stimulation by a noxious or non-noxious stimulus.

96. **The correct answer is A.** Neurapraxia is a benign injury, usually caused by compression or prolonged retraction. Neurapraxia consists of a temporary failure of conduction stimuli. Spontaneous recovery from neurapraxia usually occurs within 4 weeks. Axonotmesis is caused by partial severance or crushing of the nerve. It is a more severe injury than neurapraxia. While the general structure of the nerve remains intact, there is a loss of continuity of some axons, which then undergo Wallerian degeneration. Conduction failure is prolonged. Initial symptoms of returning sensation occur 5 to 11 weeks after injury. Patients often experience hypoesthesia, which may be accompanied by persistent dysesthesias. Neurotmesis is the complete severance or internal physiologic disruption of all the nerve layers (epineurium, perineurium, endoneurium). Neurotmesis is characterized by total conduction block of all impulses. Total numbness for 12 weeks or longer is likely because of neurotmesis. Hyperpathia is characterized by an exaggerated subjective painful response to any stimulus. Allodynia, a subclass of hyperesthesia, describes pain because of a stimulus that normally does not provoke pain.

97. **The correct answer is C.** Antibiotic prophylaxis is recommended for end-stage renal disease patients undergoing hemodialysis. Typical streptococcal and staphylococcal infections associated with dental bacteremia can contaminate dialysis access sites (shunts or fistulas). It is recommended that oral surgery procedures be performed the day after dialysis. Therefore, it is best to coordinate treatment with the patient's physician. End-stage renal disease patients do require special considerations to their care. It is correct to consult with a patient's physician. Current recommendations are for oral surgery procedures to be performed on the day after dialysis, and antibiotic prophylaxis will likely be required. This patient is a candidate for surgical implant therapy, so long as the patient's

physician is consulted, and special therapeutic conditions are met to minimize risk.

98. **The correct answer is A.** Elective surgical procedures such as implantology should be delayed until after delivery when the mother's health is at her normal state. It is preferred that the mother not be breastfeeding because of the possible effects of anesthesia and medications on the infant. This patient is 9-weeks pregnant. Therefore, she is in her first trimester of pregnancy. The first trimester begins at conception and continues through the 11th week or day 70. The second trimester is from day 70 to 154. The third trimester is from day 154 to delivery. The period between days 18 and 60 is the time where the human embryo is most vulnerable to teratogenic insult. Therefore, risk to the fetus is greatest during this period. Many physiologic changes occur in pregnancy. By the third trimester, the vena cava and aorta can be compressed by the uterus with the patient in the supine position. This can result in the supine hypotensive syndrome. Invasive dental therapy during the third trimester poses the greatest risk to the mother. Elective restorative and periodontal treatment can be performed during the second trimester. However, invasive elective procedures such as implantology should be delayed until after delivery. It is important to remember that dental treatment for a pregnant patient who is experiencing pain or infection should not be delayed until after delivery. Maxillary and mandibular third molar teeth are the most often impacted teeth. Next in frequency are the maxillary canine teeth, mandibular bicuspid teeth, maxillary bicuspid teeth, and maxillary second molar teeth. Impactions of first molars and incisors are relatively uncommon. This patient's surgical plan will most likely involve surgical removal of the impacted tooth, bone grafting procedures, and dental implant placement. It is best to wait until after delivery to undergo such extensive, elective dental treatment.

99. **The correct answer is B.** Acetaminophen is the analgesic and antipyretic of choice in pregnancy. Acetaminophen is considered a pregnancy category B drug.

The following Food and Drug Administration (FDA) categories of prescription drugs can be used as a reference:

Pregnancy Category A	Adequate and well-controlled human studies have failed to demonstrate a risk to the fetus in the first trimester. (And there is no evidence of risk in later trimesters.) The probability of fetal harm seems remote
Pregnancy Category B	Animal studies indicate no fetal risk, and there are no adequate, well-controlled human studies to demonstrate risk. OR Animal studies show an adverse effect on the fetus, but adequate, well-controlled human studies do not show a risk to the fetus in any trimester
Pregnancy Category C	Teratogenic or embryocidal effects are shown in animals. No controlled studies have been performed in either animals or humans. Potential benefits versus risks must be assessed to warrant use of the drug in pregnant women
Pregnancy Category D	Positive evidence of human fetal risk exists based on adverse reaction data from investigational or marketing experience or studies, but potential benefits may outweigh potential risks in certain situations
Pregnancy Category X	Studies or experience have shown fetal risk that clearly outweighs any possible benefit for use in pregnant women

Adapted from Pregnancy categories for prescription. *FDA Drug Bull* 1979;9:23–24, www.fda.gov.

Aspirin is a pregnancy category D drug. Its use is considered unsafe during pregnancy. Acetaminophen is a better choice for treatment of mild-to-moderate pain in this patient.

Codeine is considered a pregnancy category C drug. Codeine use during the first trimester has been associated with congenital abnormalities such as cleft lip and palate. Acetaminophen is a better choice for the treatment of this patient's mild-to-moderate postoperative pain.

Hydromorphone is a pregnancy category C drug. However, this patient's mild-to-moderate pain will likely respond to acetaminophen.

This patient is pregnant, and appropriate pain medication can be used. The safest medication should be chosen for the clinical situation. This patient is experiencing mild-to-moderate pain 1 week after dental implant placement. She will likely respond well to acetaminophen.

100. The correct answer is B. The geriatric patient group can be divided into three categories: the elderly (ages 65–74 years), the aged (ages 75–84 years), and the very old (ages 85 and older).

Diseases or conditions contraindicating dental implants in the elderly patient include:

- Dementia
- Diabetes mellitus (poorly controlled)
- Cardiac infarction
- Hemorrhage syndromes
- Psychosis
- Cerebral stroke
- Epilepsy
- Extreme dyskinesia
- Hepatic cirrhosis
- Cortisone-medication effect
- Radiation effects
- Alcoholism
- Cardiovascular transplant

Hypertension is not considered a contraindication for the placement of dental implants in the elderly. Normal blood pressure (BP) is defined as systolic BP less than 120 mm Hg and diastolic BP less than 80 mm Hg. Prehypertension is defined as systolic BP 120 to 139 mm Hg, or diastolic BP 80 to 89 mm Hg. Stage 1 hypertension is defined as systolic BP 140 to 159 mm Hg or diastolic BP 90 to 99 mm Hg. Stage 2 hypertension is classified as a systolic BP $\geq$ 160 mm Hg or diastolic BP $\geq$ 100 mm Hg.

Hypercholesterolemia increases a patient's risk of cardiovascular disease (i.e., atherosclerosis). Hypercholesterolemia is not considered a contraindication for the placement of dental implants in the elderly.

Atrial fibrillation is the most common cardiac arrhythmia. During atrial fibrillation, the atrial muscles fibrillate rather than contract with coordination. Many patients with atrial fibrillation will be treated with anticoagulants by their primary medical doctors or cardiologist. Careful coordination and communication is necessary between the implant surgeon and prescribing physician. The patient may be advised to discontinue anticoagulant use prior to implant placement and resume the anticoagulant after surgery. Local measures should be taken to ensure adequate hemostasis at the surgical site. Atrial fibrillation is not considered a contraindication for the placement of dental implants in the elderly.

101. The correct answer is D. As a general rule, one should always use the largest possible implant diameter. Larger diameter implants offer greater surface area for osseointegration, and thus provide greater implant stability. Because of their reduced mechanical stability, small-diameter implants are used only in cases with a low mechanical load. The diameter of the implant does, in fact, affect the stability of the implant fixture. The wider (larger) diameter implants provide greater surface area for osseointegration, and therefore provide greater stability. An implant must never be placed into (or too close to) vital structures such as the inferior alveolar nerve.

102. The correct answer is A. Because the implant shoulder is the largest part of the implant, it is used as the point of reference for measuring the mesiodistal distance. A minimal distance of 1.5 mm is recommended between the implant shoulder and the adjacent tooth at bone level. A distance of 1.0 mm is too small between the implant shoulder and the adjacent tooth at bone level. A distance of 0.5 mm is too small between the implant shoulder and the adjacent tooth at bone level. A distance of 3.0 mm will not damage the implant or the adjacent tooth because this value is greater than the recommended minimal distance of 1.5 mm at bone level.

103. **The correct answer is C.** The recommended orofacial implant position is contingent upon a minimum of 1.0-mm thickness of facial and palatal bone. 1.0 mm of facial or palatal bone is recommended to ensure stability of the hard and soft tissues. If the facial or palatal bone wall width is less than 1-mm thick, augmentation procedures are indicated. Ideally, the axis of the implant should be angulated so that the screw channel of a screw retained restoration is located behind (palatal) to the incisal edge of an implant placed in the anterior region. 0.5 mm is too thin amount of bone to adequately support the implant. To ensure predictability of hard and soft tissue stability, a minimum of 1.0-mm thickness of bone is recommended on the facial and palatal aspects of the implant. 0.25 mm is definitely too thin amount of bone to adequately support the implant fixture. Such a thickness is likely to result in fenestration.

2.0 mm is greater than the 1.0 mm minimum thickness required facial and palatal to the implant fixture. While 2.0 mm would adequately support the implant fixture, the question asks for the minimum thickness of bone. Therefore, the correct answer is 1.0 mm.

104. **The correct answer is B.** It is recommended that implant insertion torque should not exceed 35 Ncm. 45 and 50 Ncm exceed the recommended maximum torque for implant insertion. 25 Ncm is not the maximum torque allowed for implant placement. Implant insertion can occur using a torque up to 35 Ncm, and a maximum of 15 rpm using the implant handpiece. Always follow the manufacturer's recommendations for implant placement.

105. **The correct answer is A.** The "second-stage" implant surgical procedure traditionally involves the placement of the healing abutment (healing cap). This is the second surgical procedure in a second-stage implant surgery model. During the first implant surgery, the implant fixture is placed into the bone, and a cover screw is inserted. The full thickness mucoperiosteal flaps are sutured closed, and submucosal healing occurs. After the healing period, a second surgical procedure is required to un-cover the implant, remove the cover screw, and place the healing abutment. The healing abutment will extend transmucosally, allowing for soft tissue sculpturing. Torque testing of the implant *fixture* can help determine if the implant has achieved stability in bone. It can be done during the second-stage surgical procedure. However, torque testing of the implant *cover screw* is not a part of the second-stage surgical procedure. Placement of the cover screw would occur during the first stage of a traditional, second-stage implant surgery model. In a single-stage procedure, the implant healing abutment would be placed immediately, and no cover screw would be utilized. Placement of the implant fixture occurs during the first surgery of a second-stage implant.

106. **The correct answer is A.** Estimates of the time remaining in oxygen E-cylinders can be approximated using the following formula:

$$(psi \times F)/L/min = \text{Time remaining in minutes}$$

Where F for E-cylinders $= 0.3$

In this case, $(1,000 \times 0.3)/10 = 30$ min

Portable E-cylinders of oxygen should be replaced when their content is below 1,000 psi.

107. **The correct answer is B.** Supplemental oxygen can be safely administered to patients with COPD. The current thinking is that one can provide whatever concentration of supplemental oxygen that is required to maintain the patient's oxygen saturation above 90% as measured by pulse oximeter. Generally, this can be accomplished by nasal cannula.

108. **The correct answer is A.** Arthrocentesis. This is the indicated therapy for recent onset of unilateral failure of translation because of abnormal relationship of the articular disk to the mandibular condyle because of inflammation from functional loading. Arthroscopic surgery (answer choice B) is used to visualize intraarticular pathology such as adhesions, synovitis, osteoarthritis, disk displacement, and disk perforation but is not the treatment once a diagnosis is made. All other answers involve occlusal

adjustment, which has not been proven to be the etiology is any type of TMJ disorder.

109. **The correct answer is B.** This is a nerve-related TMJ disorder that is usually described as stabbing, burning, shocking pain that is provoked by wind, tactile, or thermal stimulation. Myofascial pain dysfunction or MPD primarily affects muscles of mastication and is often stress related. Osteoarthritis is a degenerative joint disease and does not present as described in the question. TMJ ankylosis is most commonly caused by trauma and results in fusion of the condyle, disk, and TMJ fossa. Disk displacement would most likely cause the patient to have trouble opening and/or closing, which is not apparent in this situation.

110. **The correct answer is A.** The maximum amount of 2% lidocaine with 1:100,000 epinephrine that can be administered to a healthy 150-lb man is 477 mg or roughly 13 dental cartridges. Therefore, this patient would be able to receive eight or more carpules in addition to the six he has already received. Therefore, six carpules is the correct answer.

111. **The correct answer is A.** For coronal fracture of a root, the correct treatment is the removal of coronal segment and pulpectomy. Rigid splint (B) is indicated for 2 to 3 months in patients who fracture apical and mid-root portions of the root. Occlusal adjustment (C) is only indicated if needed in cases of subluxation, luxation, avulsion, and alveolar process fracture. Extraction (D) is indicated if greater than one-third of the root is fractured and pulp is exposed.

112. **The correct answer is C.** It is contraindicated to place implants immediately after extraction of teeth in a region of active infection. At least 8 weeks should pass before placing the implant. Oral bisphosphonates (answer choice B) are not a contraindication to implant placement, although IV bisphosphonates may be. Not enough bone height (answer choice A) is incorrect because the patient has 9 mm of vertical height and needs 8 mm at least. Osteoporosis (answer choice D) and type II diabetes (answer choice E) are not contraindications as long as they are controlled.

CHAPTER 4

Orthodontics

1. A 12-year-old boy was classified as having class II division 2 malocclusion. What position would you suspect the patient's maxillary centrals and laterals are in?

   A. Maxillary centrals tipped palatally and in retruded position; maxillary lateral tipped labially and mesially
   B. Maxillary centrals tipped palatally and in retruded position; maxillary lateral tipped palatally
   C. Maxillary centrals tipped labially and in protruded position; maxillary lateral tipped labially and mesially
   D. Maxillary centrals tipped labially and in protruded position; maxillary lateral tipped palatally

2. How would you classify the occlusion below?

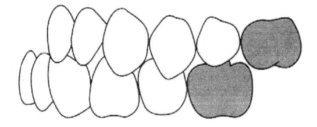

   A. Class III malocclusion, also known as distoclusion
   B. Class II malocclusion, also known as mesioclusion
   C. Class III malocclusion, also known as mesioclusion
   D. Class II malocclusion, also known as distoclusion
   E. Class I malocclusion

3. In a pseudo–class III malocclusion, the patient has the ability to:

   A. Bring the mandible back with strain so that the mandibular incisors touch the maxillary incisors
   B. Bring the mandible forward without strain so that the mandibular incisors touch the maxillary incisors
   C. Bring the mandible forward with strain so that the mandibular incisors touch the maxillary incisors
   D. Bring the mandible back without strain so that the mandibular incisors touch the maxillary incisors

4. This is the most innermost point on contour of mandible between incisor tooth and bony chin. This landmark is known as:

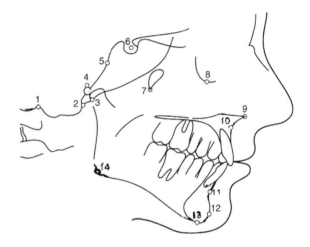

   A. #11—point B
   B. #11—point A
   C. #10—point A
   D. #13—pogonion
   E. #12—menton

5. When the lines connecting sella–nasion and gonion–menton meet, they create an angle that helps to determine the malocclusion. What type of anterior vertical dimension and malocclusion correlates with this steep angle?

   A. Long anterior vertical dimension and a deep-bite malocclusion.
   B. Short anterior vertical dimension and an open-bite malocclusion.
   C. Short anterior vertical dimension and a deep-bite malocclusion.
   D. Long anterior vertical dimension and an open bite malocclusion.

6. A 35-year-old man presents for an evaluation. Upon examination, you notice that the patient's

buccal cusps of the lower posterior teeth occlude buccal to the buccal cusps of the upper posterior teeth on the left and the right side. What treatment should be rendered to correct this malocculsion?

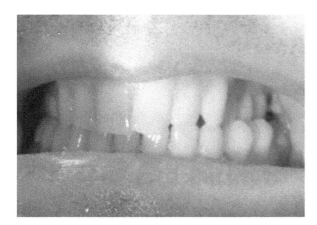

A. Surgery
B. Rapid maxillary expander
C. Quad helix expander
D. W-arch
E. Do nothing, it will eventually rectify by itself

7. This has been adapted as the best horizontal orientation that assesses lateral representation of the skull. Which of the following cephalometric landmarks make up this plane when a line is drawn to connect them?

A. Sella and nasion
B. Gonion and gnathion
C. Porion and orbitale
D. Spheno-occipital synchondrosis and anterior nasal spine (ANS)

8. A 37-year-old Caucasian man has SNA angle of 88 degrees. What does SNA angle of 88 degrees indicate regarding the patient's occlusion?

A. Maxillary retrusion
B. Maxillary protrusion
C. Class I skeletal pattern
D. Mandibular prognathism
E. Mandibular retrognathism

9. Which headgear has an extraoral component that is supported by chin and forehead and is used in skeletal class III malocclusions to protract the maxilla?

A. Cervical-pull headgear
B. Straight-pull headgear
C. High-pull headgear
D. Reverse-pull headgear

10. Functional appliances have dental and skeletal effect and can be tissue-borne or tooth-borne. Which of the following appliances is tissue-borne?

A. Bionator
B. Frankel functional appliance
C. Herbst
D. Edgewise appliance

11. A 14-year-old girl demonstrates a deviation in maxillary and mandibular midlines as the patient closes and does not have smooth closure to centric occlusion. What type of crossbite, if any, does the patient demonstrate?

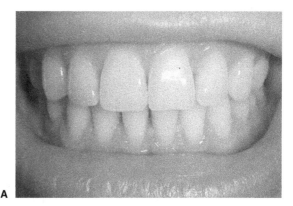

A

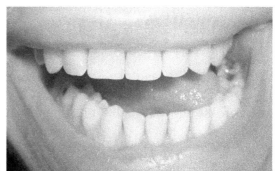

B

A. Skeletal crossbite
B. Dental crossbite
C. Functional crossbite
D. This is not an example of a crossbite.

Orthodontics

12. A 15-year-old patient presents for orthodontic treatment with the cephalometric radiograph shown below. Upon examination, the patient does not have an open bite. What is the most likely cause for the malocclusion?

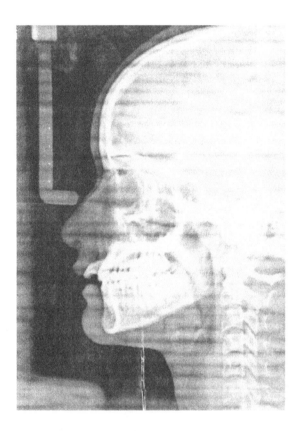

A. Thumb sucking
B. Tongue thrusting
C. Lower lip sucking
D. Skeletal in origin

13. A 14-year-old boy is ongoing a comprehensive orthodontic treatment and presents for a regular orthodontic visit. Upon intraoral examination, the physician finds a fistula above tooth #9 and takes a radiograph, which is shown below. What is the next best step of treatment for this patient?

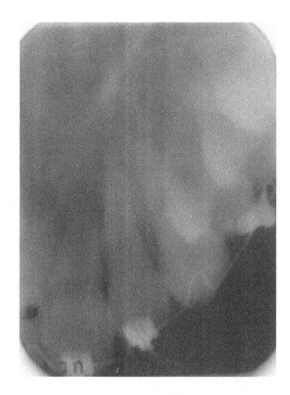

A. Disengage and remove the archwire and send the patient for endodontic evaluation.
B. Continue with orthodontic treatment and send the patient for an endodontic evaluation after the comprehensive treatment is complete.
C. Do not disengage the wire from the brackets, leave as is, and send the patient for endodontic evaluation.
D. Continue with the orthodontic treatment, but disengage tooth #9 and send patient for endodontic evaluation.

14. A 10-year-old girl has teeth #12, #13, #14, and #15 in crossbite. The orthodontist has placed a palatal expander as part of her treatment. Which of the following statements are correct?

A. After activation is complete, the expander remains in the mouth for at least 3 months.
B. After activation is complete, the expander can be taken off right away.
C. The expander is activated once a day by the patient.
D. The expander is never activated by the patient, only by the physician.
E. The expander is activated 0.5 mm each turn.
F. The expander is activated 1 mm each turn.

15. A 20-year-old man is finishing his comprehensive orthodontic treatment that involved a rotated tooth #7. What is the next step of treatment?

    A. Perform circumferential supracrestal fibrotomy prior to removal of orthodontic appliances.
    B. Perform circumferential supracrestal fibrotomy after removal of orthodontic appliances.
    C. Perform circumferential subcrestal fibrotomy prior to removal of orthodontic appliances.
    D. Perform circumferential subcrestal fibrotomy after removal of orthodontic appliances.
    E. Circumferential fibrotomy should not be performed.

16. What site is responsible for mandibular vertical growth and how will this site affect the facial height during puberty?

    A. Coronoid process, increase in posterior facial height
    B. Coronoid process, no change in posterior facial height
    C. Body of mandible, no change in posterior facial height
    D. Condylar cartilage, increase in posterior facial height
    E. Condylar cartilage, no change in posterior facial height
    F. Ramus of the mandible, increase in posterior facial height

17. Which process does mandibular growth follow?

    A. Reposition occurring at the posterior surface of the ramus and apposition of bone occurring along the posterior surface of the ramus as well
    B. Reposition occurring at the anterior surface of the ramus and apposition of bone occurring along the anterior surface of the ramus as well
    C. Reposition occurring at the posterior surface of the ramus and apposition of bone occurring along the anterior surface of the ramus

    D. Reposition occurring at the anterior surface of the ramus and apposition of bone occurring along the posterior surface of the ramus

18. What is the most common cause of an anterior crossbite of maxillary teeth in young children?

    A. Oral habits
    B. Trauma to the incisors
    C. Jaw size discrepancies
    D. Prolonged retention of primary teeth
    E. All of the above

19. In orthodontic therapy, adult patients in comparison with adolescent patients:

    A. Need less periodontal maintenance during comprehensive orthodontic treatment
    B. Are more compliant
    C. Are less concerned with esthetic
    D. Are more prone to decalcification stains on enamel

20. A 7-year-old boy was previously diagnosed with marked "bowing of the femurs" and decreased radiographic bone opacity. What disease does this patient have? What would you notice upon the examination of this patient's oral cavity and intraoral radiographs?

    I.   Hyperthyroidism
    II.   Rickets
    III. Scurvy
    IV.   Missing or delayed tooth eruption
    V.   Premature exfoliation of primary teeth
    VI.   Normal eruption pattern

    A. III and VI
    B. III and V
    C. I and VI
    D. I and V
    E. II and IV
    F. II and V

21. All these conditions are associated with supernumerary teeth *except*:

    A. Gardner syndrome
    B. Down syndrome
    C. Ectodermal dysplasia
    D. Cleidocranial dysplasia
    E. Sturge–Weber syndrome

22. A 10-year-old boy presents with severe crowding. The patient has a bilateral class I malocclusion and discrepancy in all four quadrants of 5 mm. As a part of the comprehensive orthodontic treatment, this patient needs several teeth extracted. Permanent incisors and the first permanent molars are the only permanent teeth erupted. Which teeth need to be extracted to correct the malocclusion?

    A. Permanent lateral incisor → primary canine → primary first molars
    B. Primary first molars → permanent first premolars → permanent second premolars
    C. Primary canines → primary first molars → primary second molars
    D. Primary first molars → primary second molars → permanent first premolars
    E. Primary canines → primary first molars → permanent first premolars

23. Interarch elastics are sometimes used as an aid tool in treatment of malocclusions. What malocclusion is being treated with the help of the interarch elastic mentioned below?

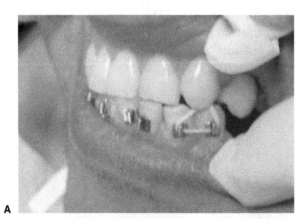

A

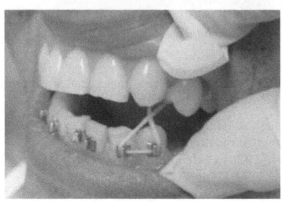

B

A. Anterior open bite
B. Class I
C. Class II
D. Unilateral crossbite

24. What is the most efficient way to move teeth, reinforce anchorage, and avoid friction in the appliance system?

    A. Apply gentle constant force.
    B. Incorporate springs into archwire.
    C. Incorporate interarch elastic.
    D. Bond magnets to individual teeth.
    E. All of the above

25. There are multiple forces being applied to teeth #8 and #9 by the step bend between two teeth. What type of force is being applied to each tooth?

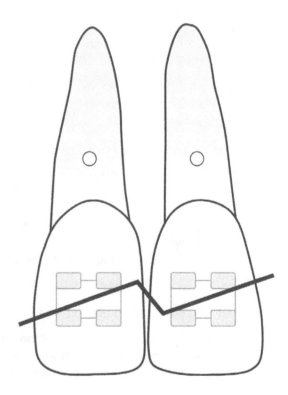

A. Teeth #8 and #9 are being intruded.
B. Teeth #8 and #9 are being extruded.
C. Tooth #8 is being intruded and #9 is being extruded.
D. Tooth #8 is being extruded and #9 is being intruded.
E. Teeth #8 and #9 are being rotated.

26. A 5-year-old girl has her molar occlusion in flush terminal plane. What is most likely to be her occlusion at age 10 with proper adequate space management?

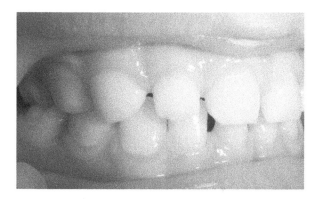

A. Class I
B. Class II division 1
C. Class II division 2
D. Class III

27. Physiologic age of the patient can be determined by examining the ossification pattern of:

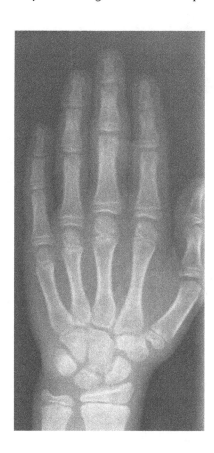

A. Carpal bones of the wrist
B. Metacarpals of the hands
C. Phalanges of the fingers
D. All of the above

28. What type of tooth movement does the diagram below represent?

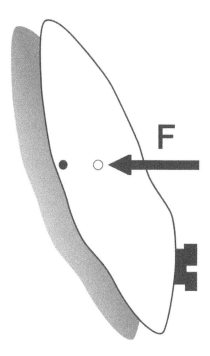

A. Rotation
B. Translation
C. Tipping
D. Intrusion
E. Extrusion

29. What is the condition that may complicate molar uprighting?

A. Open bite
B. Presence of periodontal disease
C. Extruded maxillary and mandibular molars
D. Molar having short roots
E. All of the above

30. Which of the following malocclusions is the easiest to maintain after orthodontic treatment?

A. Expansion
B. Rotation
C. Anterior crossbite
D. Generalized spacing
E. Generalized crowding

31. Which is a true statement about edgewise brackets?

    A. The magnitude of the forces generated in the faciolingual and occlusogingival direction is dependent on the bracket slot size.
    B. Twin bracket is used to gain more rotational control.
    C. Single-wing bracket is used to gain more rotational control.
    D. All statements above are true.

32. Why would an orthodontist place a nonrigid archwire at the beginning of treatment?

    A. The appliance may break if a rigid archwire is placed.
    B. The nonrigid archwire is more pliable, which is needed in the initial stages of treatment of malocclusions.
    C. The rigid archwire may become permanently deformed if placed at the beginning of treatment.
    D. All of the above are correct.

33. Which statement is true regarding Invisalign treatment?

    A. Aligners are worn 24 hours a day and taken off for eating, drinking, and oral hygiene.
    B. Change set of new aligners every two weeks.
    C. Focus is esthetic and functional alignment without utilization of complex orthodontic auxiliary treatments.
    D. Treatment is focused on straightforward cases (20 aligners or less).
    E. All of the above are true.

34. Which case would satisfy the Invisalign criteria?

    A. More than 2 mm crowding between any two anterior teeth
    B. Class III bilateral molar relationship
    C. Patient with moderate to severe periodontal disease
    D. A 9-year-old patient
    E. Patient must have fully erupted second molars.

35. A 24-year-old woman presented to an orthodontist's office to fix the spaces between her teeth. Intraoral examination shows class I molar oc-clusion. The patient does not want "a mouth full of metal." What is the best treatment option for this patient?

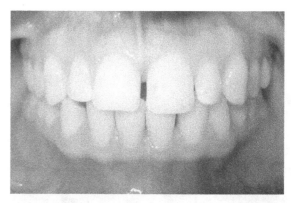

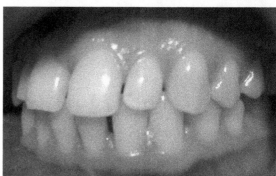

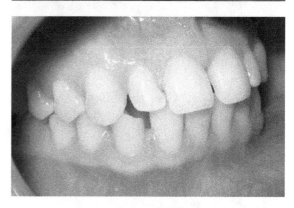

    A. Place brackets only on anterior teeth.
    B. Place brackets on the lingual surface.
    C. Treat her mild spacing with the Invisalign product.
    D. Refer her to a specialist for possible placement of laminates.

36. This is a stress–strain graph. Each letter is an important part of the elasticity curve. What do the letters X, Y, and Z represent, pertaining to the graph below?

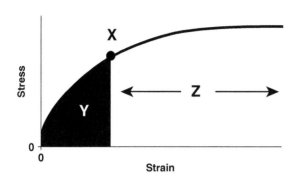

I.   X = Plastic limit
II. X = Elastic limit
III. Y = Module of plasticity
IV. Y = Module of elasticity
V.   Z = Plastic range
VI. Z = Elasticity range

A. I, III, and VI
B. I, IV, and V
C. I, IV, and VI
D. II, III, and V
E. II, III, and VI
F. II, IV, and V

37. What are the determining factors of the load–deflection rates of wires?

A. Modules of elasticity
B. Length of wire
C. Cross-sectional area
D. All of the above

38. What type of tooth movement are open-coil springs used for?

A. Close spaces between teeth
B. Upright teeth
C. Intrusion
D. Translation

39. When is the best time to refer a patient to an orthodontist for the maximum improvement with minimum treating time?

A. At approximately age 3, when all the primary teeth are present
B. At approximately age 7, when there is mixed dentition
C. At approximately age 13, when all the permanent dentition is present
D. All of the above are correct.

Refer to this picture for questions 40–44.

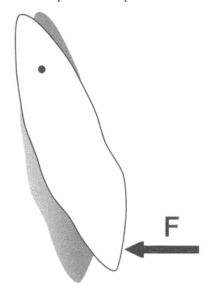

40. What type of movement is shown above?

A. Rotation
B. Translation
C. Tipping
D. Intrusion
E. Extrusion

41. What will be detected in the dark zones after light continuous force is applied for a few minutes?

A. Osteoclasts
B. Osteoblasts
C. Both osteoblasts and osteoclasts
D. Neither osteoblasts nor osteoclasts
E. Cyclic adenosine monophosphate (cAMP)

42. What will be detected in the dark zones with application of light continuous force for 4 hours?

A. Osteoclasts
B. Osteoblasts
C. Both osteoblasts and osteoclasts
D. Neither osteoblasts nor osteoclasts
E. cAMP

43. What will be detected in the dark zones with application of light continuous force for 2 days?

A. Osteoclasts
B. Osteoblasts
C. Both osteoblasts and osteoclasts
D. Neither osteoblasts nor osteoclasts
E. cAMP

44. What will be detected in the dark zones with application of heavy continuous force for 4 hours?

    A. Increase in cAMP levels
    B. Cell differentiation
    C. Cell death
    D. Release of prostaglandins and cytokines

45. Methods employed in orthodontic treatment to align a crowded dentition include:

    A. Extraction of teeth
    B. Expansion of arches
    C. Distalization of teeth
    D. Interproximal reduction of teeth
    E. All of the above

46. Which of the following will require the most force to move tooth #27?

    A. Tipping
    B. Translation
    C. Root uprighting
    D. Rotation
    E. Extrusion
    F. Intrusion

47. Below are the indications for using bands instead of brackets, *except* for:

    A. Patient with amelogenesis imperfecta
    B. Teeth with long clinical crowns
    C. Patient with cuspal interference
    D. Teeth that will need both lingual and labial attachment

48. Which one of the following statements is true about primate space in the primary dentition?

    A. Primate space is located between canine and first molar in the mandibular arch.
    B. Primate space is located between canine and first molar in the maxillary arch.
    C. It should be present in permanent teeth.
    D. It should be present in permanent teeth and deciduous teeth.

49. A 10-year-old girl presents to the office requesting to close her diastema. What is the correct treatment for this patient?

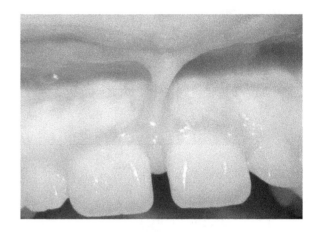

    A. Perform a frenectomy prior to orthodontic treatment and after maxillary canines erupt.
    B. Perform a frenectomy prior to orthodontic treatment and before maxillary canines erupt.
    C. Perform a frenectomy after orthodontic treatment and after maxillary canines erupt.
    D. Perform a frenectomy after orthodontic treatment and before maxillary canines erupt.
    E. Do not perform a frenectomy, and proceed with the orthodontic treatment.

50. Which one of the following statements is false about headgear?

    A. Headgear is typically used in skeletal class II.
    B. Headgear needs to be worn 10 to 14 hours per day to be effective.
    C. Treatment length is 6 to 18 months.
    D. Headgear can be used in adult patients.
    E. All of the above statements are false.
    F. All of the above statements are true.

51. The wrist–hand radiograph is used by orthodontists to predict the time of the pubertal growth spurt and thus jaw growth. What is examined in the wrist–hand radiograph?

    A. Carpal bones of the wrist
    B. Metacarpal bones of the hand
    C. Phalanges of the fingers
    D. All of the above

52. What is the most common site to find a supernumerary tooth?

    A. Distal to the third molars
    B. Between the central incisors
    C. Between the central and lateral incisors
    D. Inferior border of the mandible

53. Which of the following is not considered a method of closing a diastema?

    A. Posterior bite plate
    B. Lingual arch with finger spring
    C. Hawley appliance with finger spring
    D. Cemented orthodontic bands with inter-tooth traction

54. Which of the following is used to maintain the space of one prematurely missing primary molar?

    A. Lingual holding arch
    B. Distal shoe
    C. Band and loop
    D. A and B
    E. B and C

55. A pediatric patient has premature loss of tooth #A, but tooth #B is present, and #3 has not erupted yet. What is the best space maintainer for this situation

    A. Hawley with finger spring
    B. Hawley without finger spring
    C. Distal shoe
    D. Nance appliance

56. When is a Nance appliance indicated?

    A. Bilateral loss of primary maxillary molars
    B. Bilateral loss of primary mandibular molars
    C. Loss of one primary molar
    D. To control thumb-sucking behavior

57. What percent of the population is in class I occlusion?

    A. Less than 5%
    B. 25%
    C. 50%
    D. 70%

58. The mesiobuccal cusp of the maxillary first molar is between the mandibular first molar and mandibular second molar. What classification of occlusion is this?

    A. Class I
    B. Class II division 1
    C. Class II division 2
    D. Class III

59. In class II occlusion, in what relationship is the maxillary canine to the mandibular teeth?

    A. Mesial to the embrasure between mandibular canine and mandibular first premolar
    B. Between the mandibular canine and mandibular first premolar
    C. Distal to the embrasure between the mandibular canine and mandibular first premolar
    D. Lingual to the mandibular canine

60. The left molar is in a class II relationship, whereas the right molar is in a class I relationship.

    A. Class II division 1 subdivision left
    B. Class II division 1 subdivision right
    C. Class II division 1 subdivision 1
    D. Class I division 2 subdivision left

61. What is the sequence of treatment for an impacted maxillary canine?

    A. Extract overretained primary tooth, surgically expose canine, place bracket, pull into arch through keratinized tissue.
    B. Surgically expose canine, place bracket, extract overretained primary tooth once canine has been pulled into arch as far as possible.
    C. Extract overretained primary tooth, surgically expose canine, place bracket, pull into arch through alveolar mucosa.
    D. Wait for canine to descend so that it is visible through palatal tissue, place bracket, extract overretained primary tooth, pull canine into arch through keratinized tissue.

62. What is the name given to the line connecting the upper border of the external auditory canal and the lower orbital rim?

    A. Frankel plane
    B. Frankfort plane
    C. Posselt envelope of motion
    D. Sagittal plane
    E. Angle plane

63. Identify pogonion on the lateral cephalometric tracing.

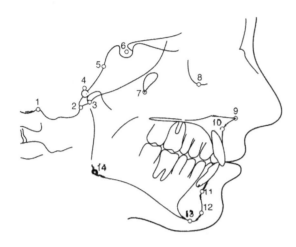

A. 1
B. 11
C. 12
D. 13

64. Spacing is normal throughout the anterior section of the primary dentition. The spaces are called primate spaces and are found:

A. Between the lateral incisors and canines in the maxilla
B. Between the canines and first molars in the mandible
C. Between the lateral incisors and canines in the mandible
D. A and B
E. B and C

65. On the lateral cephalometric radiograph, the craniometric point orbitale refers to:

A. Lowest point on the inferior margin of the orbit
B. Most anterior point on anterior wall of the orbit
C. Highest point on the superior margin of the orbit
D. Most posterior point on posterior wall of orbit

66. Identify basion on the lateral cephalometric tracing.

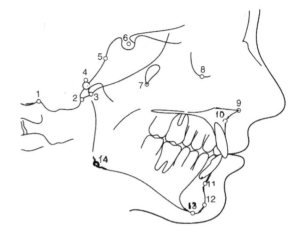

A. 2
B. 14
C. 6
D. 7

67. Which is represented by #9 on the lateral cephalometric radiograph?

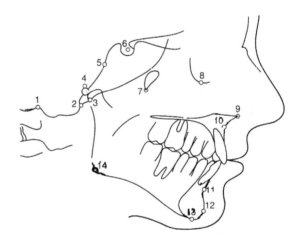

A. ANS
B. Point A
C. Point B
D. Menton
E. Pogonion

68. Where is nasion found on the lateral cephalometric radiograph?

A. The point of intersection between the shadow of the zygomatic arch and the posterior border of the ramus
B. Anterior point of the intersection between the nasal and frontal bones

C. Intersection between the occipital and ba-sisphenoid bones

D. Between the menton and pogonion

69. Which is the goal of molar uprighting?

A. Better lifetime of restorations due to improved direction and distribution of occlusal forces

B. Better periodontal prognosis

C. Easier access should endodontic/prosthetic treatments become necessary

D. Better alveolar contour

E. All of the above

70. What are the properties of an ideal archwire?

A. High strength

B. Low stiffness

C. High range

D. High formability

E. All of the above

71. Which of the following alloys is not currently used in archwires?

A. Nickel and titanium

B. Copper, tin, and titanium

C. Beta titanium (titanium and molybdenum)

D. Stainless steel and cobalt chromium

72. Which of the following is not a possible negative sequella associated with orthodontic treatment?

A. Root resorption with fast tooth movement or prolonged treatment

B. Development of gingivitis

C. Xerostomia

D. Decalcification of enamel around brackets/bands

73. Why is a palate expander kept in the patient's mouth 3 to 6 months after expansion is completed?

A. To give patients time to improve oral hygiene

B. To allow for bone fill/reorganization in the midpalatal suture region

C. To allow third molars to erupt

D. To prevent derangement of the temporomandibular joint (TMJ)

74. A patient's maxillary and mandibular midlines are not coincident, and there is a mandibular shift noted as the patient closes his mouth. What type of crossbite is likely in this patient?

A. Functional

B. Skeletal

75. Which of the following are types of removable retainers?

A. Lingual bonded retainer

B. Hawley retainer

C. Essix retainer

D. A and B

E. B and C

F. All of the above

76. What is the drawback of a palatal bonded retainer?

A. Occlusal interference

B. Aesthetics

C. Patient compliance

D. Ability to prevent relapse of midline diastemas

77. What are the properties of the alveolar ridge?

A. It exists to support teeth.

B. It does not form if a tooth fails to erupt.

C. It resorbs after a tooth is extracted.

D. It grows in height and length.

E. All of the above

78. When is postorthodontic circumferential supracrestal fibrotomy indicated?

A. To prevent mesial drift of the mandibular incisors

B. To prevent maxillary lateral incisors from relapsing into their previously rotated position

C. To maintain the buccal plate after movement of an impacted canine

D. To control thumb-sucking behavior

79. Which is the normal relationship between primary molars?

A. Flush terminal plane

B. Mesial step

C. Distal step

Orthodontics

80. The distal step relationship in primary molars often translates to which classification of occlusion in the permanent molars?

    A. Class I
    B. Class II
    C. Class III

81. Which of the following are considered systemic causes for delayed tooth eruption?

    A. Hereditary gingival fibromatosis
    B. Down syndrome
    C. Rickets
    D. All of the above

82. An orthodontist has moved the crown of tooth #8 in one direction, whereas the roots were displaced in the opposite direction about an axis of rotation. This is the definition of:

    A. Tipping
    B. Bodily movement
    C. Rotation
    D. Extrusion

83. Which orthodontic force moves the tooth into the socket along the long axis of the tooth?

    A. Extrusion
    B. Intrusion
    C. Torque
    D. Tipping

84. Which cells are pivotal for the process of tooth movement through bone?

    A. Red blood cells and white blood cells
    B. Osteoclasts and osteoblasts
    C. Neutrophils
    D. Oligodendroglia

85. What are the average distances of mandibular leeway space and maxillary leeway space per side, respectively?

    A. 2.5 mm, 1.5 mm
    B. 3 mm, 4 mm
    C. 3 to 4 mm, 2 to 2.5 mm
    D. 5 to 6 mm, 4 to 5 mm

86. Which of the following scenario is a serial extraction indicated in?

    A. Loss of primary incisors due to early childhood caries
    B. Severe class I malocclusion in mixed dentition stage, with insufficient arch length
    C. Congenitally missing maxillary lateral incisors
    D. To prevent mesial drift and subsequent crowding of mandibular incisors after all permanent teeth have erupted

87. Which of the following conditions is not associated with supernumerary teeth?

    A. Gardner syndrome
    B. Cleidocranial dysplasia
    C. Hyperthyroidism
    D. Down syndrome
    E. Sturge–Weber syndrome

88. Serial extraction refers to the orderly removal of selected primary and permanent teeth in patients with severe arch length discrepancy. Which teeth are extracted, and in what order?

    A. Primary canines, primary first molars, permanent first premolars
    B. Primary canines, primary first molars, primary second molars
    C. Primary first molars, primary second molars, permanent first premolars
    D. Primary first molars, permanent first premolars

89. What is not included in a routine set of orthodontic diagnostic records?

    A. Intraoral photographs
    B. Computed tomography of the temporomandibular joint
    C. Panoramic radiograph
    D. Impressions for dental casts of both arches
    E. Wax or polyvinyl siloxane record of occlusion
    F. Lateral cephalometric radiograph

90. Which of the following bones is formed by intramembranous ossification?

    A. Maxilla
    B. Mandible
    C. Femur
    D. Ethmoid
    E. Temporal

F. A and B
G. C, D, and E
H. A and E
I. All of the above

91. Bone grows by the addition of new layers on previously formed layers. What is this process called?

    A. Endochondral growth
    B. Appositional growth
    C. Intramembranous growth
    D. Interstitial growth

92. What is the normal overjet in class I occlusion?

    A. –2 mm
    B. 0 mm
    C. 1 to 2 mm
    D. 4 mm

93. Bimaxillary protrusion is a profile type that provides more space to accommodate teeth and alleviate crowding. The clinical picture of bimaxillary protrusion is:

    A. The mandibular teeth lean buccally
    B. The maxillary teeth lean buccally
    C. The teeth in both arches lean buccally
    D. The teeth in both arches lean lingually

94. When is it preferable to use bands instead of brackets in orthodontic treatment?

    A. To resist breakage in areas of heavy mastication or occlusal interference
    B. When both labial and lingual attachment are needed
    C. For teeth with short clinical crowns
    D. For tooth surfaces that are incompatible with bonding
    E. All of the above

95. How is the edgewise appliance different from the Begg appliance?

    A. The slot is horizontally positioned in the edgewise appliance.
    B. No wires are necessary.
    C. The slots are vertically positioned in the edgewise appliance.
    D. The edgewise appliance is made of porcelain instead of metal.

96. What is the purpose of mixed dentition analysis?

    A. To predict the number of hours per day the patients must wear their headgear appliance.
    B. To predict the amount of spacing or crowding that will be present after the permanent teeth erupt.
    C. To predict the need for a space maintainer if the primary second molar is lost prematurely.
    D. To determine the type of retainer necessary for the patient.

97. What is the mechanism of action of headgear?

    A. Used in skeletal class II patients to hold the growth of the maxilla back while allowing growth of the mandible to catch up.
    B. Used in skeletal class III patients to protract the maxilla
    C. Used in class I malocclusion patients
    D. A and B
    E. B and C
    F. All of the above

98. The norm for SNA is 82 ± 2 degrees in the Caucasian population. What does an SNA value of 85 in a Caucasian patient indicate?

    A. Maxillary prognathism
    B. Maxillary retrognathism
    C. Mandibular prognathism
    D. Mandibular retrognathism

99. What does an ANB angle of 2 to 4 degrees indicate?

    A. Class I skeletal pattern
    B. Class II skeletal pattern
    C. Class III skeletal pattern

100. ANB is a measurement gathered from a lateral cephalometric radiograph, used to determine the magnitude of the skeletal jaw discrepancy. How is ANB determined?

    A. SNA minus SNB
    B. SNA plus SNB
    C. ANS-Me minus SNB
    D. SN-MP minus SNB

Orthodontics

101. All of the following are analyses commonly used to study cephalometric radiographs *except* one:

    A. Steiner
    B. Wits
    C. Downs
    D. COGS
    E. Richards

102. If a person has a severe skeletal class II malocclusion, one would typically expect to see this manifest clinically with a:

    A. Severe underbite
    B. Severe overjet
    C. A protuberant chin
    D. Tooth decay
    E. Excessive occlusal wear

103. What is a TAD?

    A. Transmural advancement device
    B. Temporary anchorage device
    C. Topical anesthetic distributor
    D. Training assessment for dentistry
    E. Torque application distributor

104. A "Bolton discrepancy" refers to:

    A. The amount of overjet
    B. The amount of overbite
    C. The difference in size between the maxillary and mandibular teeth
    D. The difference in transverse width between the maxilla and the mandible
    E. The difference in anteroposterior length between the maxilla and the mandible

105. A rapid palatal expander (RPE) is not effective in creating skeletal expansion in adults. After the fusion of the mid-palatine suture during adolescence, an RPE will produce dental tipping rather than true skeletal expansion.

    A. Both statements are TRUE.
    B. Both statements are FALSE.
    C. The first statement is TRUE, the second is FALSE.
    D. The first statement is FALSE, the second is TRUE.

106. What percentage of the population manifests class II malocclusion?

    A. 70%
    B. 25%
    C. Less than 5%
    D. Less than 1%

107. Class II division 1 subdivision right means:

    A. The right molar is in a class II relationship, whereas the left molar is in a class I relationship.
    B. The right molar is in a class I relationship, whereas the left molar is in a class II relationship.
    C. Both molars are in class I relationship, whereas maxillary incisors are in linguoversion.
    D. Both molars are in class II relationship, whereas maxillary incisors are in labioversion.

108. Each of the following statements is correct about pseudo–class III malocclusion *except*:

    A. It describes a situation where the patient adopts a jaw position upon closure which is forward to normal.
    B. A pseudo–class III patient typically presents with an edge-to-edge bite.
    C. This patient cannot bring the mandible back without strain; and therefore, the mandibular incisors will not touch the maxillary incisors.
    D. This is a milder form of the true class III malocclusion.

109. Crowding of the permanent incisors in the early mixed dentition typically results in crowding in the permanent dentition.

    The premature loss of the primary canines, particularly in the mandibular arch is indicative of incipient malocclusion.

    A. Both statements are TRUE.
    B. Both statements are FALSE.
    C. The first statement is TRUE, the second is FALSE.
    D. The first statement is FALSE, the second is TRUE.

110. Each of the following speech sounds are correctly linked to their related malocclusion *except*:

A. "s," "z": anterior open bite, large gap between incisors
B. "t," "d": lingually positioned maxillary incisors
C. "f," "v": skeletal class II
D. "th," "sh," "ch": anterior open bite

111. Each of the following is a contraindication to molar uprighting *except* one. Which one is this EXCEPTION?

A. High mandibular plane
B. Presence of root resorption
C. Severe lingual inclination of the tooth in addition to mesial tipping
D. Occlusal plane discrepancy
E. Presence of periodontal disease
F. Low mandibular plane

112. Adequate space should be provided in the arch before attempting to pull an impacted tooth into position.

During surgical exposure, flaps should be reflected so that the impacted tooth is pulled into unkeratinized tissue.

A. Both statements are TRUE.
B. Both statements are FALSE.
C. The first statement is TRUE, the second is FALSE.
D. The first statement is FALSE, the second is TRUE.

113. Which of the following is an application of cephalometric radiographs?

A. It is the only method to determine the Angle classification.
B. It can be used to analyze treatment results.
C. It is the only reliable method to determine which teeth to extract.
D. It is the only radiograph that determines the status of wisdom teeth.
E. It is used to determine the exact inclination and location of an impacted tooth.

114. A flat mandibular plane angle correlates with a long anterior vertical dimension and an anterior open-bite malocclusion because cephalometrically, the mandibular plane angle is measured at the intersection formed by mandibular plane and the sella–nasion line.

A. Both the statement and the reason are correct and related.
B. Both the statement and the reason are correct but NOT related.
C. The statement is correct, but the reason is NOT.
D. The statement is NOT correct, but the reason is correct.
E. NEITHER the statement NOR the reason is correct.

115. Porion is located:

A. In the center of external auditory canal
B. Below the external auditory canal
C. In front of the external auditory canal
D. Behind the external auditory canal
E. On the outer upper margin of the external auditory canal

116. All of the following are indications for removable appliances *except*:

A. Limited tipping movement
B. Retention after comprehensive treatment
C. Growth modification during mixed dentition
D. Close extraction spaces fully

117. Which one of the following is a disadvantage of removable appliances versus fixed appliances?

A. Cannot achieve two-point tooth contact, therefore, making bodily tooth movement impossible
B. Improved hygiene
C. Increased patient comfort
D. Decreased chair time

118. Each of the following statements about headgear is correct *except*?

A. Headgear needs to be worn 10 to 14 hours/day to be effective.
B. High-pull headgear places a distal and intrusive force on maxillary molars.
C. Cervical-pull headgear places a distal and intrusive force on maxillary molars.
D. Reverse-pull headgear is used in class III malocclusions to protract the maxilla.

Orthodontics

119. An example of a tissue-borne functional appliance is:

    A. Bionator
    B. Herbst
    C. Frankel
    D. Forsus

120. Functional appliances are designed to modify growth during mixed dentition.

    Functional appliances have a dental effect only.

    A. Both statements are TRUE.
    B. Both statements are FALSE.
    C. The first statement is TRUE, the second is FALSE.
    D. The first statement is FALSE, the second is TRUE.

121. Which of the following is NOT a negative sequellae associated with orthodontic treatment?

    A. Orthodontic appliances decrease the risk of gingivitis.
    B. Prolonged orthodontic treatment is associated with root resorption.
    C. Prolonged orthodontic treatment is associated with decalcification stains on enamel.
    D. Orthodontic appliances may increase the risk of gingivitis due to irritation to gingiva or mucosa.

122. In straight-wire appliance:

    A. Torque in bracket slots compensate for mesial and distal inclination of teeth.
    B. Angulation of bracket slot relative to the long axis of the tooth allow for facial or lingual inclination of the teeth.
    C. Variation in bracket thickness compensates for incisal or gingival positioning of teeth.
    D. The brackets are designed with a built-in prescription to eliminate wire bends.

123. Each of the following statement is indication for using bands instead of brackets except:

    A. In heavy mastication areas
    B. In situations where only lingual attachments are needed

    C. In teeth with short clinical crowns
    D. In amelogenesis imperfecta cases
    E. In patients with stainless steel crowns

124. All of the following statements regarding crossbite are true except:

    A. A skeletal crossbite has smooth closure to centric occlusion.
    B. A functional crossbite manifests as a deviation in upper and lower midline as the patient closes.
    C. Posterior crossbites may be associated with mandibular shifts.
    D. Mild anterior crossbites can be corrected at later stages of treatment.
    E. After RPE is used, it must remain intraorally for 3 to 6 months for bone to form in the midpalatal suture region

125. All of the following statements regarding open bite are true except:

    A. Maxillary constriction usually seen in open-bite cases results from increased pressure on the mylohyoid muscles from finger sucking.
    B. The resultant maxillary constriction seen in open-bite cases tends to cause bilateral crossbites.
    C. If the finger-sucking habit involves the hand resting on the chin, mandibular growth can get retarded producing a class II retrognathic profile.
    D. Compensatory tongue thrust habit is often observed in patients with open bite.
    E. Combined orthodontic and surgical treatment is required in patients who show an excess of anterior vertical facial height, steep mandibular plane angle, or long lower facial heights.

126. Which of the following is NOT a treatment modality for open-bite cases?

    A. Tongue crib
    B. RPE
    C. Posterior bite plates
    D. High-pull headgear
    E. Straight-pull headgear

127. The correct name of the appliance below is:

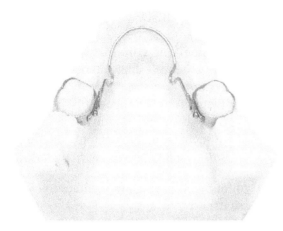

A. Tongue crib
B. Bluegrass appliance
C. Transpalatal bar
D. Lower lingual holding arch

128. All of the following statements regarding types of space maintainers are true *except*:

A. Band and loop appliance prevents mesial migration of primary second molar after unilateral loss of primary first molar.
B. Distal shoe appliance prevents mesial migration of primary second molar after unilateral loss of primary first molar.
C. A Nance appliance is used to prevent mesial rotation and mesial drift of permanent maxillary molars when primary maxillary molars have been bilaterally lost.
D. Premature loss of a primary canine may be due to arch length deficiency, and it results in lingual collapse of mandibular anterior.

129. Early loss of primary second molar leads to mesial tipping and rotation of permanent first molars.

When primary second molars are lost, no space maintenance is necessary.

A. Both statements are TRUE.
B. Both statements are FALSE.
C. The first statement is TRUE, the second is FALSE.
D. The first statement is FALSE, the second is TRUE.

130. The correct name of the following appliance is:

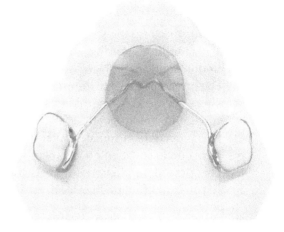

A. Nance
B. Band and loop
C. Distal shoe
D. Transpalatal bar

131. All of the following are examples of removable retainers *except*:

A. Wrap-around
B. Hawley
C. Essix
D. Bonded lingual wire

132. Which of the following statements is NOT a rationale for retention?

A. To minimize changes due to growth
B. To maintain teeth in unstable conditions
C. To allow for reorganization of the gingival and periodontal tissues
D. The occlusal result of hard tissue is modified and maintained by retention.

133. Retention can be accomplished with either fixed or removable retainers.

Anterior crossbite is retained after orthodontic correction by the overjet achieved during treatment.

A. Both statements are TRUE.
B. Both statements are FALSE.
C. The first statement is TRUE, the second is FALSE.
D. The first statement is FALSE, the second is TRUE.

134. Which of the following statements are correct regarding postorthodontic circumferential supracrestal fibrotomy?

A. It is indicated for rotated maxillary lateral incisors because the supraalveolar tissue is significantly responsible for relapse of orthodontically rotated teeth.
B. The incision is made at the crest of the bone where all the collagen fibers are inserted into the root of the tooth.
C. This procedure eliminates potential for relapse due to collagen fiber retraction.
D. This procedure allows new fibers to form that will help retain the tooth in its new position.
E. All of the above are correct.

135. A distal step means:

A. Edge-to-edge position of cusps of permanent maxillary and mandibular first molars, leading to Angle class II malocclusion
B. Distal of maxillary first molars is mesial to the distal of mandibular molars, leading to Angle class II malocclusion
C. Distal of maxillary first molars is distal to the distal of mandibular molars, leading to Angle class II malocclusion
D. Incisal edge of maxillary incisors is distal to the incisal edge of mandibular incisors.

136. The maxillary primate space is located between lateral incisors and canines.

The mandibular primate space is located between canines and first premolars.

A. Both statements are TRUE.
B. Both statements are FALSE.
C. The first statement is TRUE, the second is FALSE.
D. The first statement is FALSE, the second is TRUE.

137. Which one of the following are causes of a diastema:

A. Tooth size discrepancy
B. Mesiodens
C. Abnormal frenum attachment
D. Normal stage of development
E. All of the above

138. All of the following are correct with regards to treatment of a diastema *except*:

A. Spaces will always close as permanent canines erupt.
B. Diastema of 2 mm or less usually closes spontaneously if lateral incisors are in good position.
C. Teeth should be aligned first if the diastema is caused by an abnormal frenum.
D. In such cases, a frenectomy should be performed after canines have erupted.

139. All of the following are methods to close a diastema *except*:

A. Lingual arch with finger spring
B. Hawley appliance with finger spring
C. Cemented orthodontic bands with intertooth traction
D. Using an Essix appliance

140. All of the following statements are true *except*:

A. Nonnutritive sucking habit leads to malocclusion only if it continues during the mixed dentition stage.
B. Adenoids are a definite etiologic agent in a "long-face" pattern of malocclusion
C. Tongue trust swallow originates from the need to attain an oral seal, especially in anterior open bite cases.
D. Tongue trust swallow is considered the result of displaced incisors, not the cause.

141. All of the following statements are true *except*:

A. Intramembranous ossification takes place in membranes of connective tissue.
B. Osteoprogenitor cells in the membrane differentiate into osteoblasts.
C. The maxilla and mandible are formed via endochondral ossification.
D. Short and long bones and ethmoid, sphenoid, and temporal bones are formed via endochondral ossification.

142. Growth of bone occurs via appositional growth phenomenon and interstitial growth phenomenon.

Growth of cartilage occurs via appositional growth only.

A. Both statements are TRUE.
B. Both statements are FALSE.
C. The first statement is TRUE, the second is FALSE.
D. The first statement is FALSE, the second is TRUE.

143. Minor imperfections in the occlusion can trigger clenching and grinding and lead to temporomandibular disease or disorder (TMD).

Condylar cartilage a critical growth center of the mandible.

A. Both statements are TRUE.
B. Both statements are FALSE.
C. The first statement is TRUE, the second is FALSE.
D. The first statement is FALSE, the second is TRUE.

144. What is the single most important indicator of joint function?

A. Right and left excursions
B. Protrusion
C. The amount of maximum opening
D. Absence of pain

145. Orthodontic extractions (premolars) cause TMD.

TMD symptoms can disappear during orthodontic treatment.

A. Both statements are TRUE.
B. Both statements are FALSE.
C. The first statement is TRUE, the second is FALSE.
D. The first statement is FALSE, the second is TRUE.

146. What are the general TMD classifications?

A. Internal joint pathology and disk displacements
B. Disc displacements and myofascial pain
C. Disc fractures and muscle fatigue
D. Internal joint pathology and myofascial pain

147. What causes disc displacement and the sound of "popping" after trauma to the joints?

A. Fractured condylar head
B. Stretched or torn ligaments opposing the action of pterygoid muscle
C. A and B
D. None of the above

148. All of the following are true in regards to growth of the mandible *except*:

A. Resorption of bone occurs along the anterior surface of the ramus.
B. Apposition of bone occurs along the posterior surface of the ramus.
C. Growth at the mandibular condyle during puberty usually results in increased posterior facial height.
D. The main growth thrust of the condyle is upward and forward to fill in the resultant space to maintain contact with the base of the skull.

149. In both arches, the permanent incisor tooth buds lie buccal and apical to primary incisors.

The permanent mandibular canines erupt more facially but most often in line compared with primary mandibular canines.

A. Both statements are TRUE.
B. Both statements are FALSE.
C. The first statement is TRUE, the second is FALSE.
D. The first statement is FALSE, the second is TRUE.

150. Which one of the following is a systemic cause of failure or delayed tooth eruption?

A. Abnormal position of the crest
B. Supernumerary teeth
C. Dilacerated roots
D. Hereditary gingival fibromatosis
E. Congenital absence

151. Which of the following is correct regarding ectopic eruption?

    A. Most likely to occur in the eruption of maxillary first molars and mandibular incisors.
    B. Much more common in the maxilla.
    C. Treatment of ectopically erupting molar entails placing a brass wire between primary second molar and permanent first molar to tip it distally.
    D. Ectopic eruption of mandibular lateral incisors may lead to transposition of lateral incisor and canine.
    E. All of the above

152. What is the gender predilection for supernumerary teeth in the permanent dentition?

    A. 2:1 male:female
    B. 2:1 female:male
    C. 4:1 male:female
    D. 4:1 female:male

153. Which of the following conditions is associated with multiple supernumerary teeth?

    A. Diabetes
    B. Hyperthyroidism
    C. Gardner syndrome
    D. Rickets

154. All of the following statements regarding serial extraction are correct *except*:

    A. The indication is in severe class I malocclusion in mixed dentition with insufficient arch length.
    B. The extraction sequence is primary canine, primary first molar, and permanent first premolar.
    C. Extract first premolars after permanent canines erupt.
    D. One should always use a lingual arch in mandible and Hawley appliance in maxilla for support and retention.

155. The maxillary leeway space is bigger than mandibular leeway space, this will help with achievement of class I occlusion via late mesial shift of permanent first molars.

    A. Both the statement and the reason are correct and related.
    B. Both the statement and the reason are correct but NOT related.
    C. The statement is correct, but the reason is NOT.
    D. The statement is NOT correct, but the reason is correct.
    E. NEITHER the statement NOR the reason is correct.

1. **The correct answer is A.** In class II division 2, it is typical for maxillary centrals to have linguoversion, whereas maxillary laterals are tipped in the labial mesial direction. Class II division 1 typically has maxillary centrals tipped palatally and in a retruded position. Maxillary laterals are also tipped palatally.

2. **The correct answer is C.** The image shows a dentition in class III malocclusion, which is known as mesioclusion. Class II, not class III, is known as distoclusion. While the statement in answer choice D is true, to classify malocclusion as class II: the first mandibular molar needs to be distal to the first maxillary molar. Class I malocclusion has the mesiobuccal cusp of the maxillary first molar interdigitating with the buccal groove of the first mandibular molar.

3. **The correct answer is D.** Pseudo–class III patients adopt a closed-jaw position that is forward to normal and typically presents with an edge-to-edge bite. Bringing the mandible back with strain so that the mandibular incisors touch the maxillary incisors depicts a patient who has class III malocclusion. Bringing the mandible forward without strain so that the mandibular incisors touch the maxillary incisors depicts a class I malocclusion. Bringing the mandible forward with strain so that the mandibular incisors touch the maxillary incisors depicts a class II malocclusion.

4. **The correct answer is A.** Point B is also known as supramentale; #10 is point A; #12 is pogonion; #13 is menton.

5. **The correct answer is D.** The mandibular plane angle is a line connecting gonion – gnathion (menton), and the sella–nasion. Mandibular plane angle determines open- or deep-bite malocclusion by its measurement. A steep angle signifies a long vertical dimension with an open-bite malocclusion. A steep angle signifies a long vertical dimension with an open-bite malocclusion, not deep-bite malocclusion. When the mandibular plane angle is flat, it signifies a short vertical dimension with a deep-bite malocclusion. Although answer choice C is a correct statement, the question was asking for a *steep* angle.

6. **The correct answer is A.** The patient presented with a bilateral posterior crossbite, and since the patient is 35 years of age, the sutures have closed and the maxilla and mandible stopped growing. Surgery is one of the best treatment options to correct a crossbite.

   A rapid maxillary expander is an appliance that is used for a skeletal expansion of the upper arch in the primary or mixed dentition, in cases where the upper arch is very narrow and/or crossbite exists.

   The quad helix expander is a fixed, spring-loaded orthodontic appliance that uses four helical springs and is used primarily to expand the maxillary dental arch, in cases where it is very narrow and/or crossbite exists. It is utilized at an early stage of development to guide growth.

   The W-arch is a fixed appliance constructed of steel wire soldered to molar bands. The W-arch is a form of rapid palatal expander (RPE) that is used for a skeletal expansion of the upper arch in the primary or very early mixed dentition, in cases where the upper arch is very narrow and/or crossbite exists. It is utilized at an early stage of development to guide growth.

   Bilateral posterior crossbite is corrected only with orthodontic intervention.

7. **The correct answer is C.** This plane is known as the Frankfort-horizontal plane, which is constructed by drawing a line connecting porion and orbitale. Sella–nasion line makes the mandibular plane angle when intersected with the mandibular plane and is also used to establish the vertical position of the mandible. Gonion and gnathion lines create the mandibular plane. There is no plane connecting the spheno-occipital synchondrosis and anterior nasal spine (ANS).

8. **The correct answer is B.** SNA angle is the inferior–posterior angle between S–N line to

N–A line. It shows the anterior–posterior position of the maxilla in relation to cranial base. The adult norm is 82 ± 4 degrees. SNA angle greater than 86 degrees is indicative of a maxillary prognathism. SNA angles less than 78 degrees indicate maxillary retrusion. SNA angles of 2 to 4 degrees indicate a class I skeletal pattern. SNA angle is not indicative of mandibular position. Angle SNB is used to evaluate the anteroposterior position of the mandible.

9. **The correct answer is D.** Reverse-pull headgear (also known as Delaire-type facemask) is used to place forward traction against the maxilla. Cervical-pull headgear consists of a neck strap connected to a face bow and places a distal and extrusive force against the maxillary molars and maxilla. Straight-pull headgear is similar to cervical-pull headgear but places the force in a straight distal direction. High-pull headgear consists of a head cap connected to a face bow and places a distal and intrusive force on the maxillary molars and maxilla.

10. **The correct answer is B.** Frankel functional appliance is the only tissue-borne appliance that alters mandibular posture and contour of facial soft tissue. Bionator is a tooth-borne appliance and advances mandible to an edge-to-edge position to stimulate mandibular growth for correction of class II malocclusion. The Herbst appliance is a tooth-borne appliance and splints maxillary and mandibular framework together via pin that holds the mandible forward. An edgewise appliance is a tooth-borne appliance with horizontally positioned slot.

11. **The correct answer is C.** A crossbite is clinically observed when teeth are on the wrong side of the opposing dentition. If there is no evidence of a discrepancy in the upper and lower midlines when the mandible is at rest but a deviation of the mandible toward the side of the crossbite is noted when teeth are brought into occlusion and do not have smooth closure to centric occlusion, the malocclusion should be considered functional in origin.

A crossbite is clinically observed when teeth are on the wrong side of the opposing dentition. Skeletal crossbite is observed when there is a deviation in maxillary and mandibular midlines as the patient closes and has a smooth closure to centric occlusion. Skeletal crossbite results from a discrepancy in the structure of the mandible or maxilla.

Dental crossbite is observed when a maxillary anterior tooth is lingual to the mandibular anterior teeth.

Answer choice D is an example of a functional crossbite.

12. **The correct answer is C.** Lower lip sucking presents with closed bite in addition to features of thumb sucking. In this case, one can clearly see that the lower lip can fit in the space between upper and lower incisors.

Thumb sucking causes malocclusion characterized by flared and spaced maxillary incisors, lingually positioned lower incisors, anterior open bite, and a narrow upper arch.

Tongue thrust swallow does not always imply an altered rest position or a malocclusion and does not cause an open bite. The maxillary anterior teeth are severely protruded in this case, which is typically not a result of a tongue thrust habit.

This patient has a normal maxilla to mandible relationship; therefore, this malocclusion is not skeletal in origin.

13. **The correct answer is C.** Sometimes, there is a loss of tooth vitality during orthodontic treatment. Usually, there is a history of trauma to the tooth; however, poor control of orthodontic force may also be the cause of the periapical pathology in this case. Do not disengage the wire from the brackets, leave as is, and send the patient for endodontic evaluation is the correct choice because the wire stabilizes the tooth.

Disengagement and removal of the archwire may cause the teeth to relapse and move toward their original position.

Orthodontic treatment should be paused, rather than continued or discontinued, because any changes in pressure may lead to deleterious effects to tooth #8. An endodontic evaluation should be obtained as soon as possible. Disengagement of the wire from tooth #9 may cause the tooth to extrude and become unstable.

14. **The correct answer is A.** After the activation is complete, the expander remains in the mouth for at least 3 to 6 months for proper bone formation in the midpalatal suture region. The expander is activated twice a day by the patient and is activated 0.25 mm each turn.

15. **The correct answer is A.** Supraalveolar tissue is responsible for the relapse of orthodontically relapsed teeth. Circumferential supracrestal fibrotomy should be performed prior to removal of orthodontic appliances, which eliminates the potential for relapse due to collagen fiber retraction. New fibers will form that will aid in retention of the tooth in its new location.

16. **The correct answer is D.** The major site of mandibular vertical growth is condylar cartilage, which provides space between the jaws into which the teeth erupt. Growth of the condyle during puberty usually results in the increase in posterior facial height.

17. **The correct answer is D.** The mandible grows by reposition and opposition processes. Reposition occurs at the anterior surface of the ramus and apposition of bone occurs along the posterior surface of the ramus.

18. **The correct answer is E.** Anterior crossbite of one or more of the permanent incisors is often associated with prolonged retention of primary teeth, as well as poor oral habits and trauma to incisors.

19. **The correct answer is B.** Adult patients tend to be more compliant with treatment than are adolescents. All patients need periodontal maintenance during comprehensive orthodontic treatment because fixed appliance makes it more difficult to maintain the same oral health. There is no significant difference between adult and adolescent patients with respect to their concern for esthetics. Adult and adolescent patients are equally predisposed to decalcification stains on enamel.

20. **The correct answer is E.** The data presented in the question are indicative of rickets disease secondary to vitamin D deficiency, which presents with missing or delayed eruption. Scurvy results from dietary deficiency of water-soluble vitamin C. There may be gingival involvement, which includes swelling, friability, bleeding, secondary infection, and loosening of teeth. Hyperthyroidism is the result of increased secretion of thyroxine (T4) by the thyroid gland and usually presents with premature exfoliation of primary teeth.

21. **The correct answer is C.** Ectodermal dysplasia is usually associated with oligodontia (congenitally missing one or more teeth) and other missing ectodermal derivatives such as hair and nails.

    Although supernumerary or extra teeth can incidentally be found in healthy children; they are much more common in children with Gardner syndrome, Down syndrome, cleidocranial dysplasia, and Sturge–Weber syndrome. The most common site for these is between central incisors (mesiodens).

22. **The correct answer is E.** Serial extraction is the orderly removal of selected primary and permanent teeth in a predetermined sequence, which is as follows: primary canines → primary first molars → permanent first premolars.

23. **The correct answer is D.** Interarch forces have side effects, such as widening or constriction of the dental arches and alteration of the occlusion; therefore, it is best used in treatment of unilateral crossbite.

24. **The correct answer is E.** All of the above statements are correct. Gentle constant force must be applied for the survival of cells in the periodontal ligament (PDL). Incorporation of springs into the archwire eliminates the difficulty in anchorage control caused by frictional resistance. Reinforcement of anchorage can be produced by using interarch elastic. Magnets in attraction or repulsion could generate forces of the magnitude needed to move teeth and would have the advantage of providing predictable force levels without direct contact or friction.

25. **The correct answer is C.** A step bend between two teeth produces intrusive force on tooth #8 and extrusive force on tooth #9.

Orthodontics

26. **The correct answer is A.** Flush terminal plane is the normal primary molar teeth relationship. This causes edge-to-edge position of cusps of permanent maxillary and mandibular first molars. When mandibular molars drift forward, the flush terminal plane becomes class I occlusion.

The primary molars have to be in distal step relationship to classify for class II occlusion. Deviation I and II are determined by the anterior maxillary to mandibular teeth only.

The primary molars have to be in mesial step relationship to be classified as class III occlusion.

27. **The correct answer is D.** All of the above statements are correct. Hand–wrist radiographs are used by some investigators to judge the skeletal age and development of the patient because physical maturity and skeletal development correlate well with jaw growth.

28. **The correct answer is B.** White circles indicate the center of resistance at the starting tooth position. Shaded circles show the center of resistance moved in the direction of the force. A force through the center of resistance causes all points of the tooth to move the same amount in the same direction. This type of movement is called *translation* or *bodily movement*. Rotation is the movement of a tooth around its longitudinal axis. Tipping is the movement of a tooth in any direction while its apex remains in almost the original position. Intrusion is the movement of the tooth in an inward direction. Extrusion is the movement of teeth beyond the natural occlusal plane that may be accompanied by a similar movement of investing tissues.

29. **The correct answer is E.** All of the above statements are correct. Slow progress in molar uprighting in an adult patient is most likely due to occlusal interferences, such as extruded maxillary and mandibular molar with an open bite already present. Presence of periodontal disease or short clinical crown is not favorable for orthodontic treatment.

30. **The correct answer is C.** Corrected anterior crossbite is best retained by the normal incisor relationship.

When expansion has been completed, a 3-month period of retention with the appliance in place is recommended. A fixed appliance can be removed, but a removable retainer that covers the palate is often needed as further insurance against early relapse.

When rotation has been completed, circumferential supracrestal fibrotomy should be performed prior to removal of orthodontic appliances, which eliminates the potential for relapse due to collagen fiber retraction. New fibers will form that will aid in retention of the tooth in its new location.

When treatment for generalized crowding or spacing has been completed, either a fixed or removable appliance is needed to prevent relapse.

31. **The correct answer is D.** All of the statements are true regarding edgewise appliances. The magnitude of the forces generated in the faciolingual and occlusogingival direction is dependent on the bracket slot size. Both bracket types (twin bracket and single-wing bracket) are used to gain more rotational control.

32. **The correct answer is D.** All of the above statements are true. There are many irregularities in malocclusions, and a rigid appliance may break or create permanent deformation in the archwire. If a rigid wire is used, the patient may be in a lot of pain.

33. **The correct answer is E.** All of the above statements are true. Aligners are worn 24 hours a day and taken off for eating, drinking, and oral hygiene. Change your set of new aligners every 2 weeks. The focus of Invisalign treatment is on aesthetic and functional alignment without utilization of complex orthodontic auxiliary treatments. Treatment is focused on straightforward cases requiring 20 or fewer aligners.

34. **The correct answer is E.** Eruption is a change in vertical movement—aligners made before all the teeth are fully erupted (excluding third molar) will not fit, because they are not made to accommodate the erupting molar.

To satisfy the Invisalign criteria, there must be less than 2 mm crowding between any two anterior teeth. There also must be ideal class I molar relationship.

Thin tissue that is prone to recession is not favorable for any regular orthodontic treatment, including Invisalign. Mild horizontal bone loss does not mean that the patient is a poor candidate for Invisalign. However, patients should be warned of possible risks that may occur during treatment.

The patient must be at least 14 years of age and should not have a mixed dentition. The aligners will not fit in the process of primary teeth exfoliation and permanent teeth eruption.

35. **The correct answer is C.** Although all choices are acceptable, the best option is treatment with Invisalign (the patient does not want the conventional braces, and she is very concerned about her smile).

36. **The correct answer is F.** Stress–strain curve is like a spring. X represents the elastic limit, the point at which permanent deformation occurs. Y represents the stiffness (modulus of elasticity), the ration of load to deflection. Z represents plastic range, the amount of deformation or strain a wire can undergo between the elastic limit and the ultimate strength. Ultimate strength of the material is the maximum load at which point the material will fracture.

37. **The correct answer is D.** All the choices are correct. The type of wire used is determined by its modulus of elasticity. The main two types of wires used are the nickel titanium and stainless steel. The length of wire is directly proportional to the springiness and indirectly proportional to the strength. The cross-sectional area of wire is indirectly proportional to the springiness and directly proportional to the strength.

38. **The correct answer is B.** When an open spring is compressed, it has a tendency to reopen, causing an uprighting of the tooth that it is attached to (e.g., making room for an implant on site #19, where tooth #18 has displaced mesially and tooth # 20 distally). The closed coil spring is used to close spaces, given its natural recoil tendency once it is placed on teeth in open

position. Springs are not able to make intrusive tooth movement, are usually not used in translation, and alone could not accomplish this type of tooth movement.

39. **The correct answer is B.** The American Association of Orthodontists recommends an orthodontic screening examination by age 7 (may be performed by a general dentist).

Three-year-old children may not have all the primary teeth yet, which makes them poor candidates for orthodontic treatment. Thirteen-year-old patients are not at their prime age for an orthodontic treatment.

40. **The correct answer is C.** During tipping, the crown and the apex move in opposite directions, creating two areas of compression: the cervical area on the side toward which the tooth is tipping and the apical region on the side opposite from which the tooth crown is moving. The tension areas are located on the opposite sides of where the compression occurs. Rotation is the movement of a tooth around its longitudinal axis. A force through the center of resistance causes all points of the tooth to move the same amount in the same direction. Intrusion is the movement of the tooth in an inward direction. Extrusion is the movement of teeth beyond the natural occlusal plane that may be accompanied by a similar movement of investing tissues.

41. **The correct answer is D.** Neither osteoblasts nor osteoclasts are located in the dark zones after a force is applied for a few minutes. Blood flow is altered and oxygen tension begins to change, leading to release of prostaglandins and cytokines. Osteoclasts and osteoblasts remodel bony socket, which induces tooth movement at approximately second day after a continuous light force is applied to a tooth. There is an increase in cyclic adenosine monophosphate (cAMP) level along with cellular differentiation within the periodontal ligament in approximately 4 hours after an application of continuous light force to a tooth.

42. **The correct answer is E.** There is an increase in cAMP level along with cellular differentiation

within the periodontal ligament in approximately 4 hours after an application of continuous light force to a tooth. Osteoclasts and osteoblasts remodel the bony socket, which induces tooth movement at approximately the second day after a continuous light force is applied to a tooth.

43. **The correct answer is A.** Resorption of alveolar bone is represented by the dark areas (known as *compression areas of the periodontal ligaments*). Osteoclasts are usually found in these areas. Osteoclasts and osteoblasts remodel bony socket, which induces tooth movement at around second day after a continuous light force is applied to a tooth. Osteoblasts are present only on the opposite surface of a root that is undergoing bodily movement and appear on the second day of continuous light force application. Along the tension front, a different type of activity occurs as the fibers are under tension and the bone quickly activates; here, bone is stimulated to begin formation. There is an increase in cAMP levels along with cellular differentiation within the periodontal ligament, in approximately 4 hours after an application of continuous light force to a tooth.

44. **The correct answer is C.** The amount of force (heavy or light) determines the biological pathway of tooth movement and the formation or lack of formation of a hyalinized zone with undermining resorption. With an application of heavy continuous force, the cell death is observed in the compressed area. Increased cAMP levels are detectable within 4 hours of continuous light force application to the tooth. There is cellular differentiation within periodontal ligament in approximately 4 hours of continuous light force application to the tooth. Few minutes of light continuous force application usually leads to release of prostaglandins and cytokines.

45. **The correct answer is E.** All of the methods mentioned are employed in orthodontic treatment to align a crowded dentition. The extraction of first premolars to relieve the crowding (in case of severe crowding) is known as *serial extraction*. For example, palatal arch can be lengthened to make room for proper eruption of teeth with palatal expander. Distalization is a process of tipping a crown of the tooth distally to create space. Interproximal reduction is a process of removing a small portion of tooth enamel interproximally to create space and align teeth.

46. **The correct answer is B.** Tooth movement such as translation requires the most force (70–120 gm). Tooth movements in descending order of requiring force are:
    I.   Translation
    II. Root uprighting
    III. Tipping, rotation, and extrusion require similar force application
    IV. Intrusion

47. **The correct answer is B.** Patients with short clinical crowns have an indication to use a band instead of a bracket. Patients with amelogenesis imperfecta have tooth surface that is incompatible with successful bonding for the placement of brackets. Therefore, the use of bands is indicated. Patients with cuspal interference or who experience heavy masticatory forces require band placement rather than brackets to better resist breakage. Patients with teeth requiring both lingual and labial attachment have an indication for a band placement.

48. **The correct answer is A.** Generalized spacing of primary teeth is required for proper alignment of the permanent incisors. The primate space is located between lateral incisor and canine in the maxillary arch, and between the canine and first molar in the primary dentition of the mandibular arch. It should be present in deciduous teeth. The primate space should not be present in permanent teeth, and if there is spacing, then an orthodontic appliance should be placed to close it.

49. **The correct answer is C.** In this case, a diastema is caused by a low frenum attachment. Teeth should be aligned orthodontically, followed by a frenectomy after maxillary canines erupt, because spaces tend to close as permanent canines erupt.

50. **The correct answer is F.** Headgear is typically used in skeletal class II growing patients to hold the growth of the maxilla back and to allow the mandible to catch up. To be effective, it needs to be worn 10 to 14 hours per day for 6 to 18 months depending on the case. Adults can wear orthodontic headgear for maintenance of anchorage.

51. **The correct answer is D.** The hand–wrist radiographs can help pinpoint a child's skeletal age and the areas examined are the carpal bones of the wrist, metacarpal bones of the hand, and phalanges of the fingers. Orthodontists compare a hand–wrist radiograph with a picture atlas of wrist bones at various radiographic developmental stages. This is used to help predict the child's next growth spurt.

52. **The correct answer is B.** The most common supernumerary tooth is the mesiodens, which is a peg-like tooth that occurs between the central incisor. This occurs in 0.15% to 1.9% of the population.

53. **The correct answer is A.** Posterior bite plates are used in correcting an anterior open bite. Lingual arch with finger spring appliance, Hawley appliance with finger spring, and cemented orthodontic bands with intertooth traction are all methods that can be used to close a diastema.

54. **The correct answer is E.** Both distal shoe and band and loop are appliances used to maintain the space of one prematurely missing primary molar. Lingual holding arch is used to maintain the spaces for bilateral or multiple missing primary teeth.

55. **The correct answer is C.** A distal shoe is indicated when the primary second molar is lost prior to eruption of the permanent first molar.

56. **The correct answer is A.** Nance appliance is best used to maintain the space for bilateral loss of primary maxillary molars. A lingual holding arch is best used to maintain the space when bilateral primary mandibular molars are lost. A distal shoe or band and loop can be used to maintain the space of one loss primary

molar. To control thumb-sucking behavior, a crib should be used.

57. **The correct answer is D.** Approximately 70% of the population is in class I occlusion. Approximately 25% of the population is in class II occlusion, and less than 5% of the population is in class III occlusion.

58. **The correct answer is D.** In a class III occlusion, the mesiobuccal cusp of the maxillary first molar is posterior to the buccal groove of the mandibular first molar. In class I occlusion, the mesiobuccal cusp of the maxillary first molar is lined up with the buccal groove of the mandibular first molar. In class II division 1, the mesiobuccal cusp of the maxillary first molar falls between the mandibular first molar and the mandibular second premolar. (THINK: The whole maxilla is more forward of where it should be.) In class II division 2, the relationship between the first molars is the same as in class II division 1. The difference here is that the maxillary central incisors are tipped palatally, and the maxillary lateral incisors are tipped buccally and mesially.

59. **The correct answer is C.** In a class II occlusion, the maxillary canine would be mesial to the embrasure between the mandibular canine and the mandibular first premolar. In a class I occlusion, the maxillary canine is in the embrasure between the mandibular canine and mandibular first premolar. In a class III occlusion, the maxillary canine is distal to the embrasure between the mandibular canine and mandibular first premolar. A maxillary canine that is lingual to the mandibular canine signifies skeletal arch discrepancy between the maxilla and mandible.

60. **The correct answer is A.** Subdivision is added to the classification when only one side of the dental arch has a malocclusion and according to the side of the dental arch the malocclusion is found on. Even though one side of the arch is normal (class I), the classification is named for the abnormal (class II). The malocclusion (class II) is on the left, so it is subdivision left. Subdivision is always followed by either left or

Orthodontics

right, as it refers to the side of the arch the malocclusion is found on.

61. **The correct answer is A.** A space should be established in the arch prior to pulling the canine into position. It is also best to pull an impacted canine into position through keratinized mucosa, not alveolar mucosa. And if treatment is delayed, a canine is more likely to ankylose instead of erupting on its own through the palate.

62. **The correct answer is B.** Frankfort plane is the line on the lateral cephalogram connecting the upper border of the external auditory meatus and the lower orbital rim. The posselt envelope of motion is a diagram that shows the shape of the pathway the mandible makes during functioning.

63. **The correct answer is C.** Pogonion is the craniometric point that is the most forward-projecting point on the anterior surface of the chin.

64. **The correct answer is D.** Primate space is found between the lateral incisors and canines in the maxilla and between the canines and first molars in the mandible.

65. **The correct answer is A.** Orbitale is the craniometric point that is the lowest point on the inferior orbital margin.

66. **The correct answer is A.** Basion is the craniometric point that is the midpoint of the anterior border of the foramen magnum.

67. **The correct answer is A.** ANS is the craniometric point that is the anterior extremity of the intermaxillary suture.

68. **The correct answer is A.** Nasion is the anterior point of the intersection between the nasal and frontal bones on the lateral cephalometric radiograph. Articulare is the point of intersection between the shadow of the zygomatic arch and the posterior border of the ramus. Spheno-occipital synchondrosis is the intersection between the occipital and basisphenoid bones. Gnathion is the point on the lateral cephalo-

metric radiograph that is between menton and pogonion.

69. **The correct answer is E.** As per answers.

70. **The correct answer is E.** As per answers.

71. **The correct answer is B.** Copper, tin, and titanium alloy are not used for orthodontic archwires. Commonly used alloys for orthodontic wire fabrication are made out of nickel and titanium alloys, titanium and molybdenum alloys, and stainless steel and cobalt chromium alloys.

72. **The correct answer is C.** Common causes of xerostomia include medications, cancer therapy, Sjögren syndrome, stress nutritional deficiencies, and nerve damage. Orthodontic treatment does not cause xerostomia but can have other common negative sequelae such as root resorption, development of gingivitis, and decalcification of enamel around orthodontic appliances.

73. **The correct answer is B.** A palate expander is kept in the patient's mouth for 3 to 6 months after expansion to allow for bone formation in the midpalatal suture region. Third molars erupt at approximately the age of 18 years. Traditional palate expansion cannot be completed at this age, unless it is surgically assisted, because the midpalatal suture is already closed.

74. **The correct answer is A.** A skeletal crossbite has smooth closure to centric occlusion whereas there tends to be shift when it is a functional crossbite.

75. **The correct answer is E.** Orthodontic retainers are custom-made devices used to hold teeth in position after realignment or surgery and usually made of wires or clear plastic. The Hawley retainer is a removable retainer made of a metal wire that surrounds the teeth and is anchored in an acrylic arch that sits in the palate or lingual walls of the mouth. The Essix retainer, a vacuum-formed retainer, is a clear retainer that fits over an entire arch of teeth or only from the canine to canine and is removable. The lingual bonded retainer is fixed and consists of a passive wire bonded to the tongue side of the incisors.

76. **The correct answer is A.** Benefits of the palatal bonded retainer include aesthetics as it is hidden from sight in the palate, increased patient compliance as it is fixed, and ability to prevent relapse of the midline diastemas.

77. **The correct answer is E.** An alveolar ridge is one of the two ridges on the maxilla and on the mandible that contain the alveoli of the teeth. It fails to form if a tooth fails to erupt, resorbs after a tooth is extracted, and can grow in height and length.

78. **The correct answer is B.** The supracrestal circumferential fibrotomy is used to prevent maxillary lateral incisors from pure rotational relapse.

79. **The correct answer is A.** The normal relationship of primary molars is one in which the maxillary and mandibular molars are in a flush terminal plane. After the eruption of the permanent first molars, there is an early mesial shift with the closing of the mandibular primate space, and after the exfoliation of the primary molars, a late mesial shift develops and the leeway space is closed. As a result of the early and late mesial shifts, a class I molar relationship develops.

80. **The correct answer is B.** The primary dentition equivalent of Angle class II relationship is the distal step. A mesial step relationship corresponds to Angle class I. An equivalent to a class III relationship is almost never seen in the primary dentition and the normal pattern of craniofacial growth in which the mandible lags behind the maxilla.

81. **The correct answer is D.** Disturbances in tooth eruption are commonly due to mechanical interferences by supernumerary teeth, crowding, odontogenic tumors and cysts, eruption sequestrum, or local causes such as gingival fibromatosis. A number of systemic disease and syndromes can also affect the delayed tooth eruption and shedding of primary teeth, such as rickets, cleidocranial dysplasia and Down syndrome.

82. **The correct answer is A.** As per the question.

83. **The correct answer is B.** Intrusion is when the tooth is moved into the socket along the long axis of the tooth, whereas extrusion is the opposite, in which the tooth is moved out of the socket along the long axis of the tooth. Torque movement is used to tip a tooth buccal lingually or mesial distally about an axis of rotation.

84. **The correct answer is B.** Osteoclasts and osteoblasts are vital to bone resorption and formation as a tooth is moved orthodontically. Oligodendroglia is a type of glial cell found in the brain.

85. **The correct answer is A.** Leeway space is the space differential between the primary posterior teeth (i.e., primary canine to primary second molars) and their replacement teeth (i.e., permanent canine to permanent second premolar). It spans approximately 2.5 mm per side in the mandibular arch and 1.5 mm per side in the maxillary arch.

86. **The correct answer is B.** Serial extractions are employed for selected patients with straightforward crowding such as moderate class I malocclusion in mixed dentition stage due to insufficient arch length. It is a planned sequence of extractions that begins initially with the deciduous canine and then the deciduous first molars. This is designed to allow crowded incisor segments to align spontaneously during the mixed dentition by shifting labial segment crowding to the buccal segments where it could be dealt with by premolar extractions.

87. **The correct answer is C.** Supernumerary teeth are commonly associated with the following: Gardner syndrome, cleidocranial dysplasia, Down syndrome, and Sturge–Weber syndrome. Hyperthyroidism is associated with early exfoliation of primary teeth.

88. **The correct answer is A.** Serial extractions are employed for selected patients with straightforward crowding such as moderate class I malocclusion in mixed dentition stage due to insufficient arch length. It is a planned sequence of extractions that begins initially with the deciduous canine and then the deciduous

first molars. This is designed to allow crowded incisor segments to align spontaneously during the mixed dentition by shifting labial segment crowding to the buccal segments where it could be dealt with by premolar extractions.

89. **The correct answer is B.** Routine set of orthodontic diagnostic records include radiographs such as panoramic and lateral cephalometric radiographs, impressions for dental casts of both arches, and occlusion records. Computed tomography or magnetic resonance imaging of the temporomandibular joints are not routinely indicated unless the patient has symptoms of dysfunction of that joint that may be related to internal joint pathology.

90. **The correct answer is F.** Maxilla and mandible bones are formed by intramembranous ossifications. Femur, ethmoid, and temporal bones are formed by endochondral ossification.

91. **The correct answer is B.** Appositional bone growth is when bone grows by the addition of new layers on previously formed layers. Endochondral ossification is when a bone is formed through replacement of a cartilage template by a bone matrix. Intramembranous ossification is the direct ossification of embryonic connective tissue.

92. **The correct answer is C.** Normal overjet in class I occlusion is 1 to 2 mm. An overjet of 4 mm will tend to be class II occlusion. An overjet of –2 mm will tend to be class III occlusion.

93. **The correct answer is C.** Bimaxillary protrusion is a relatively forward position, or prognathism, of the maxillary and mandibular teeth, alveolar processes, or jaws. This provides space to accommodate teeth and alleviate crowding.

94. **The correct answer is E.** As per answer choices. Tooth surfaces such as a stainless steel crown or in cases of amelogenesis imperfecta are incompatible with bonding.

95. **The correct answer is A.** The edgewise appliance is a fixed, multibanded orthodontic appliance that uses an attachment bracket slot that receives a rectangular archwire horizontally that can be used to control tooth movement in all three planes of space. The Begg appliance is an orthodontic appliance based on a modified ribbonarch attachment, and the slots are positioned vertically.

96. **The correct answer is B.** Mixed dentition space analyses form an essential part of diagnostic procedure. It helps to assess the amount of space required for the alignment of unerupted permanent teeth in a dental arch. Inappropriate and not valid analysis could lead to extractions that can negatively alter a patient's soft tissue facial profile.

97. **The correct answer is D.** When used in skeletal class II patients, high pull, cervical pull, and reverse straightpull headgears apply forces distally to the maxilla/maxillary teeth to hold the growth of the maxilla back are used. When used in a skeletal class III patient, a reverse-pull headgear force is used.

98. **The correct answer is A.** Maxillary prognathism with the norm of SNA 82 ± 2 degrees has an SNA >84 degrees. Maxillary retrognathism would have an SNA <80 degrees if the SNA is 82 ± 2 degrees. Mandibular prognathism would be an SNB >82 degrees and mandibular retrognathism would be an SNB <78 degrees if the SNB norm is 80 ± 2 degrees.

99. **The correct answer is A.** ANB has a norm of 2 to 4 degrees. It tells us what the maxillary and mandibular skeletal base discrepancies are. A large value, such as 8 degrees, would indicate a large maxillary protrusion and a negative value would indicate a mandibular prognathism.

100. **The correct answer is A.** ANB can be determined by subtracting SNB from SNA or by straight measurements with the three craniometric points.

101. **The correct answer is E.** There is no Richard analysis of cephalometry. Other analyses are very commonly used by orthodontists to analyze cephalometric radiographs.

102. **The correct answer is B.** Skeletal class II malocclusions are frequently accompanied by excessive overjet.

103. **The correct answer is B.** Temporary anchorage device. It is a small implant that can be used for additional anchorage to assist in tooth movement during orthodontic treatment.

104. **The correct answer is C.** A Bolton discrepancy is typically referred to as a "tooth size discrepancy" and measures the difference in tooth size between the maxillary and mandibular dental arches.

105. **The correct answer is A.** Both statements are true. RPEs are commonly used in children because the halves of the palate can still be separated with relative ease. RPEs are much less effective in older teenagers and adults because of the fusion of the midpalatine suture. The halves of the palate cannot usually move apart, so the pressure from the RPE has a greater effect on the dentition instead. This can cause the tipping of posterior teeth rather than true skeletal expansion.

106. **The correct answer is B.** On the basis of the recent National Health and Nutrition Estimates Survey III of the U.S. population among white, black, and Hispanic races, 25% of the population manifests a class II malocclusion. 70% of the population manifests class I malocclusion. Less than 5% of the population manifests class III malocclusion.

107. **The correct answer is A.** Answer B is incorrect because the subdivision describes the side where the malocclusion occurs. Answer C is incorrect because both molars cannot be in class I when the question statement says it is class II. Answer D is incorrect because subdivision means malocclusion has occurred only on one side of the dental arch.

108. **The correct answer is C.** Answer C is a false statement because pseudo–class III patients **can** bring the mandible back without strain to a position where mandibular and maxillary incisors can touch. The typical reason that

pseudo–class III patients slide the mandible forward is to avoid interferences and achieve maximal intercuspation. These patients can often be guided back to a normal jaw position once the interference is removed.

109. **The correct answer is A.** The first statement is true because arch perimeter increases slightly after the eruption of the incisors, but after this stage of dental development, arch length reduces as a result of the loss of E space. Hence, any crowding of the permanent incisors in the early mixed dentition typically results in crowding in the permanent dentition.

The second statement is true because the premature loss of the primary canines is indicative of insufficient arch size in the anterior region. During eruption of the lateral incisors, the crown of the laterals impinges on the roots of the primary canines and causes them to resorb. When the canine is shed, the midline will shift in the direction of the lost tooth. This causes lateral and lingual migration of the mandibular incisors.

110. **The correct answer is C.** Answer C is a false statement because difficulty in pronouncing sounds "f" and "v" are associated with skeletal class III cases. An anterior crossbite of multiple teeth does not allow for maxillary incisors to touch the lower lip, which is a position needed to create these sounds.

111. **The correct answer is F.** Answer A is incorrect because in patients with high mandibular plane angle, unsuccessful molar uprighting can lead to an increased open bite and loss of anterior guidance.

Answer B is incorrect because any orthodontic movement in teeth with existing root resorption can lead to more resorption.

Answer C is incorrect because correcting the lingual inclination can lead to bite opening.

Answer D is incorrect because occlusal plane discrepancy (i.e., extruded maxillary and mandibular molars) will only pose more problems in terms of deficient occlusal clearance needed to upright a molar.

Answer E is incorrect because any orthodontic movement in teeth with existing periodontal disease can lead to more compromised periodontal conditions.

Answer F is a false statement because patients with low mandibular plane angle are the best candidates in which to upright molars, since these patients usually present with a deep overbite. Molar uprighting can help "open up" and correct their occlusion.

112. **The correct answer is C.** The first statement is correct because without adequate space provided, only crowding will be introduced into the system, which will hinder the path of eruption of the impacted tooth.

The second statement is incorrect because impacted teeth should be pulled into keratinized tissue, and not alveolar mucosa, to ensure adequate periodontal support.

113. **The correct answer is B.** Superimposition of cephalometric radiographs taken before, during, and after treatment will show changes in jaw and tooth positions that have occurred due to orthodontic therapy and orthognathic surgery.

Answer A is incorrect because Angle classification can usually be determined from cast models, photographs, or clinical examination of the patient.

Answer C is incorrect because the decision to extract teeth is the result of a comprehensive evaluation of the patient's complete record in combination with clinical presentation of the patient in addition to patient preferences.

Answer D is incorrect because the status of the wisdom teeth can usually be determined via Panorex radiogram or orthopantogram.

Answer E is incorrect because the exact location of an impacted tooth is best studied through Cone Beam CAT Scans.

114. **The correct answer is D.** The statement is not correct because a steep mandibular plane angle correlates with a long anterior vertical dimension and an anterior open bite. The reason is also correct.

115. **The correct answer is E.** Porion is located on the outer upper margin of the external auditory canal.

116. **The correct answer is D.** Answer D is false because bodily tooth movement is required to close extraction spaces fully for which full orthodontic treatment with fixed appliances is necessary.

117. **The correct answer is A.** Answer A is correct because removable appliances can accomplish only tooth tipping.

Answer B is incorrect because improved hygiene is one of the advantages of removable appliances

Answer C is incorrect because increased patient comfort is one of the advantages of removable appliances.

Answer D is incorrect because decreased chair time is one of the advantages of removable appliances.

118. **The correct answer is C.** Answer C is false because cervical-pull headgear produces a distal and extrusive force on the maxillary molars and maxilla.

119. **The correct answer is C.** Answer A is incorrect because the Bionator is a tooth-borne functional appliance.

Answer B is incorrect because the Herbst is a tooth-borne functional appliance.

Answer D is incorrect because the Forsus is a tooth-borne functional appliance.

120. **The correct answer is C.** The first statement is correct. The second statement is incorrect because functional appliances used during mixed dentition have both dental and skeletal effects.

121. **The correct answer is A.** Answer A is correct because orthodontic appliances increase the risk of gingivitis due to irritation of gingiva or mucosa.

122. **The correct answer is D.** Answer A is incorrect because torque in bracket slots compensate for facial and lingual inclination of the teeth.

Answer B is incorrect because angulation of bracket slot relative to the long axis of the teeth allow for proper positioning of the tooth roots.

Answer C is incorrect because variation in bracket thickness compensates for the varying thickness of individual teeth.

123. **The correct answer is B.** Answer B is a false statement because bands are used in cases where both lingual AND buccal attachments are needed. Bands are preferably used in heavy mastication areas or areas with cuspal interference to reduce chance of breakage. Bands are preferably used in cases with short clinical crown. Bands are preferably used in patients with amelogenesis imperfect since tooth surfaces are incompatible with successful bonding. Bands are preferably used in patients with stainless steel crowns since crown surfaces are incompatible with successful bonding.

124. **The correct answer is D.** Answer D is a false statement because mild anterior crossbites need to be corrected in the first stage of treatment (as soon as possible), as the transverse dimension is the first to stop growth.

125. **The correct answer is A.** Answer A is a false statement because maxillary constriction usually seen in open-bite cases result from increased pressure on the buccinators muscles from finger sucking.

126. **The correct answer is E.** Answer A is incorrect because habit-breaking appliances can help with treatment of open-bite cases.

Answer B is incorrect because RPE can help with treatment of open-bite cases to correct narrow maxillas.

Answer C is incorrect because posterior bite plates can help with treatment of open-bite cases by discouraging posterior teeth from erupting further and encouraging anterior teeth to erupt more and close the bite.

Answer D is incorrect because high-pull headgear places a distal and intrusive force on the molars. The intrusive force will discourage molars from erupting more.

Answer E is correct because straight-pull headgear places a horizontal force on the molars, neither intruding nor extruding the molars. This does not help with the correction of open-bite in any way.

127. **The correct answer is D.** The image pictured is that of a lower lingual holding arch.
Correct picture of tongue crib:

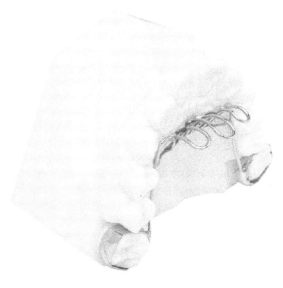

Correct picture of Bluegrass appliance:

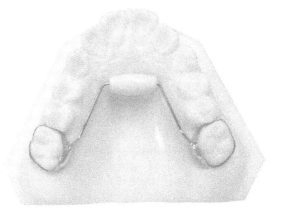

Correct picture of transpalatal bar:

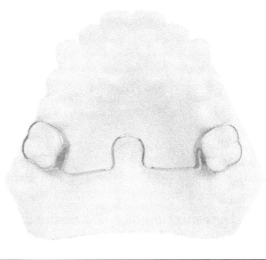

Orthodontics

128. **The correct answer is B.** Answer B is a false statement because distal shoe appliance is usually used when primary second molar is lost prior to the eruption of the permanent first molar.

129. **The correct answer is C.** Early loss of primary second molars leads to the most rapid loss of arch perimeter due to mesial tipping and rotation of the permanent first molar; therefore, space maintenance is always needed until arrival of the second premolar.

130. **The correct answer is A.** Nance orthodontic appliance.

Correct picture of band and loop:

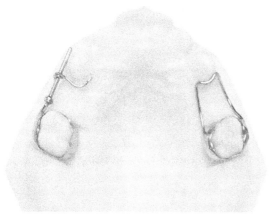

Correct picture of distal shoe:

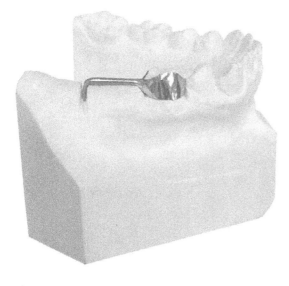

131. **The correct answer is D.** A bonded lingual retainer is fixed.

Correct picture of wrap-around retainer:

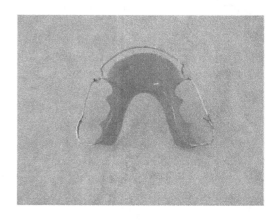

Correct picture of Hawley:

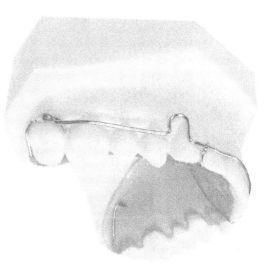

Correct picture of Essix:

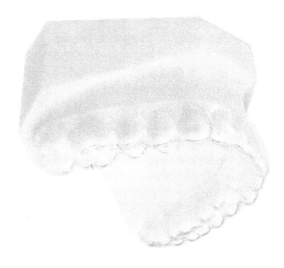

Correct picture of Bonded lingual wire:

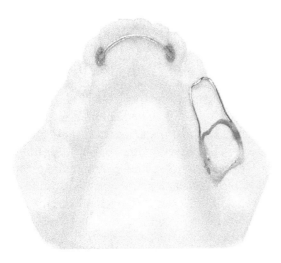

132. **The correct answer is D.** Answer D is a false statement because the occlusal result of hard tissue is modified by orthodontic treatment.

133. **The correct answer is C.** The first statement is true. The second statement is false because anterior crossbite is retained after orthodontic correction by the overbite achieved during treatment.

134. **The correct answer is E.** All of the above are true statements about the postorthodontic circumferential supracrestal fibrotomy.

135. **The correct answer is B.** Answer A is incorrect because an edge-to-edge position is the flush terminal plane, which is the normal relationship of maxillary and mandibular first molars. This leads to class I Angle classification due to early mesial shift of mandibular molars in relation to maxillary molars.

Answer B is correct because the more forward position of the maxillary first molar in relation to mandibular molar often leads to Angle class II malocclusion.

Answer C is incorrect because the more backward position of the maxillary first molar in relation to mandibular molar often leads to Angle class III malocclusion.

Answer D is incorrect because distal step is a term involving primary molars and has nothing to do with incisors.

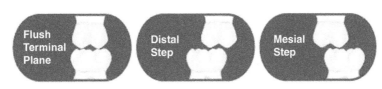

1. **Flush terminal plane:** The distal surfaces of maxillary and mandibular primary second molars lie in the same vertical plane.
2. **Distal step:** The distal surface of the mandibular primary second molar is distal to that of the maxillary primary second molar.
3. **Mesial step:** The distal surface of the mandibular primary second molar is mesial to that of the maxillary primary second molar.

136. **The correct answer is A.** Both statements are true.

137. **The correct answer is E.** All of the above are causes of diastemas.

138. **The correct answer is A.** Answer A is a false statement because not all spaces always close. The greater the spacing, the less likely the diastema space will close on its own.

139. **The correct answer is D.** Answer D is a false statement because Essix is a passive appliance.

140. **The correct answer is B.** Answer B is a false statement because studies show that the majority of the "long-face" population has no nasal obstruction.

141. **The correct answer is C.** Answer C is a false statement because the maxilla and mandible are formed via intramembranous ossification.

Orthodontics

142. **The correct answer is B.** Both statements are false.

Growth of bone occurs only via appositional growth phenomenon where new layers are added to those previously formed. Cartilage grows via both appositional and intramembranous growth phenomena. In appositional growth, recruitment of fresh cells, chondroblasts, perichondral stem cells, and the addition of new matrix to the surface takes place. In interstitial growth, mitotic division of and deposition of more matrix around the existing chondrocytes already established in the cartilage occur. This does not occur in bone growth.

143. **The correct answer is B.** The first statement is false because if this were true, it would mean that there is an indication to treat everyone's occlusion to perfection to avoid possibility of developing facial muscle pain. The number of people with moderate degrees of malocclusion (50–75% of the population) is far more than the number of people with TMD (5–30% depending on which symptoms are examined). Therefore, it seems unlikely that occlusion alone is enough to cause hyperactivity of the oral musculature. Usually, a reaction to stress is involved. There are some people with very poor occlusion who have no muscle pain. Some types of malocclusion (especially posterior crossbite with a shift on closure) correlate positively with TMD, whereas others do not. So, for the majority of people, there is no association between malocclusion and TMD. On the other hand, if a patient does respond to stress by increased oral muscle activity, improper occlusal relationships may make the problem more severe and difficult to control. Therefore, malocclusion coupled with pain and spasm in the muscles of mastication may indicate a need for orthodontic treatment as an adjunct to other treatment for the muscle pain. But orthodontics as a primary treatment process is almost never indicated. If the problem is a pathologic process within the joint itself, improving the dental occlusion may or may not help the patient adapt to the necessarily altered joint function.

Myofascial pain develops when muscles are overly fatigued and tend to go into spasm. It is all but impossible to overwork the jaw muscles to this extent during normal eating and chewing. To produce myofascial pain, the patient must be clenching or grinding the teeth for many hours per day, presumably as a response to stress. Great variations are seen in the way different individuals respond to stress, both in the organ system that feels the strain (those who develop an ulcerated colon rarely have TMD) and in the amount of stress that can be tolerated before symptoms appear (tense individuals develop stress-related symptoms before their relaxed colleagues do). For this reason, it is impossible to say that occlusal discrepancies of any given degree will lead to TMD symptoms. It is possible to demonstrate that some types of occlusal discrepancies predispose patients who clench or grind their teeth to the development of TMD symptoms. It must be kept in mind that it takes two factors to produce myofascial pain: an occlusal discrepancy and a patient who clenches or grinds the teeth.

The second statement is false because in some difficult births, the use of forceps to the head to assist in delivery might damage either or both joints. At least in theory, heavy pressure in the area of the joints could cause internal hemorrhage, loss of tissue, and a subsequent underdevelopment of the mandible. At one time, this was a common explanation for mandibular deficiency. If the cartilage of the mandibular condyle were an important growth center, the risk from damage to a presumably critical area would seem much greater. In light of the current understanding that the condylar cartilage is not critical for proper growth of the mandible, it is not as easy to blame underdevelopment of the mandible on birth injuries. It is interesting to note that although the use of forceps in deliveries has decreased considerably over the last 50 years, the prevalence of class II malocclusion due to mandibular deficiency has not decreased.

144. **The correct answer is C.** Answer C is correct because jaw function is more than temporomandibular (TM) joint function, but evaluation of the TM joints is an important aspect of the diagnostic workup. As a general guideline, if the mandible moves normally, its function is

not severely impaired, and by the same token, restricted movement usually indicates a functional problem. For this reason, the most important indicator of joint function is the amount of maximum opening.

145. **The correct answer is D.** The first statement is false because it is possible that functional problems related to malocclusion would appear as TMD. Little or no data support the idea that orthodontic treatment is needed at any age to prevent the development of TMD.

The relationship, if any, between TMD and premolar extraction is difficult to assess because data from well-controlled studies are not available. There is simply no evidence to support the allegation that premolar extraction causes TMD.

In the late 1980s, it was claimed by some dentists that extraction of upper first premolars would later lead to TMD problems. The theory was that retracting the upper incisors would inevitably lead to incisor interferences, and this would cause TMD. The claim was never supported by any evidence, and research data have refuted it.

The second statement is true because the extent to which TMD symptoms in many adults disappear when comprehensive orthodontic treatment begins can be surprising. TMD symptoms disappear long before the occlusal relationships have been corrected. The explanation is that orthodontic treatment makes the teeth sore, grinding or clenching sensitive teeth as a means of handling stress does not produce the same subconscious gratification, the parafunctional activity stops, and symptoms vanish. The changing occlusal relationships also contribute to breaking up the habit patterns that contributed to the muscle fatigue and pain. At the end of orthodontic treatment, however, even if the occlusal relationships have been significantly improved, clenching and grinding tend to recur. Use of interocclusal splints may be helpful in these situations.

146. **The correct answer is D.** Answer D is correct because patients with TMD can be divided into two large groups: those with internal joint pathology, including displacement or destruction of the intraarticular disk, and those with symptoms primarily of muscle origin, caused by spasm and fatigue of the muscles that position the jaw and head. Because muscle spasm and joint pathology can coexist, the distinction in many patients is difficult. Nevertheless, the distinction is important when orthodontics will relieve TMD symptoms in a patient who has internal joint problems or other nonmuscular sources of pain. Those who have myofascial pain/dysfunction, on the other hand, may benefit from improved occlusal relationships. Almost all people develop some symptoms of degenerative joint disease as they grow older, and it is not surprising that the jaw joints are involved sometimes. Arthritic involvement of the TMJ is most likely to be the cause of TMD symptoms in patients who have arthritic changes in other joints of the body. A component of muscle spasm and muscle pain should be suspected in individuals whose only symptoms are in the TMJ, even if radiographs show moderate arthritic degeneration of the joint.

147. **The correct answer is B.** Answer B is correct because displacement of the disk can arise from a number of causes. One possibility is trauma to the joint, such that the ligaments that oppose the action of the lateral pterygoid muscle are stretched or torn. In this circumstance, muscle contraction moves the disk forward as the mandibular condyles translate forward on wide opening, but the ligaments do not restore the disk to its proper position when the jaw is closed. The result is a click upon opening and closing, as the disk pops into place over the condylar head as the patient opens, but is displaced anteriorly on closure. The click and the symptoms associated with it can be corrected if an occlusal splint is used to prevent the patient from closing beyond the point at which displacement occurs.

148. **The correct answer is D.** Answer D is a false statement because the main growth thrust of the condyle is upward and backward to fill in the resultant space to maintain contact with the base of the skull.

149. **The correct answer is D.** Answer D is correct because in both arches, the permanent incisor tooth buds lie lingual and apical to primary incisors.

150. **The correct answer is D.** Hereditary gingival fibromatosis is a generalized condition.

    Answers A, B, C, and E are incorrect because they are the localized causes of local delayed tooth eruption.

151. **The correct answer is E.** All of the above are true statements.

152. **The correct answer is A.** There is no significant sex distribution in primary supernumerary teeth. However, males are affected approximately twice as frequently as females in the permanent dentition.

153. **The correct answer is C.** Gardner syndrome, also known as *familial colorectal polyposis*, is an autosomal dominant disease characterized by gastrointestinal polyps, multiple osteomas, skin and soft tissue tumors, and dental abnormalities such as multiple supernumerary teeth.

154. **The correct answer is C.** Answer C is a false statement because the whole point of serial extraction is to extract the first premolar before the permanent canine erupts. The crowding is, therefore, corrected when the canine is guided to erupt into the premolar space.

155. **The correct answer is D.** The maxillary leeway space is smaller than mandibular leeway space; therefore, the mandibular permanent first molars shift mesially more than maxillary permanent first molars, which in turn helps with achievement of a class I occlusion.

CHAPTER 5

Pediatric Dentistry

1. A 20-month-old female presents with her mother to your office for her first check-up. Her mother is concerned because her daughter only has a few erupted teeth. Upon examining the patient, which teeth should you expect to find?

    A. Primary centrals and laterals only
    B. Primary centrals, laterals, canines
    C. Primary centrals, laterals, first molars, second molars
    D. Primary centrals, laterals, first molars
    E. Primary centrals, laterals, first molars, canines

2. A 5-year-old girl lives in an area with 0.4 ppm F in the city drinking water. How much supplemental fluoride should you prescribe for the patient to consume the optimal amount of fluoride?

    A. 0
    B. 0.25 mg
    C. 0.33 mg
    D. 0.5 mg
    E. 1.0 mg

3. A child presents to your office after a fall from a tree, during which his primary maxillary central incisor was avulsed. The mother has brought the tooth in a cup of milk and says the fall occurred 2 hours ago. What is the best treatment for this patient?

    A. Replant the tooth, stabilize the tooth for 1 to 2 weeks at which time a pulpotomy should be performed
    B. Replant the tooth, stabilize for 1 to 2 weeks, and then perform a pulpectomy
    C. Replant tooth, stabilize for 1 to 2 weeks, and begin apexification if pulp necrosis is evident
    D. Take a radiograph, irrigate socket, do not re-plant tooth

4. A 6-year-old child presents with a Class I fracture to a tooth with an immature apex. What is the treatment of choice for this patient?

    A. Restore tooth
    B. Place calcium hydroxide to exposed dentin, restore tooth
    C. Perform pulpotomy, then temporarily restore

    D. Perform pulpectomy, place stainless steel crown
    E. Extract tooth, place space maintainer

5. A disease process is characterized by painful, bleeding gingival tissue, punched out erosions covered by gray pseudomembrane, blunting of interproximal papillae, and a fetid odor. Treatment usually comprises debridement, mouth rinses, and antibiotics. This description is associated with which of the following conditions that may exist in teenagers?

    A. Aggressive periodontitis
    B. Acute necrotizing ulcerative gingivitis
    C. Primary herpetic gingivostomatitis
    D. Severe gingivitis
    E. Early childhood caries

6. How much fluoride, in ppm, is contained in commonly used toothpastes?

    A. 1,000 ppm
    B. 5,000 ppm
    C. 9,000 ppm
    D. 12,300 ppm

7. Fordyce granules are:

    A. Epithelial inclusion cysts
    B. Found on the buccal and lingual aspects of the alveolus
    C. Ectopic sebaceous glands
    D. Remnants of the dental lamina

8. As compared with permanent teeth, primary teeth have:

    A. Pulp horns further away from the tooth surface
    B. Smaller pulp relative to crown size
    C. Thicker and shorter roots
    D. Increased number of accessory canals in pulpal floor

9. The calcification of maxillary and mandibular permanent first molars occurs at what age?

    A. 3 to 4 months
    B. Birth

C. 10 to 12 months

D. 1.5 to 2 years

10. The definition of primate space is:

A. The space mesial to the mandibular primary canines and distal to the maxillary primary canines

B. The space distal to the mandibular primary canines and distal to the maxillary primary canines

C. The space mesial to the maxillary primary canines and distal to the mandibular primary canines

D. The space mesial to the maxillary primary canines only

11. What amount of fluoride should be prescribed to a 4-year old child who lives in a community with 0.4 ppm fluoridated water?

A. 0

B. 0.25

C. .5

D. 1.0

E. 0.85

12. A tooth has a periapical radiolucency with normal periodontal probing depths except at the mesiobuccal (MB) line angle it probes to the apex. The tooth tests nonvital. What is the most likely classification of the lesion?

A. Periodontal

B. Endodontic

C. Primarily periodontal with secondary endodontic involvement

D. Primarily endodontic with secondary periodontal involvement

E. True combined lesion

13. Which of the following is a contraindication to the use of an electric pulp tester?

A. A pediatric patient

B. A patient with a recent MI

C. A patient with a cardiac pacemaker

D. A patient with recent trauma

E. A patient with a large metal restoration

14. Which of the following factors is the least likely to cause an instrument separating inside a root canal?

A. Overuse of the instrument

B. Excessive force

C. Filing a dry canal

D. Manufacturing defects

E. Using larger files before smaller ones fit loosely

15. Which of the following is true of apexogenesis?

A. It is nonvital pulp therapy

B. Its objective is to artificially close the root apex

C. It is indicated for a tooth with damaged radicular pulp

D. It is indicated for an immature avulsed tooth

E. Endodontic therapy can be performed more effectively following apexogenesis

16. Fluoride varnish (5% sodium fluoride in a resin vehicle) is the preferred choice of pediatric dentistry for in-office fluoride delivery for which of the following reasons?

A. Ease of delivery

B. Measured maximum dose/exposure to fluoride ion

C. Stays on enamel surfaces longer than any other fluoride product/longer contact time

D. Can be used more frequently for high-risk patients

E. All of the above

17. Which of the following antimicrobial therapies can be utilized for high-caries-exposed patients?

A. Xylitol gums, lozenges, mints, rinses, sprays

B. ART restorative techniques

C. Stannous fluoride

D. Fluoride varnish therapy at high-frequency intervals

E. All of the above

18. According to the American Academy of Pediatric Dentistry Guidelines, the following restorative materials for a high-caries experience patient are recommended:

A. Composite resin

B. Glass ionomer or resin modified GI

C. Stainless steel crown

D. B and C only

E. All of the above

19. Which of the following combinations is correct regarding local anesthesia and pediatric dentistry?

    A. Short-acting local anesthetics, that is, ones without epinephrine should be avoided
    B. Articaine can be used to locally infiltrate the mandibular primary posterior teeth
    C. Increasing the epinephrine dose above 1:100,000 should be avoided
    D. A and C only
    E. All of the above

20. Avulsed teeth, pimary-permanent should be treated as follows:

    A. Primary: reimplanted/Permanent: reimplanted
    B. Primary: reimplanted and splinted/Permanent: reimplanted and splinted
    C. Primary: no reimplantation/Permanent: reimplanted and splinted rigidly
    D. Primary: no reimplantation/Permanent: reimplanted and splinted flexibly for 14 days maximum
    E. Primary: no reimplantation/Permanent: reimplanted and splinted flexibly

21. A mother brings her son to your office for his 1-year-old dental appointment. You notice that there is a problem with the shape of his teeth. The problem probably occurred in what stage of development?

    A. Initiation
    B. Proliferation
    C. Differentiation
    D. Apposition
    E. Calcification

22. You are counting the teeth of a 5-year old, and there are 20 crowns, but when you look at the radiograph, there are only 19 roots. This is most likely:

    A. Fusion
    B. Concrescence
    C. Gemination
    D. Attrition
    E. There is no problem

23. A child comes to your office and has a bilateral cleft lip. This is classified as what class?

    A. Class I
    B. Class II
    C. Class III
    D. Class IV
    E. There is no classification for bilateral cleft lip

24. A child was brought to your office after tooth #E fell out when he tripped and fell playing outside. Mom says the tooth has been out for only 15 minutes and she put it in milk right away and came to your office. The tooth looks viable and clean. You should:

    A. Reimplant the tooth immediately since it has been less than 1/2 hour
    B. Clean the tooth with normal saline then reimplant the tooth since it has been less than 1/2 hour
    C. Reimplant the tooth and splint it. Have the child follow-up in 2 weeks
    D. Reimplant the tooth, perform a pulpotomy, splint, and follow-up in 1 week
    E. Do not reimplant tooth

25. A 5-year old who lives in a nonfluoridated area should receive how much fluoride supplementation?

    A. This child does not need fluoride supplementation
    B. 0.25 mg
    C. 0.5 mg
    D. 1.0 mg

26. At what age can one expect eruption of a maxillary permanent canine in an individual with an ideal eruption sequence?

    A. 7 to 8 years
    B. 8 to 9 years
    C. 9 to 10 years
    D. 10 to 11 years
    E. 11 to 12 years

27. When recommending a storage medium for avulsed teeth, order the following from most favorable to least favorable.

    A. Cold milk, Hank's balanced salt solution, saliva, water
    B. Hank's balanced salt solution, cold milk, saliva, water

C. Hank's balanced salt solution, cold milk, water, saliva

D. Cold milk, Hank's balanced salt solution, water, saliva

E. Saliva, Hank's balanced salt solution, cold milk, water

28. The amount of articaine in a 1.7-mL cartridge of articaine HCL 4% with epinephrine 1:100,000 is:

A. 34 mg
B. 36 mg
C. 54 mg
D. 68 mg
E. 72 mg

29. Basic pediatric behavior management techniques include all of the following *except*:

A. Voice control
B. Tell-show-do
C. Hand over mouth exercise (HOME)
D. Positive reinforcement
E. Distraction

30. Which of the following is not a factor in a caries-risk assessment tool?

A. Previous caries experience
B. Socioeconomic status of caregiver
C. Exposure to fluoride
D. Eruption sequence
E. Level of mutans streptococci

1. **The correct answer is E.** By 19 months, a child should have mandibular and maxillary central and lateral incisors, all first molars, and all canines. According to answer choice A, primary central and laterals should be found by 7 months of age. Answer B is incorrect also in terms of sequence—if the canines were present, the first molars should also be present. By the time the second molars erupt, the canines should already be present in the mouth. Primary centrals, laterals, and first molars should erupt by 15 months of age.

2. **The correct answer is B.** In a population with 0.3- to 0.6-ppm fluoride in the drinking water, a 0.25-mg supplement is the recommended amount. According to answer choice A, no fluoride supplements are recommended from birth to 6 months, in populations where 0.6 ppm or more is present, or for a patient aged 6 months to 3 years in a 0.3- to 0.6-ppm fluoridated area. 0.33 mg is not included as a recommended amount of fluoride supplementation. 0.5 mg is the recommended dose for a child aged 3 to 6 years in an area of less than 0.3-ppm fluoridation, and for 6- to 16-years old in a 0.3- to 0.6-ppm area. 1.0 mg is recommended for a child aged 6 to 16 years in a population with less than 0.3-ppm water fluoridation.

3. **The correct answer is D.** A primary tooth has a poor prognosis if replantation is attempted; therefore, primary teeth are very rarely replanted. A radiograph should be taken to visualize if any fragments of the tooth remain. If the tooth was a permanent tooth, the tooth may be replanted, splinted, and then root canal therapy (RCT) performed after 7 to 10 days. If the apices of the tooth are open, the tooth should be monitored and apexification procedures should begin if there is evidence of an infected pulp. As explained before, if the tooth was permanent with closed apices, the steps indicated in answer choice B should be followed. This answer choice is the best treatment if a permanent tooth was avulsed that had open apices and evidence of an infected pulp.

4. **The correct answer is A.** Class I fracture involves only the enamel of the tooth. Smoothing out the rough edges of the enamel and restoring with a permanent restoration is the only treatment necessary for this tooth. In Class II fracture, this may be covered with calcium hydroxide or glass ionomer and restored as there will be much more substantial dentin exposure. No pulpotomy is necessary since there was no pulp exposure (as in a Class III fracture) and the pulp is still vital. As in answer choice C, the pulp is still healthy, so a pulpectomy is not necessary. An stainless steel crown (SSC) is also not necessary if only a minimal amount of enamel has been lost. In Class IV fracture, a pulpectomy and an SSC are both necessary as the entire crown has been lost. There is no indication for extraction of a tooth that has a healthy pulp, no fracture present, and may be restored with a permanent restorative material.

5. **The correct answer is B.** Acute necrotizing ulcerative gingivitis may occur in both adults and teenagers and is also known as Vincent's infection, Vincent's angina, or trench mouth. This is a painful condition that reacts well to debridement, hydrogen peroxide rinses, and antibiotics and is caused by fusiform, spirochetes, and *Prevotella intermedia*. Aggressive periodontitis may be localized or general and is associated with *Actinobacillus actinomycetemcomitans*. It is marked by rapid loss of attachment and bone (in the localized form, on the first permanent molars and permanent incisors) and increased plaque and calculus. Treatment usually includes surgery and antibiotics for the permanent dentition. Primary herpetic gingivostomatitis is caused by the Herpes simplex virus, and the primary form usually involves children under the age of 3. The primary form is usually subclinical. Gingivitis in children is very common and may be treated with oral hygiene instruction and more parental supervision. There is no loss of attachment associated with gingivitis, though there may be bleeding on probing. Early childhood caries is rampant decay that is usually associated with letting a child sleep with

a bottle filled with sugary liquids and/or milk. The teeth most usually affected are the maxillary incisors. Parents should be educated as to encouraging their children to drink from a cup before their first birthday and to not allow them to constantly be drinking from a bottle or to sleep with a bottle.

6. **The correct answer is A.** Answer B is incorrect; 5,000 ppm is the amount contained in 1.1% NaF foam that is delivered in a tray. Answer C is incorrect; 9,000 ppm is the amount contained in 2% NaF that is delivered in gel form. Answer D is incorrect; 12,300 ppm is the amount contained in 1.23% APF that is delivered in gel or foam form.

7. **The correct answer is C.** Answer A is the definition of Epstein's Pearls. Answer B is descriptive of Bohn's Nodules. Answer D is descriptive of a dental lamina cyst.

8. **The correct answer is D.** Answer A is incorrect. The pulp horns of primary teeth are closer to the outer surface of the tooth than those in permanent teeth. Answer B is incorrect. Primary teeth have larger pulp to crown ratios than permanent teeth. Answer C is incorrect. Primary molars have longer and thinner roots than those of permanent molars.

9. **The correct answer is B.** Answer A is the calcification time of maxillary and mandibular canines. Answer C is the calcification time of maxillary and mandibular lateral incisors. Answer D is the calcification time of maxillary and mandibular first premolars.

10. **The correct answer is C.** Answer A is incorrect. The space mesial to the mandibular canine is not included in the primate space. Answer B is incorrect. The space distal to the maxillary canine is not included in the primate space. Answer D is incorrect. The space distal to the mandibular canine is also included in the definition of primate space.

11. **The correct answer is B.** When fluoride in water is below 0.3 ppm, for age 0 to 6 months, no supplement is needed; for 6 months to 3 years, 0.25 mg/day of fluoride supplement; for 3 to 6 years, 0.5 mg/day of fluoride supplement; and for 6 to 16 years, 1.0 mg/day of fluoride supplement is recommended. When fluoride is between 0.3 and 0.6 ppm, for age 0 to 6 months, no supplement is needed; for age 6 months to 3 years, no supplement is needed; for age 3 to 6 years, 0.25 mg/day of fluoride supplement is needed; and for age 6 to 16 years, 0.5 mg/day of fluoride is needed. When fluoride is above 0.6 ppm, no supplements are needed for all ages.

12. **The correct answer is D.** The inflammatory process of an endodontic lesion may create a sinus tract along the periodontal ligament (PDL) space, which clinically appears as a narrow, deep pocket. Therefore, choice D is correct. Choice A is wrong because periodontal lesions usually have broad-based pocket formation, not narrow, and usually have a history of periodontal disease and are vital. Choice B is wrong because there is a probing depth to the apex; therefore, there must be some type of periodontal involvement. Choice C is wrong because there is no broad-based pocketing and no history of extensive periodontal disease. Choice E is wrong because true combined lesions are very rare and would have signs of periodontal involvement, that is, wide-based pocketing.

13. **The correct answer is C.** An electric pulp tester may interfere with some cardiac pacemakers and is therefore contraindicated in a patient with a pacemaker. Answer choice A is wrong because electric pulp testing is not a reliable test in pediatric patients but is not contraindicated. Answer choice B is wrong because there is no contraindication to the use of an electric pulp tester in a patient with a recent MI, although endodontic therapy is contraindicated. Answer choice D is wrong because recent trauma may cause a false negative response to electric pulp testing but is not a contraindication. Choice E is wrong because a metal restoration may give a false positive response to electric pulp testing but is not contraindicated.

14. **The correct answer is D.** Although manufacturing defects can cause instruments to separate in a canal, they are very rare and much less likely to cause separation than the other answer choices.

15. **The correct answer is E.** One of the objectives of apexogenesis is to allow for safer and more effective endodontic therapy. Choice A is wrong because apexogenesis is vital pulp therapy. Choice B is wrong because apexogenesis encourages natural root lengthening, root wall thickening, and apical closure. Choice C is wrong because apexogenesis is indicated in teeth with damaged coronal pulp but healthy radicular pulp. Choice D is wrong because apexogenesis is indicated for an immature tooth but contraindicated for an avulsed tooth.

16. **The correct answer is E.** All of the above is the correct answer as fluoride varnish is quickly becoming the choice of pediatric dentists because it is a premeasured dose, so overdose is impossible; the fluoride is delivered via a resin carrier so ingestion is greatly reduced and adhesion is greatly increased; because of these benefits, it is perfect for high-caries risk patients and should be used safely on more frequent intervals to reduce enamel damage, enhance enamel remineralization, and decrease pathogenic bacteria.

17. **The correct answer is E.** All of the above is the correct answer because xylitol has been extensively shown to affect pathogenic bacteria cell walls, thus reducing pathogenic bacteria viability; ART techniques can be used as a therapy to enhance enamel/dentin before final restorations; stannous fluoride also inhibits proper cell wall biology of pathogenic bacteria; and fluoride varnish also can enhance enamel and cause pathogenic bacteria reductions.

18. **The correct answer is D.** The AAPD guidelines suggest avoiding resin-based composite material in high-caries patients. Resin composite has significant shrinkage and is not suited to pediatric restorations in high-risk patients. Glass ionomer and resin-based GI has fluoride release and bonds chemically to enamel and dentin without significant shrinkage. Stainless steel crowns provide 360-degree coverage from microbial contamination when properly fit and cemented using glass ionomer cement. Stainless steel crowns are the gold standard for any high-risk pediatric patient with multiple cavitated surfaces.

19. **The correct answer is E.** Pediatric anesthesia is important to master. Understanding that dosage and toxicity are different in children as compared with adults is paramount. Dosage and toxicity are directly related to epinephrine (EPI) concentration as increasing EPI decreases the speed of systemic uptake. To avoid local anesthesia (LA) toxicity in children, a concentration of 1:100,000 EPI should not be exceeded. Avoid using 1:50,000 concentrations. Another potentially fatal mistake is to use LA without any EPI. This can cause too rapid systemic uptake of LA. Children have increased heart rates inherently; thus, faster systemic uptake of drugs and LA without EPI will be released too fast into the systemic circulation. Articaine has been shown in the literature and extensive European and Canadian use to provide pulpal anesthesia following mandibular infiltrations in the posterior, including second primary molars. Articaine can potentially eliminate the dreaded "Missed" block.

20. **The correct answer is D.** Avulsed primary teeth should not be reimplanted as it can result in damaging the permanent tooth bud or follicle. Permanent teeth need to be reimplanted as soon as possible with best results if reimplanted within 30 minutes. Flexible splinting is preferred for 14 days or less; rigid splinting seems to not mimic the flexibility of the PDL and inhibits proper healing.

21. **The correct answer is B.** Proliferation (cap stage) is the formation of shape of tooth and enamel organ. Bud stage is the interaction of oral epithelium and dental lamina. Bell stage is the differentiation into specific tooth and tissue types, histodifferentiation. Apposition cells begin depositing their corresponding tissues. Primary teeth begin calcification during second trimester.

22. **The correct answer is C.** Gemination is when two crowns are on a single root; therefore, the root count would be one less than the crown count. Fusion appears as a large crown; usually, there are two roots, so the root count would be normal and crown count would be one less. This is a form of fusion; the cementum is in contact. Attrition is physiologic wear of the incisal and

occlusal surfaces. There is a problem with the count.

23. **The correct answer is D.** Class I—unilateral notching of the vermilion not extending to lip. Class II—same as Class I but extending to lip but not to floor of the nose. Class III—Class II and extending to floor of the nose. Class IV—any bilateral cleft of the lip.

24. **The correct answer is E.** Never reimplant primary teeth—risk of ankylosis and affecting permanent tooth eruption. A to D—these are wrong choices because you never want to reimplant primary teeth no matter how soon or clean the tooth is. For a permanent tooth that has avulsed, you want to reimplant as soon as possible and splint for 1 to 2 weeks.

25. **The correct answer is C.** When fluoride in water is below 0.3 ppm, for age 0 to 6 months, no supplement is needed; for 6 months to 3 years, 0.25 mg/day of fluoride supplement; for 3 to 6 years, 0.5 mg/day of fluoride supplement; and for 6 to 16 years, 1.0 mg/day of fluoride supplement is recommended. When fluoride is between 0.3 and 0.6 ppm, for age 0 to 6 months, no supplement is needed; for age 6 months to 3 years, no supplement is needed; for age 3 to 6 years, 0.25 mg/day of fluoride supplement is needed; and for age 6 to 16 years, 0.5 mg/day of fluoride is needed. When fluoride is above 0.6 ppm, no supplements are needed for all ages.

26. **The correct answer is E.** Eleven to 12 years is the age when one can expect the eruption of a maxillary permanent canine in an individual with an ideal eruption sequence. The most favorable eruption sequence in the permanent dentition is: Maxilla: 61245378 Mandible: 61234578. Note the difference in the eruption sequence with regards to the permanent canines (3s).

27. **The correct answer is B.** Hank's balanced salt solution, cold milk, saliva, water. Extra-oral dry time and root development are major determinants of reimplantation prognosis. Preservation of PDL fibers is key to success. The best medium is one that does not destroy tissue. Water is hypotonic and causes cell lysis.

28. **The correct answer is D.** Sixty-eight milligram. 4% = 4,000 mg/100 mL = 40 mg/1 mL. 68 mg = 1.7 mL.

29. **The correct answer is C.** Hand over mouth exercise. According the AAPD Reference Manual, voice control, tell-show-do, positive reinforcement, and distraction are all acceptable basic behavior management techniques. Hand over mouth, while previously utilized with success, is no longer mentioned in the AAPD Clinical Guidelines. This technique has fallen out of favor because of lack of parental acceptance.

30. **The correct answer is D.** Eruption sequence. All of the other answers have been shown to have a direct impact on caries risk.

CHAPTER 6

Endodontics

1. A patient received a large MOD composite restoration 1 week ago. She is now experiencing intense, spontaneous pain, with exacerbation of symptoms occurring when she applies heat or cold or when she eats sweets. The pulpal diagnosis is:

   A. Pulp necrosis
   B. Acute periapical periodontitis
   C. Reversible pulpitis
   D. Traumatic occlusion
   E. Irreversible pulpitis

2. A 12-year-old boy has arrived in your office after a fall that fractured tooth #9 up to the gingival margin on the mesial aspect with a pulp exposure. What is the appropriate treatment?

   A. Extraction
   B. Pulpotomy
   C. Direct pulp cap
   D. Root canal therapy
   E. Apexogenesis

3. Root canal therapy was completed on a nonvital tooth that suffered trauma 5 years prior. At the time of obturation, the tooth exhibited a periapical radiolucency on radiographic examination. Radiographically, healing should be visualized in:

   A. 1 week
   B. 6 weeks
   C. 1 month
   D. 6 months
   E. 1 year

4. A patient presents with a chief complaint of pain in the upper right quadrant. Cold test produces a response lingering for 1 minute on tooth #4. In addition, tooth #4 is sensitive to percussion with the blunt end of an instrument. What is the pulpal and periapical diagnosis?

   A. Irreversible pulpitis, normal periapex
   B. Irreversible pulpitis, acute apical periodontitis
   C. Reversible pulpitis, acute apical periodontitis

   D. Necrotic pulp, chronic apical periodontitis
   E. Necrotic pulp, acute apical periodontitis

5. You have been treating a patient in your practice for 20 years. As your patient has aged, numerous changes have occurred in his pulp tissues. All of the following can be associated with age-related changes to the dental pulp *except*:

   A. Decreased cellular elements
   B. Pulp stone formation
   C. Radiographic obliteration of the pulp space
   D. Increased response to electric pulp testing
   E. Decreased vascularity

6. A patient presents to your office with a chief complaint of dull, diffuse pain in the lower right quadrant. The nerve fibers responsible for this sensation are:

   A. Myelinated A fibers
   B. Unmyelinated A fibers
   C. Myelinated C fibers
   D. Unmyelinated C fibers
   E. Subodontoblastic plexus of Raschkow

7. On physical and radiographic examination, your patient presents with DO decay and a gingival swelling at tooth #28. The conical defect on the tooth probes more than 12 mm on the buccal aspect and does not respond to electrical pulp testing. There is no mobility, and this condition is localized to the affected tooth. The periapical radiograph shows destruction of the periodontium from the level of the gingival sulcus to the apex of the tooth. Proper treatment of this condition includes:

   A. Endodontic treatment only
   B. Endodontic treatment followed by periodontal treatment
   C. Periodontal treatment only
   D. Periodontal treatment followed by endodontic treatment
   E. Extraction

8. Your patient presents with diffuse pain in her upper right quadrant. She is unable to determine the offending tooth. She states that the pain is

exacerbated when she drinks cold liquids but not with mastication. Tooth #4 has an existing MOD amalgam restoration, as does tooth #5. All other teeth in the quadrant are free of restorations and caries. What is the appropriate first-line diagnostic pulp test?

A. Electric pulp test
B. Heat test
C. Cold test
D. Test cavity
E. Percussion test

9. All of the following factors may affect endodontic anesthesia *except*

A. Fatigue
B. Anxiety
C. Tissue inflammation
D. Tooth type
E. Previous unsuccessful anesthesia

10. You have placed files in all three canals located in tooth #19 during a root canal procedure to obtain measurement. Upon taking the first radiograph, the two files in the distal canal are superimposed. For your second radiograph, you move the cone to the mesial. The resulting image shows both files in the distal canal. The file that has moved to the mesial is positioned:

A. Mesially
B. Distally
C. Buccally
D. Lingually
E. Cannot be determined

11. You are instrumenting a canal with a size 30, 25 mm k-type file. What does each of the sizes denote, respectively?

A. The length of the file and the diameter of the tip of the file
B. The diameter of the tip of the file and the length of the file
C. The taper of the file and the length of the file
D. The diameter of the tip of the file and the taper of the file
E. The length of the file and the taper of the file

12. An Asian patient presents to your office with pain bilaterally in her lower second premolars. Both teeth are sensitive to percussion and show periapical radiolucencies on radiographic examination. The teeth do not respond to either cold or electric pulp tests. There is an irregular bulge on the occlusal surfaces of each tooth. The most likely diagnosis is:

A. Irreversible pulpitis
B. Dens invaginatus
C. Dens evaginatus
D. Pulp stones
E. Internal resorption

13. When instrumenting and subsequently obturating a root canal, the length should be determined by the:

A. Anatomic apex
B. Apical foramen
C. Apical constriction

14. The endodontic access form is triangular in shape for which of the following teeth?

A. Maxillary central incisor, mandibular central incisor, and maxillary lateral incisor
B. Mandibular central incisor, maxillary first molar, and maxillary first premolar
C. Maxillary canine, maxillary first premolar, and maxillary lateral incisor
D. Maxillary second molar, mandibular first molar, and maxillary lateral incisor
E. Maxillary central incisor, maxillary first molar, and maxillary second molar

15. Root canal therapy is completed on a mandibular first molar and closed temporarily with a cotton pellet and a temporary sealing material, with plans for a definitive restoration to be placed as soon as possible. What is the most important factor in ensuring the success of the procedure?

A. Type of definitive restoration
B. Marginal integrity of definitive restoration
C. Type of temporary sealing material
D. Placement of a post
E. Type of sealer used during obturation

Endodontics

16. A patient presents to your office for an emergency visit with a chief complaint of constant, severe throbbing pain in the upper right quadrant for 2 days that has kept him awake at night and is not relieved by over-the-counter pain medications. He is unable to discriminate which tooth is causing the pain and is visiting your office for the first time on the basis of the referral of another one of your patients. What is the correct sequence for your initial diagnosis?

 1. Extraoral examination
 2. Elicit details about the history of the chief complaint
 3. Pulp vitality testing
 4. Obtain a full medical and dental history
 5. Radiographic interpretation

 A. 1, 2, 3, 4, 5
 B. 5, 1, 2, 3, 4
 C. 4, 1, 2, 5, 3
 D. 4, 2, 1, 3, 5
 E. 1, 4, 2, 5, 3

17. You have initiated root canal therapy on a patient when he suddenly experiences sudden pain during working length determination, begins to hemorrhage, and detects a burning sensation when you attempt to irrigate with sodium hypochlorite. What is the most likely cause of these symptoms?

 A. Inadequate straight line access
 B. Root canal contamination
 C. Root perforation
 D. Incomplete canal debridement
 E. Ledging

18. During instrumentation of tooth #19, you realize that you are unable to negotiate your file to the complete working length. The procedural error that has occurred is most likely:

 A. Ledging
 B. Instrument separation
 C. Vertical root fracture
 D. Inadequate straight line access
 E. Furcation perforation

19. During instrumentation of the mesial root of tooth #30, your file separates and remains stuck in the canal. In an attempt to remedy this procedural error, you attempt to bypass and remove the instrument. If you are unable to remove the instrument, what should your next step be?

 A. Extract the tooth
 B. Perform a root amputation
 C. Perform a bicuspidation of the tooth
 D. Prepare and obturate up to the separated instrument
 E. Obturate the distal canals only

20. One of the most serious procedural errors that can occur during root canal therapy is instrument aspiration. What is the most important precaution an operator can take to prevent instrument aspiration?

 A. Proper rubber dam isolation
 B. Only use rotary files
 C. Use adequate lubrication during instrumentation
 D. Recapitulate between each file
 E. Irrigate often with sodium hypochlorite

21. A patient presents to your office for initial examination. A root canal procedure had been completed on tooth #3 a year prior. Upon clinical examination, you observe a narrow periodontal pocket measuring the full length of your probe in the area of the mesial root. Upon radiographic examination, you detect a J-shaped radiolucency surrounding the mesial root. Your initial diagnosis is:

 A. Incomplete debridement of the mesial root
 B. Ledging of the mesial root
 C. Underobturation of the mesial root
 D. Periodontal abscess
 E. Vertical fracture of the mesial root

22. You completed a root canal procedure on tooth #9 approximately 6 months ago. Your patient is still reporting persistent symptoms of acute apical pathosis including sensitivity on mastication and a dull ache, and the periradicular radiolucency that was visible on your obturation radiograph has not appeared to decrease in size. The most likely reason for the persistence of these symptoms is:

 A. Phantom tooth pain
 B. Root canal failure

C. Trigeminal neuralgia
D. Traumatic occlusion
E. Myofascial pain

23. After completion of root canal therapy, you recall your patient to evaluate the treatment outcome. What are the criteria for successful root canal therapy?

1. Absence of pain
2. Absence of swelling
3. Sinus tract healing
4. No residual probing defects
5. Resolution or healing of periapical lesions

A. 1, 3, 5
B. 1, 2, 4, 5
C. 2, 3, 4
D. 1, 2, 3, 4, 5
E. 1, 2, 3, 4

24. Retrograde (apical resection surgery) treatment is considered over orthograde treatment (root canal retreatment) for patients by their dentist after their root canal therapy is considered to have failed. When should retrograde treatment be performed over orthograde treatment?

A. When an expensive, yet coronally sealed restoration would have to be refabricated to accommodate orthograde treatment
B. When a patient is anxious about traditional retreatment procedures
C. If the goal of treatment is to eliminate microorganisms from the root canal system
D. When the root canal filling materials are easy to remove
E. If the treating dentist prefers surgical intervention

25. An 8-year-old patient presents to your office for an emergency visit with a traumatic exposure of tooth #9. The treatment of choice for this patient is:

A. Root-end closure procedure/apexification
B. Traditional root canal therapy
C. Vital pulp therapy/apexogenesis
D. Partial pulpectomy
E. Temporization and reevaluation in 1 week

26. A 4-year-old child has fallen and hit his central incisor. Over time, the tooth has become increasingly more discolored and does not resolve. The most likely cause of the discoloration is:

A. Endemic fluorosis
B. Systemic drugs
C. Enamel hypocalcification
D. Intrapulpal hemorrhage
E. Amelogenesis imperfecta

27. Following obturation, sealer was left in the coronal pulp chamber of tooth #9, and the conservative access was filled with a composite restoration. This could most likely result in:

A. Root canal failure
B. Discoloration of the tooth
C. Vertical root fracture
D. Inadequate coronal seal
E. Bacterial leakage

28. A patient presents to your office with a discolored tooth #24 that was treated with root canal 4 years before. The material of choice for an internal bleaching procedure is:

A. Hydrogen peroxide
B. Carbamide peroxide
C. Sodium perporate

29. Incision for drainage will release exudates from a soft tissue swelling, reducing irritants and pain from pressure buildup. What are the ideal conditions under which to perform an incision for drainage?

A. A tooth with reversible pulpitis and pain on mastication
B. A necrotic tooth with an indurated swelling at the apex
C. A necrotic tooth with a fluctuant swelling at the apex
D. A tooth with irreversible pulpitis and pain on percussion
E. A necrotic tooth with spontaneous pain but no swelling

30. A patient presents to your office for an initial maintenance visit and you prescribe a full series of radiographs. During interpretation, you note as an incidental finding a periapical radiolucency on the mesial root of tooth #19. The tooth is restored with an intact amalgam MO restoration with intact margins and no signs of leakage or recurrent caries. The tooth is asymptomatic and responds normally to all vitality testing. Your patient has indicated a history of cancer in his medical history. The proper course of action in this case is:

    A. Pulpotomy
    B. Biopsy the lesion
    C. Root canal therapy
    D. Extraction

31. When making a diagnosis, the primary goal of your diagnostic tests is to reproduce the chief complaint. You test the suspected tooth for percussion sensitivity and palpation sensitivity. Your positive percussion findings can be interpreted as follows:

    A. The tooth is nonvital and should be treated with root canal therapy.
    B. There is inflammation in the PDL.
    C. There is inflammation in the PDL and the surrounding periodontium.
    D. There is a root fracture present.
    E. The tooth is necrotic.

32. When making a diagnosis as to the vitality of a tooth, you employ the electric pulp tester. You obtain a measurement that suggests the tooth is necrotic. With this information alone, you can determine that:

    A. The tooth is necrotic.
    B. Further testing is necessary to make a definitive diagnosis.
    C. The tooth needs root canal therapy.
    D. The tooth has an inflamed PDL.
    E. The tooth has calcified canals.

33. A patient presents to your office with pain in tooth #12. You perform a cold test with Endo Ice to determine vitality. If the tooth has irreversible pulpitis, the cold test will result in:

    A. No response to the cold test

B. Severe pain that disappears 1 to 2 seconds after removing the cold
C. Mild to moderate pain that disappears 1 to 2 seconds after removing the cold
D. Moderate to severe pain that lingers after removing the cold

34. You are doing a deep occlusal preparation on tooth #30. The tooth was asymptomatic prior to treatment. All caries have been removed, but you notice a pinpoint mechanical pulpal exposure. Hemorrhage is easily stopped. The treatment of choice is:

    A. Pulpotomy
    B. Indirect pulp cap
    C. Root canal therapy
    D. Direct pulp cap
    E. Amalgam restoration

35. The outline form of the access cavity of which of the following teeth is trapezoid in shape?

    A. Maxillary first molar and mandibular first molar
    B. Mandibular first molar and maxillary second molar
    C. Maxillary first molar and maxillary second premolar
    D. Mandibular second premolar and maxillary second molar
    E. Mandibular first molar and mandibular second molar

36. A patient presents to your office with a fractured tooth #9. The fracture involves enamel, dentin, and pulp. This fracture can be classified as:

    A. Root fracture
    B. Crown–root fracture
    C. Complicated crown fracture
    D. Uncomplicated crown fracture

37. You are halfway through the root canal treatment on tooth #30. To prevent bacterial growth in the canal between appointments, you decide to use an intracanal medication. The interappointment medicament of choice is:

    A. Sodium hypochlorite
    B. Ethylenediaminetetraacetate
    C. Chlorhexidine

D. Calcium hydroxide

E. Gutta-percha

38. A 9-year-old patient has avulsed tooth #8 in a playground accident. His mother has recovered the tooth and has called to ask how it should be stored while she gets her son to your office. The best way to store an avulsed tooth for the best prognosis is:

A. Dry

B. Tap water

C. Saline

D. Saliva

E. Milk

39. A 20-year-old male patient presents to your office with tooth #9 in his hand. It had been avulsed the day before during a camping trip and was stored dry in a plastic bag. Your treatment plan should be:

A. Perform root canal therapy and replant the tooth

B. Give your patient all of his options to replace the tooth

C. Clean the tooth and socket and replant the tooth

D. Clean the tooth and socket, replant the tooth, and splint it for a week

40. A primary tooth has an exposed vital pulp. The tooth has less than two-third of its root remaining and caries perforating the furcation. There is a succedaneous tooth forming normally apical to the tooth. The treatment of choice for this tooth is:

A. Indirect pulp cap

B. Pulp cap

C. Pulpotomy

D. Extraction

E. Root canal therapy

41. The most effective method of diagnosing the origin of fistula is:

A. Visually locating the closest tooth to the fistula

B. Percussing all of the teeth in the area of the fistula

C. Tracing the fistula with a gutta percha point in conjunction with the radiograph

D. Periodontal probing of all teeth in the area

E. Take radiograph from two different angles

42. A 35-year-old woman was in a horse back riding accident less than 1 hour ago. On clinical examination, the tooth is painful to palpation and has slight mobility. The tooth is fractured in the occlusal third and there appears to be no exposure. A periapical radiograph reveals fracture above the pulpal space and no periapical radiolucency. The treatment of choice for the asymptomatic maxillary central incisor is:

A. Root canal treatment in the occlusal segment

B. RCT in the occlusal segment and 2 weeks of passive splinting

C. RCT in both segments

D. RCT in the occlusal segment and surgical removal of the apical segment

E. No treatment at this time and continued observation

43. You are playing a soft ball game in Central Park. Your good friend is the catcher. He is not wearing a mask. A foul tip hits him in the mouth and the left central incisor is avulsed and lands in the dirt behind the home plate. Your office is 10 minutes away. The best treatment for the tooth is:

A. Scrape off all the debris and remove the contaminated periodontal ligament; then replant immediately

B. Gently clean the tooth of debris and replant

C. Gently clean the tooth and carefully remove the periodontal ligament and initiate endodontic therapy

D. Gently clean the tooth of debris with saline; carefully remove several millimeters of the apex so as not to disturb the remaining periodontal ligament

44. A new patient comes to your office. He has no adverse symptoms. On routine radiographic examination, you notice apical radiolucency on a root-canal–treated lateral incisor, which was adequately restored with a post and a PFM crown. The RCT was completed 2 years ago. The radiograph shows an adequate widening and filling of the canal. The patient has no contributory medical history. The tooth is asymptomatic. What is the likely diagnosis?

    A. Chronic apical periodontitis
    B. Foreign body reaction
    C. Apical radicular cyst
    D. Scar tissue
    E. Irreversible pulpitis

45. What should the treatment plan be?

    A. Replace the crown; retreat the canal.
    B. Perform another surgery and place another root end material.
    C. Place the patient on antibiotics to resolve the lesion.
    D. No treatment is needed.
    E. Extraction

46. When performing an endodontic re-treat procedure, gutta percha may be plasticized using each of the following *except*, which one is the *exception*?

    A. Xylol
    B. Sodium Hypochlorite
    C. Eucalyptol
    D. Chloroform

47. Transportation in the apical portion of canal walls may occur on the inner curve BECAUSE files have the tendency to return to their linear shape.

    A. Both the statement and the reason are correct and related
    B. Both the statement and reason are correct but NOT related
    C. The statement is correct, but the reason is NOT
    D. The statement is NOT correct, but the reason is correct
    E. NEITHER the statement NOR the reason is correct

48. During an intracoronal bleaching procedure the surface to which bleaching agent is applied is the?

    A. Mesial
    B. Distal
    C. Facial
    D. Lingual

49. A Hedstrom file is made by twisting a tapered or square wire into elevated cutting edges.

    It produces its cutting effect on pulling strokes only.

    A. Both statements are TRUE
    B. Both statements are FALSE
    C. The first statement is TRUE, the second is FALSE
    D. The first statement is FALSE, the second is TRUE.

50. Which of the following best illustrates the reason why calcium hydroxide is not used endodontic procedures involving the primary dentition?

    A. Can cause external resorption
    B. Promotes the formation of reparative dentin
    C. Has an alkaline pH
    D. Produces no anti-microbial effect

1. **The correct answer is E.** The classic signs of irreversible pulpitis include pain that is intense in nature that occurs spontaneously without a specific stimulus. Answer A is incorrect. A necrotic pulp indicates that the affected tooth is nonvital and would therefore have no response to heat, cold, or sweets. Answer B is incorrect. Acute apical periodontitis is a periapical diagnosis that is characterized by percussion sensitivity. Answer C is incorrect. Reversible pulpitis is usually asymptomatic, but when there are symptoms, they include sharp, transient pain with hot or cold that disappears when the stimulus is removed. Answer D is incorrect. Traumatic occlusion refers to tissue damage due to occlusal forces, and symptoms include sensitivity to percussion and tooth mobility.

2. **The correct answer is D.** At 12 years of age, the maxillary central incisors should be fully developed with closed apices. Root canal therapy is the treatment of choice as it is necessary to accommodate the post, core, and crown needed to restore the tooth to form and function. Answer A is incorrect. Extraction is the last resort treatment for a tooth that is nonrestorable. Answer B is incorrect. Pulpotomy is performed on a traumatic exposure to preserve vital pulp tissue in an immature tooth. Since the fractured tooth is mature, pulpotomy is not indicated. Answer C is incorrect. Direct pulp caps are usually reserved for small (<0.5 mm), atraumatic mechanical exposures during caries removal. Answer E is incorrect. Apexogenesis is a type of vital pulp therapy in which the pulp of an immature tooth is maintained to allow for continued dentin formation and root end closure. The tooth in this case is already fully developed.

3. **The correct answer is D.** Root canal therapy is considered successful in the absence of a periapical radiolucency. Rate and completion of healing vary depending on the size of the initial lesion but should show improvement radiographically in 6 months. Answers A, B, and C are incorrect. During this time, if the bacterial load has been decreased sufficiently, fibroblasts

and endothelial cells infiltrate, bone is replaced, cementum and dentin are repaired by cellular cementum, and the PDL is restored. Answer E is incorrect. Success is defined as elimination (or no development of) a radiolucency for at least 1 year following treatment.

4. **The correct answer is B.** Irreversible pulpitis is characterized by intense, spontaneous pain that lingers with cold stimuli. Acute apical periodontitis is characterized by sensitivity to percussion. Answer A is incorrect. The pulpal diagnosis of irreversible pulpitis is correct; however, a normal periapex would not respond to percussion with pain. Answer C is incorrect. A tooth with reversible pulpitis would not exhibit lingering pain to cold. Answer D is incorrect. A nonvital, necrotic tooth would not respond to thermal tests, and chronic apical periodontitis would not respond positively to percussion tests. Answer E is incorrect. As explained earlier, the symptoms do not describe a necrotic tooth.

5. **The correct answer is D.** The number of nerves and blood vessels in the pulp decreases with age, and this loss of sensory innervation leads to a decreased response to electric pulp testing with age. Answer A is incorrect. There is a reduction in all cell types as the pulp ages, resulting from deposition of secondary and tertiary dentin. Answer B is incorrect. Pulp stone formation increases as the pulp ages. Answer C is incorrect. Root canals decrease in diameter as a result of dentin deposition and pulp stone formation. Answer E is incorrect. Blood vessels decrease in number and undergo arteriosclerosis changes with age.

6. **The correct answer is D.** Unmyelinated nociceptive C fibers with a diameter less than 1 μm produce a pain with slow onset and a dull, diffuse quality. They are found mainly in the core of the pulp and are the most numerous nerve fibers. Answer A is incorrect. When stimulated, myelinated A fibers produce a fast, localized sharp pain sensation. Answer B is incorrect. A fibers are myelinated. Answer C is incorrect. C fibers are

unmyelinated. Answer E is incorrect. The sub-odontoblastic plexus of Raschkow is composed of the terminal portions of the A fibers as they branch off, lose their myelination, and rise to the coronal portion of the pulp around the level of the odontoblasts.

7. **The correct answer is B.** This is the classic presentation of a true endo–perio lesion. If the periodontal prognosis of the tooth is favorable, endodontics therapy should be initiated first. This will prevent drainage from the periapical lesion from interfering with the healing of the periodontal lesion. Once definitive root canal therapy has been completed, periodontal treatment should be initiated. Answer A is incorrect. If the endodontic lesion is treated without periodontal therapy following, the lesion will heal up to the base of the periodontal lesion, without further resolution. Answer C is incorrect. If the periodontal lesion is treated without the endodontic therapy, the endodontic lesion will persist, as will the periodontal defect, as the drainage from the periapical area will prevent regeneration from occurring. Answer D is incorrect. If the endodontic treatment does not precede the periodontal treatment, the periodontal treatment will not be successful. Answer E is incorrect. Extraction is the last resort treatment to be used only if the prognosis of the tooth is hopeless. Since this condition is localized and there is no mobility, the tooth should be treated.

8. **The correct answer is C.** It is helpful to attempt to elicit the painful symptom during the diagnostic process. Since cold drinks elicit pain in the patient, a cold test should be conducted prior to other vitality tests. Answer A is incorrect. Electric pulp testing may be an appropriate first test in another clinical situation. Answer B is incorrect. Since pain is not elicited by hot drinks or foods, the cold test is more appropriate. Answer D is incorrect. A test cavity is never a first-line diagnostic pulp vitality test. It is to be used only if other tests are inconclusive and a necrotic pulp is suspected. Answer E is incorrect. The patient does not report sensitivity to mastication, so percussion testing is not likely to elicit the symptom. In addition, it is not a test for pulp vitality, rather it is used to make a periapical diagnosis.

9. **The correct answer is D.** Tooth type should not affect ability to achieve profound local anesthesia. Answer A is incorrect. Often, patients receiving root canal therapy have been in severe pain for a few days, preventing them from getting adequate sleep. This can result in a decreased pain threshold. Answer B is incorrect. Many patients are fearful of root canal therapy, either as a result of a previous bad experience or because a friend or family member had a bad experience. As a result, their pain threshold is decreased. Answer C is incorrect. If the periodontium is inflamed, patients may experience hyperalgesia or a painful reaction to a normal stimulus. In addition, it has been hypothesized that because the inflamed tissue is more acidic than normal, there is less local anesthetic available in its basic form to penetrate the nerve. Answer E is incorrect. Patients who have had previous difficulty achieving anesthesia are more likely to have anxiety and, as a result, are more likely to have problems in the future with anesthesia.

10. **The correct answer is D.** We are able to determine that the mesially shifted canal is positioned lingually by using the SLOB rule. As the x-ray cone moves in the horizontal direction, the object that moves in the same direction is positioned lingually (Same, Lingual), and the object that moves in the opposite direction is positioned buccally (Opposite, Buccal). Answer A is incorrect. The two canals in the distal root of a mandibular molar are positioned buccally and lingually. Answer B is incorrect. The two canals in the distal root of a mandibular molar are positioned buccally and lingually. Answer C is incorrect. If the canal was positioned buccally, it would have moved distally, in the opposite direction of the cone. Answer E is incorrect. As was stated earlier, the SLOB rule can be used to determine the orientation of the files in the distal canal.

11. **The correct answer is B.** The first number is a measure of the diameter of the tip of the k-file (30 = 0.30 mm). The second number is a measure of the length of the k-file (25 mm). The file diameter (taper) increases at a regular rate of 0.02 mm up the shaft of the instrument in k-files. Answer A is incorrect. The value 30 is

the measure of the diameter of the tip of the file, not the length, and 25 mm is the measure of the length of the file, not the diameter of the tip. Answer C is incorrect. The taper of k-files is 0.02, not 30, although the measure of the length is 25 mm. Answer D is incorrect. While 30 is the measure of the diameter of the tip of the file, the taper of k-files is 0.02. Answer E is incorrect. The value 30 is a measure of the diameter of the tip of the file, and 0.02 would represent the taper of the file, not 25 mm.

12. **The correct answer is C.** Dens evaginatus usually presents as a tubercle, most commonly in the mandibular premolars of Asian individuals. They often contain pulp tissue, as when they fracture off or wear down as a result of attrition, the pulp may become exposed. Answer A is incorrect. This correct pulpal diagnosis for this patient is necrotic pulp, as there is no response to pulp vitality tests, and there is destruction of the periodontium. Answer B is incorrect. Dens invaginatus most commonly occurs in the lingual of maxillary lateral incisors and is an infolding rather than an outgrowth of the enamel organ. It can also result in communication between the oral cavity and the pulp and would be treated with root canal therapy as would dens evaginatus. Answer D is incorrect. Pulp stones form within the pulp, possibly as a result of irritation and are often seen as radiopaque on radiographs. Answer E is incorrect. Internal resorption occurs as a response to irritation, and it may be small and almost undetectable or so destructive that it causes root perforation.

13. **The correct answer is C.** The apical constriction, assumed to be at the junction of the cementum and the dentin, is reliably measured by apex locators and is usually 0.5 mm from the apical foramen. It is the accepted determinant for working length determination. Answer A is incorrect. The anatomic apex, which may also be called the *radiographic apex*, is the most apical portion of the root. We do not work to this length, as the apical foramen rarely coincides with the anatomic apex. Answer B is incorrect. The apical foramen is usually 0.5 mm from the radiographic/anatomic apex. Usual working length is

0.5 mm short of the apical foramen at the apical constriction.

14. **The correct answer is E.** The access form is triangular for the maxillary central incisor, the maxillary first molar, and the maxillary second molar. Answer A is incorrect. The access form for the maxillary central incisor is triangular and the access forms for both mandibular central incisor and maxillary lateral incisor are ovoid. Answer B is incorrect. The access forms for both mandibular central incisor and the maxillary first premolar are ovoid, and the access form for the maxillary first molar is triangular. Answer C is incorrect. The access forms for the maxillary canine, the maxillary first premolar, and the maxillary lateral incisor are all ovoid. Answer D is incorrect. The access form for the maxillary second molar is triangle, the access form for the mandibular first molar is trapezoidal, and the access form for the maxillary lateral incisor is ovoid.

15. **The correct answer is B.** A restoration that has a proper seal will prevent recurrent caries and bacterial recontamination of the root canal system, ensuring success of the root canal therapy. Answer A is incorrect. The type of final restoration placed after endodontic therapy is unimportant as long as the marginal integrity is maintained and proper cuspal coverage is achieved where needed. Answer C is incorrect. The type of temporary sealing material is not important, as long as the seal is tight and it is not left in for more than approximately 3 months. Answer D is incorrect. Placement of a post is used strictly as a means for retaining core material in a tooth that has lost significant coronal structure. It does not provide a coronal seal until a final restoration is placed. Answer E is incorrect. The type of sealer used during obturation does not affect the success of the procedure, the fit of the gutta percha is a more important factor in sealing the apex.

16. **The correct answer is D.** The first step in all patients' visits should be a complete review of their medical and dental history, whether it is their first visit or not. Following this, it is important to ascertain the details of their chief complaint including information about the duration and

the quality of pain and what, if any, stimuli exacerbate it. Next, an extraoral examination should be completed, noting any areas of swelling, tenderness, or lymphadenopathy. After the extraoral examination, a complete intraoral examination should be completed, including appropriate pulp vitality tests and percussion and palpation tests. Finally, a determination should be made as to what radiographs are needed, followed by interpretation. Answer A is incorrect, answer B is incorrect, answer C is incorrect, answer E is incorrect; see the earlier reasons.

17. **The correct answer is D.** Failure to direct the bur parallel to the long axis of the tooth during access preparation can result in crown or root perforation. Perforation into the PDL usually results in hemorrhage that is difficult to control. Pain may occur as the operator attempts to place an instrument through the perforation and enters the PDL. A burning sensation or a bad taste can be detected during irrigation with sodium hypochlorite as the solution exits the root canal system. Answer A is incorrect. Inadequate straight line access may be a cause of root perforation and many other procedural errors that may occur during root canal therapy, but it is not the direct cause of the listed symptoms. Answer B is incorrect. Root canal contamination would not result in the immediate symptoms but would cause more long-term problems such as intervisit emergencies or, ultimately, root canal failure. Answer D is incorrect. Incomplete root canal debridement would result in problems similar to root canal contamination. Answer E is incorrect. Ledging can result in incomplete root canal debridement and inadequate obturation, none of which would cause the listed symptoms.

18. **The correct answer is A.** To maintain the patency of the canal and to maintain the working length, it is necessary to recapitulate frequently and use irrigation and lubrication. Other causes of ledging include inadequate straight line access, retention of debris in the apical end of the canal, and excessive enlargement of curved canals. Answer B is incorrect. An instrument separation is possible but is not the best answer. An instrument that has been broken will show a blunted tip, signaling that an error has occurred. Answer C is incorrect. A vertical root fracture most often occurs during postcementation or condensation during obturation. It would not present with a sudden inability to reach working length and usually would not occur during routine instrumentation. Answer D is incorrect. Inadequate straight line access may be one of the causes of ledging but would not directly cause a sudden loss of working length. Answer E is incorrect. A furcation perforation might prevent an operator from accurately measuring working length if a file were inserted through the perforation, but it would not result in a sudden inability to reach working length.

19. **The correct answer is D.** The initial strategy for a separated instrument is to try and bypass the instrument in the same way you would bypass a ledge. If this is successful, broaches or Hedstrom files can be used in attempt to remove the separated segment. If this is possible, the canal is cleaned, shaped, and obturated to working length. If it is not possible to remove the segment, the canal is cleaned, shaped, and obturated to the new working length at the most coronal portion of the separated instrument. Answer A is incorrect. Extraction is the last resort of treatment, usually reserved for failed root canal therapy or nonrestorable teeth. The prognosis of a tooth with a separated instrument left in the canal depends on how much debridement had been finished prior to the separation, and the procedure should be deemed a failure before extraction. Answer B is incorrect. Similar to extraction, root amputation is usually reserved for cases in which root canal therapy has failed or a portion of a tooth is periodontally involved. Answer C is incorrect. Bicuspidization of a tooth, similar to root amputation, is usually not a first-line treatment for instrument separation. Answer E is incorrect. It is not acceptable to leave any canals in a root canal treated to unobturated. The treatment would be incomplete and would result in definite failure.

20. **The correct answer is A.** Aspiration of instruments can be avoided by judicious use of rubber dam isolation, which is the standard of care during root canal therapy. Answer B is incorrect.

If a tooth is properly isolated, there is no risk of instrument aspiration. Answer C is incorrect. Using proper lubrication may help to avoid instrument separation, but it will not prevent aspiration. Answer D is incorrect. Recapitulation is important in maintaining working length, not in preventing instrument aspiration. Answer E is incorrect. Frequent irrigation is necessary for complete debridement of the canals, not for the prevention of aspiration.

21. **The correct answer is E.** Narrow pockets to the level of the fracture and J-shaped or teardrop-shaped radiolucencies are indicative of vertical root fractures. The only way to definitively diagnose a vertical root fracture is to see it during an exploratory surgical procedure. The prognosis of a root with a vertical fracture is hopeless, and it should be amputated or the tooth must be extracted. Answer A is incorrect. Incomplete debridement of canals can lead to root canal failure but will not present with the narrow pocketing or J-shaped lesions of a fractured root. Answer B is incorrect. Ledging can also lead to failure if the canal has not been fully debrided or filled to original working length. Answer C is incorrect. Underobturation can result in failure if debris remains in the apical portion of the canal or the apical seal is compromised. Answer D is incorrect. A periodontal abscess does not usually present as a narrow defect to the apex of a tooth.

22. **The correct answer is B.** The persistence of swelling, sinus tracts, spontaneous or dull pain, or pain of biting, in addition to lack of resolution of periapical lesions, all indicate root canal failure. Answer A is incorrect. The more likely reason for these symptoms to remain is a failed root canal procedure. Answer C is incorrect. Trigeminal neuralgia typically presents with intense pain that is more intense than applied stimuli, referred pain, and trigger points. These are not typical presentations for failed root canal therapy. Answer D is incorrect. This is possible if the treated tooth was restored to high occlusion and the PDL was irritated; however, the more likely answer, considering the radiographic evidence, is root canal failure. Answer E is incorrect. Myofacial pain is usually not as localized as the presenting symptoms and will typically present as worse during particular times of the day, upon waking in the morning, for example.

23. **The correct answer is D.** A root canal is considered successful if there is an absence of signs and symptoms including all of those mentioned. Answer A is incorrect. If a patient is experiencing swelling or periodontal pocketing, the root canal procedure is deemed a failure. Answer B is incorrect. If a sinus tract fails to heal, the root canal therapy was not successful. Answer C is incorrect. Pain and periapical lesions that do not decrease in size are signs of root canal failure. Answer E is incorrect. In order for a root canal to be deemed a success, periapical lesions must decrease in size and/or resolve.

24. **The correct answer is A.** The decision to perform retrograde or orthograde retreatment is highly dependent on the circumstances of each individual patient. In certain circumstances, if it would be more costly and time consuming to fabricate a new restoration following conventional retreatment, it is acceptable to consider apicoectomy procedures as initial retreatment modalities. Answer B is incorrect. It is necessary to help patients deal with their anxiety, and avoidance of a procedure due to patient anxiety is not an acceptable treatment option. It is quite common for patients to have higher anxiety surrounding a retreatment procedure than an initial treatment, but it is not a reason to choose one treatment over another. Answer C is incorrect. Retrograde treatment does not function to remove microorganisms from the root canal system, orthograde treatment accomplishes this. Rather, the goal of retrograde treatment is to prevent microorganisms from leaving the root canal system. Answer D is incorrect. When root canal filling materials are easy to remove, it makes orthograde retreatment a better option than retrograde retreatment. Answer E is incorrect. Treatment is not decided on the bass of the preference of the dentist, it should be based on the best prognosis for the patient. In addition, if practitioners feel they are unable to properly perform the best procedure for the patient, the case should be referred to another practitioner who can.

Endodontics

25. **The correct answer is C.** An 8-year-old child will have maxillary central incisors with immature apices. Because this is a vital exposure, vital pulp therapy including a shallow pulpotomy should be the treatment of choice. This will result in the remaining vital pulp to continue to allow the apex to develop normally. Once the apex has formed, traditional root canal therapy should be completed. Answer A is incorrect. Root-end closure should be used only to treat nonvital teeth with immature apices because there is no possibility of further growth of the tooth structure. Answer B is incorrect. Traditional root canal therapy is not possible on a tooth with an open apex as it is hard to form an acceptable apical seal. Answer D is incorrect. A partial pulpectomy would remove vital pulp tissue from the root canal system, making continued root formation less likely. Answer E is incorrect. Temporization without a shallow pulpotomy would potentially allow for bacterial contamination of the pulp and root canal system.

26. **The correct answer is D.** Intrapulpal hemorrhage occurs as the result of injury to coronal blood vessels, usually suffered during impact to a tooth. The hemorrhaged red blood cells and their disintegration products stain the surrounding dentin, and it tends to increase over time. Answer A is incorrect. Endemic fluorosis is caused by ingestion of too much fluoride during tooth formation. Teeth may erupt with a chalky appearance, getting discolored only after they absorb stains from the oral cavity. Answer B is incorrect. Discoloration from systemic drugs, most often tetracycline, is usually bilateral and can range from yellow to dark gray depending on the exposure. Answer C is incorrect. Enamel hypocalcification usually appears as a distinct brown or white area on the crown of a tooth. Answer E is incorrect. Amelogenesis imperfecta may result in yellow or brown discolorations, usually affecting more than one tooth.

27. **The correct answer is B.** Incompletely removing the sealer or gutta percha after obturation is a common cause of tooth discoloration following root canal therapy. This dark discoloration can be prevented by maintaining pulp chamber with clean walls prior to final restorative treatment. Answer A is incorrect. As long as the coronal seal was adequate, sealer remnants in the pulp chamber would not lead to root canal failure. Answer C is incorrect. Vertical root fracture is most often caused during the placement of a post. Leaving the sealer in the chamber would not increase the chance of vertical root fracture. Answer D is incorrect. The sealer remaining in the chamber should not prevent an adequate coronal seal. Answer E is incorrect. Because it is possible to obtain a coronal seal even if the sealer is left in the chamber, it would not be the direct cause of bacterial leakage.

28. **The correct answer is C.** Sodium perborate is a powder that decomposes into hydrogen peroxide and oxygen in the presence of acid or water. It is safer and less damaging to tissues than hydrogen peroxide and is therefore the material of choice for internal bleaching. Answer A is incorrect. Hydrogen peroxide is an oxidizer that is unstable in high concentrations and tends to burn tissue. Therefore, sodium perborate is a better choice for the bleaching procedure. Answer B is incorrect. Carbamide peroxide is used for external bleaching and not for internal bleaching procedures.

29. **The correct answer is C.** When a fluctuant swelling is incised, the purulence is released immediately and a relief is felt right away. Answer A is incorrect. A tooth with reversible pulpitis and pain on mastication does not need incision for drainage or root canal therapy. Rather, the offending stimulus must be removed to relieve the symptoms. Answer B is incorrect. A necrotic tooth with an indurated swelling may be incised for drainage; however, the outcome is less predictable. Relief of pressure will most likely be felt; however, it is possible that only blood or serous fluid will be released. Answer D is incorrect. A tooth without a swelling is a contraindicated for incision for drainage. Answer E is incorrect. A tooth without swelling is a contraindicated for drainage.

30. **The correct answer is B.** All vitality testing and the lack of symptoms should lead you to determine that the tooth is vital; therefore, a periradicular lesion should not be attributed to an

infection originating in the root canal system. In addition, the patient's history of malignancy makes a biopsy the correct treatment for the undefined lesion. Answer A is incorrect. Because the tooth is vital, with no symptoms and an intact restoration, a pulpotomy should not be performed. Answer C is incorrect. Root canal therapy should not be the treatment of choice for this tooth for the same reasons as pulpotomy is not the treatment of choice. Answer D is incorrect. The tooth should not be extracted except as the last resort if the biopsy is positive for malignancy and it was determined that all of the malignant could not be removed without extraction.

31. **The correct answer is B.** The percussion test determines whether or not there is inflammation in the periodontal ligament. Answer A is incorrect. The percussion test cannot be used to determine whether a tooth is vital or not and should not be used as a test to determine whether root canal therapy is indicated as a treatment option. Answer C is incorrect. The palpation test would be used to determine whether inflammation has spread from the PDL to the surrounding periodontium. Answer D is incorrect. Although percussion sensitivity is common in the presence of a root fracture, it is not diagnostic. Answer E is incorrect. To determine the vitality of a tooth, other tests would be employed, including electric pulp testing and cold testing.

32. **The correct answer is B.** Electric pulp testing produces a high incidence of both false-positives and false-negatives. As a result, it is not a definitive test, and additional diagnostic aids should be used. Answer A is incorrect. Because electric pulp testing is not definitive, a diagnosis of necrotic at this point would be premature. Answer C is incorrect. A definitive treatment plan cannot be made until a definitive diagnosis is made. Answer D is incorrect. Electric pulp testing measures the level of stimulation for sensory nerves within the pulp, giving no information about inflammation. The proper test to diagnose inflammation in the PDL would be percussion. Answer E is incorrect. Calcified canals may lead to an electric pulp test reading that suggests necrosis but can be diagnosed only by radiographic or clinical examination.

33. **The correct answer is D.** A tooth with irreversible pulpitis will react with severe pain, reproducing the chief complaint of the patient that lingers after the stimulus is removed. Answer A is incorrect. No response to Endo Ice would indicate a necrotic pulp. Answer B is incorrect. Severe pain that does not linger after removal of the stimulus is indicative of reversible pulpitis. Answer C is incorrect. Mild to moderate pain that does not linger after removal of the stimulus is indicative of a normal pulp.

34. **The correct answer is D.** Indications for direct pulp cap therapy include permanent teeth in which there has been a pinpoint mechanical exposure of a vital, asymptomatic tooth. Bleeding must be controlled, and the pulp cap material must make direct contact with the exposure. Answer A is incorrect. A pulpotomy is indicated in primary teeth with exposed vital pulps or irreversible pulpitis. It is indicated in permanent teeth as a temporary emergency procedure to alleviate symptoms prior to conventional root canal therapy or in permanent teeth with immature apices to encourage further root development and closure. Answer B is incorrect. An indirect pulp cap is indicated on permanent teeth with immature apices if there is a carious lesion, which, if removed, will result in a pulpal exposure as long as the tooth is asymptomatic with no periapical pathology. Answer C is incorrect. Root canal therapy would be indicated in this case if the direct pulp capping procedure failed, resulting in symptoms. Answer E is incorrect. A conventional amalgam restoration may be placed only if there is no pulpal exposure.

35. **The correct answer is E.** The outline of the access cavities for both the first and second mandibular molars is trapezoid. Answer A is incorrect. The outline of the access cavity for the maxillary first molar is triangular, and the outline of the access cavity for the mandibular first molar is trapezoid. Answer B is incorrect. The outline of the access cavity for the mandibular first molar is trapezoid, and the outline of the access cavity for the maxillary second molar is triangular. Answer C is incorrect. The outline of the access cavity for the maxillary first molar is

triangular, and the outline of access cavity for the maxillary second premolar is ovoid. Answer D is incorrect. The outline of the access cavity for the mandibular second premolar is ovoid, and the outline of the access cavity for the maxillary second molar is triangular.

36. **The correct answer is C.** A complicated crown fracture involves the enamel, dentin, and pulp. Answer A is incorrect. A root fracture involves cementum, dentin, and pulp. Answer B is incorrect. A crown–root fracture involves enamel, dentin, and cementum and may or may not involve the pulp. Answer D is incorrect. An uncomplicated crown fracture involves the enamel and dentin but not the pulp.

37. **The correct answer is D.** Calcium is a white powder with a high pH and is applied to the canals between appointments as a cream mixed with sterile water. It is antibacterial and prevents bacterial growth between treatments. Calcium hydroxide is also used to encourage calcification in pulp capping, apexogenesis, and apexification procedures. Answer A is incorrect. Sodium hypochlorite is an acidic liquid that acts as a solvent on organic debris and also as an antibacterial agent. It is the irrigation solution of choice but is very caustic and can cause severe reactions if extruded past the apex. Answer B is incorrect. Ethylenediaminetetraacetate demineralizes dentin and removes inorganic material. It is used to remove the dentin smear layer and is the main ingredient in many canal lubricants. Answer C is incorrect. Chlorhexidine is an antiseptic used to inhibit bacteria but is not used as an interappointment canal medication. Answer E is incorrect. Gutta percha is an obturating material that would be used only to definitively seal a clean root canal.

38. **The correct answer is E.** Milk and Hank balanced salt solution provide the best conditions in which to store an avulsed tooth due to their osmolality. Answer A is incorrect. Storing an avulsed tooth dry would give it the worst prognosis. Answer B is incorrect. Along with dry storage, storage in tap water provides the worst prognosis for an avulsed tooth. Answer C is incorrect. If neither milk nor Hank solution were avail-able, saline would be a good storage option. Answer D is incorrect. Saliva could be used in place of saline if milk or Hank solution were not available.

39. **The correct answer is B.** A tooth that had been avulsed more than an hour earlier and not stored in an appropriate liquid medium is generally not replanted as the prognosis is very poor. Answer A is incorrect. If the tooth had been avulsed less than an hour prior and had been stored properly, root canal therapy would have been completed only after a week of splinting to reduce mobility. Answer C is incorrect. If the tooth had been avulsed less than an hour prior and had been stored properly, this would be a correct procedure, followed by flexible splinting for a week and definitive root canal therapy. Answer D is incorrect. This would have been the proper treatment plan for a tooth avulsed less than an hour prior that had been stored in the proper liquid medium.

40. **The correct answer is D.** Pulpal therapy is not indicated for this tooth, so extraction is the only viable treatment option. Answer A is incorrect. The pulp is already exposed in this case, so indirect pulp capping in no longer an option. Answer B is incorrect. Direct pulp caps are not indicated for primary teeth as the low pH of calcium hydroxide will irritate the pulp and cause internal resorption. Answer C is incorrect. Pulpotomy is contraindicated on primary teeth if more than one-third of the root has already resorbed, if there is internal resorption, if the furcation is perforated, or if there is a periradicular lesion that may damage the succedaneous tooth. Answer E is incorrect. Root canal therapy is indicated only for primary teeth when there is no evidence of a succedaneous tooth, when there is no evidence of periradicular lesions, and when treatment will not damage the succedaneous tooth.

41. **The correct answer is C.**

    A. This would be inaccurate because the fistula may be located between the teeth.
    B. This is wrong because the patient may have referred pain on adjacent teeth.

C. Although this is a good diagnostic tool to identify vertical fracture, it is not sufficient to identify the source of the fistula.

D. A fistulous tract cannot be seen on a radiograph.

42. **The correct answer is E.** The fact that the patient sustained trauma to her tooth is not an indication to initiate root canal treatment. Clinically, the tooth is not exposed. The accident happened only 1 hour ago, which is not a sufficient time for radiographic changes. Splinting is optional but not necessary since there is only slight mobility. The luxation caused inflammation around the periodontal ligament, but there is a good chance that it will resolve on its own. Observation and radiographic monitoring is the right treatment at this time.

A. Tooth is not exposed; therefore, no root canal treatment is indicated.

B. Treatment for luxated teeth is initiated with 2 weeks of passive splinting to allow for reattachment of periodontal ligament and/or ankylosis of the tooth. RCT is initiated after confirming unsuccessful reattachment and pulpal necrosis.

C. See reasons presented earlier.

D. Surgical removal of the apical segment is usually the treatment of choice in cases when infection develops or persists AFTER root canal therapy.

43. **The correct answer is B.** All the other answers call for removal of periodontal ligament, which is wrong, since it contains viable cells necessary for successful implantation. It is necessary to only gently remove gross debris.

44. **The correct answer is D.** There may be extensive bone destruction in the vicinity of the infected tooth, such as perforation of both labial and lingual cortical plates; sometimes, it takes years for the bone to fill the defect, and sometimes this does not happen at all. Instead, the area fills with scar tissue. Answer A is wrong because chronic apical periodontitis is generally a condition in which the apical portion of a tooth's root is chronically inflamed. There may be drainage through the gums from around the tooth's root.

This resolves following successful treatment of the condition with RCT. Answer B is wrong because foreign-body reaction would present with swelling, irritation, and redness in the area. Answer C is wrong because apical radicular cyst is a fluid-filled sac at the apex of the tooth following necrosis of the pulp, which usually resolves with RCT. Answer E is wrong because patient cannot have irreversible pulpitis AFTER the root canal therapy.

45. **The correct answer is D.** A complete resolution of the infection does not necessarily coincide with completion of root canal therapy. This condition will probably resolve on its own once the host immune system completely eliminates the infection. No treatment is indicated for this asymptomatic presentation. All other choices recommend a treatment much too aggressive for an asymptomatic tooth.

46. **The correct answer is B.** NaOCl is an irrigating solution. Answer A is incorrect because xylol is an aromatic isomer used as a solvent. Answers C and D are incorrect because they are organic solvents used in gutta percha removal.

47. **The correct answer is D.** Transportation will occur on the OUTER curve of canal walls, not the inner due to files returning to their linear form throughout treatment. Answers A, B, and C are incorrect because transportation occurs is the outer curve of the canal wall. Answer E is incorrect because files due have the tendency to return to their linear form.

48. **The correct answer is C.** Bleaching material is acting up facial/esthetic portion of the tooth. A, B, and D are incorrect.

49. **The correct answer is D.** Hedstrom files are made from a tapered wire only, K-files and Reamers are made from various shaped wires and use a twist-and-pull method. Answer A is incorrect because Hedstrom wires are made from a tapered wire only. Answer B is incorrect because Hedstrom wires are made from tapered wire only; second part is correct. Answer C is incorrect because Hedstrom wires are made from

tapered wire only and DO produces cutting effect only with pulling strokes.

50. **The correct answer is C.** Alkaline pH causes internal resorption in primary dentition. Answers

A, B, and D are incorrect because calcium hydroxide causes internal resorption in primary dentition, reparative dentition formation in permanent dentition, and produces an antimicrobial effect, respectively.

CHAPTER 7

Periodontics

1. Which sign or symptom is most common with a periodontal abscess?

    A. Severe throbbing pain
    B. Sinus tract in mucosa
    C. Vital tooth
    D. Deep caries

2. What Miller classification would the first and second lower premolars be classified as?

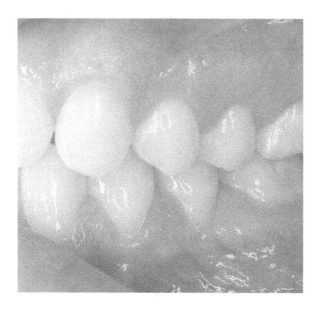

    A. Miller class II
    B. Miller class III
    C. Miller class IV
    D. Miller class I

3. What Miller classification would the lower left central incisor be classified as?

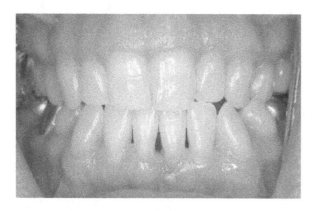

    A. Miller class II
    B. Miller class III
    C. Miller class IV
    D. Miller class I

4. What is the source of the final tissue in a free gingival graft?

    A. Stratum basal of the epithelium
    B. Adipose tissue
    C. Lamina propria of the connective tissue
    D. Stratum spinosum of epithelium

5. What is a normal hemoglobin A_{1c} ($Hb\,A_{1c}$) value in a nondiabetic person?

    A. 8–9%
    B. 3–4%
    C. 4–6%
    D. 2–3%

6. Why use a palatal approach for osseous periodontal surgery?

    A. Palatal embrasures are wider, allowing for better access to osseous surgery
    B. Less sensitivity for the patient
    C. More subgingival calculus on the palatal surfaces
    D. Less bleeding

7. Which enzyme and/or cytokine is secreted by a macrophage?

    A. Tumor necrosis factor (TNF)
    B. Transforming growth factor (TGF)
    C. Proteases
    D. All of the above

8. What is the typical dose of nitroglycerin for a patient experiencing anginal discomfort?

    A. 0.8 mg
    B. 5.0 mg
    C. 0.3 mg
    D. 3.0 mg

9. Which of the following bone grafting materials are taken from another animal species?

   A. Autografts
   B. Xenografts
   C. Alloplasts
   D. Allografts

10. Which of the following materials is not used for prefabricated posts?

   A. Stainless steel
   B. Gold-pleated brass
   C. Silver
   D. Fiber-reinforced polymers
   E. Titanium

11. According to Miller's index, a tooth has class II mobility when___

   A. Movement of greater than 1 mm in any direction
   B. Movement of greater than 1 mm in any direction and it can be depressed vertically
   C. Movement of less than 0.5 mm in any direction
   D. Movement of less than 1 mm in any direction

12. Which of the following is not a common oral manifestation of Crohn disease?

   A. Hypertrophy of the lips
   B. Hypertrophy of the gingival tissue
   C. Aphthous ulcer
   D. Cobblestone appearance of the buccal mucosa and palate
   E. Dry mouth

13. During placement of a post, what is the criterion for the post width?

   A. It should not exceed ⅓ of the root width at its narrowest location.
   B. It should not exceed ½ of the root width at its narrowest location.
   C. No criteria since post width does not affect the retention of the post.

14. If a 7-year-old patient presents with early loss of Tooth A, maxillary right second primary molar, what is the appropriate space maintainer that can be used?

   A. Nance appliance
   B. Distal shoe
   C. Band-and-loop
   D. Lower lingual arch

15. Which of the following is not a feature of primary resistance form in amalgam preparation?

   A. Maintain as much sound structure as possible
   B. Rounded axiopulpal line angle in class II preparation
   C. Vertical walls that converge occlusally
   D. Adequate thickness of amalgam

16. Which appliance is *not* used to correct class II malocclusion?

   A. Reverse-pull headgear
   B. Herbst appliance
   C. Twin block appliance
   D. Cervical-pull headgear

17. Which medicament can be used during pulpotomy procedure?

   A. Calcium hydroxide
   B. Ethylenediaminetetraacetic acid (EDTA)
   C. Mineral trioxide aggregate
   D. Flowable composite

18. A patient presents with teeth #2, 3, 4, and 14 missing. Which Kennedy classification does this partially edentulous arch belong to?

   A. Kennedy class III mod 1
   B. Kennedy class III
   C. Kennedy class I
   D. Kennedy class II mod 1

19. Allografts have the following characteristics *except*:

   A. Osteoinductive
   B. Osteogenic
   C. Osteoconductive
   D. Demineralized

Periodontics

20. A membrane is utilized in guided tissue regeneration to promote repair of intraosseous defect BECAUSE it prevents epithelial cells from contacting the root surface and forming a long junctional epithelium.

    A. Both the statement and the reason are correct and related.
    B. Both the statement and the reason are correct but NOT related.
    C. The statement is correct, but the reason is NOT.
    D. The statement is NOT correct, but the reason is correct.
    E. NEITHER the statement NOR the reason is correct.

21. Periodontitis can be associated with all of the following *except*:

    A. Bleeding upon probing
    B. Increased gingival exudate
    C. Elevated sulcular temperature
    D. Attachment and bone loss that is not progressing
    E. Enlarged gingival contours due to edema and fibrosis

22. Indications for crown lengthening include the following *except*:

    A. Esthetics
    B. Furcation involvement
    C. Delayed passive eruption
    D. Crown fracture
    E. Post or pin perforations

23. Aggressive periodontitis is always associated with poor oral hygiene. Chronic periodontitis is a condition found exclusively in older patients.

    A. Both statements are TRUE.
    B. Both statements are FALSE.
    C. The first statement is TRUE, the second is FALSE.
    D. The first statement is FALSE, the second is TRUE.

24. A patient presents with mandibular molar with furcal involvement where the bone loss is through-and-through and visible clinically. What is the Glickman classification?

    A. Class I
    B. Class II
    C. Class III
    D. Class IV
    E. Class V

25. It is important to have adequate space between a crown margin and the crest of bone to avoid impingement of the biologic width. Which of the following is NOT a limiting factor?

    A. Mobility of tooth
    B. Location of furcation
    C. Crown-to-root ratio
    D. Age of the tooth
    E. Tooth–arch relationship

26. A 44-year-old patient presents a third of the dentition with 5 mm of clinical attachment loss, bleeding upon probing, none of the teeth being mobile, and probing depths ranging between 4 and 6 mm. What is the most probable diagnosis?

    A. Localized chronic moderate periodontitis
    B. Generalized chronic severe periodontitis
    C. Localized chronic severe periodontitis
    D. Generalized chronic moderate periodontitis
    E. None of the above

27. Which of the following treatment modalities will not assist in pocket reduction?

    A. Osseous surgery
    B. Gingivectomy
    C. Apically positioned flap
    D. Guided tissue regeneration
    E. Connective tissue graft

28. Which of the following is NOT a predictable objective of periodontal surgery?

    A. Remove or eliminate the lesion
    B. Regenerate interdental papillae
    C. Promote gingival reattachment
    D. Pocket reduction
    E. Treat and/or control the etiology

29. Biofilm found on tooth surface is termed as:

    A. Enamel
    B. Dental plaque
    C. Saliva
    D. Dental caries

30. Periodontitis that does not resolve with treatment is termed as:

    A. Aggressive periodontitis
    B. Chronic periodontitis
    C. Refractory periodontitis
    D. Juvenile periodontitis

31. Radiographically, driven snow appearance is seen with:

    A. Adenomatoid odontogenic cyst
    B. Calcifying odontogenic cyst
    C. Calcifying epithelial odontogenic tumor
    D. Keratocyst

32. Increased alkaline phosphatase levels are seen with:

    A. Paget disease
    B. Hypophosphatasia
    C. Cherubism
    D. Hyperparathyroidism

33. Contrast on a radiograph is:

    A. Uneven density on a radiograph
    B. Range of densities on a radiograph
    C. Overall appearance of the radiograph
    D. Overall degree of darkening of the radiograph.

Periodontics

1. The correct answer is C.

	Pulpal Lesions (Endodontic Abscess)	Periodontal Lesions (Periodontal Abscess)
Vitality	Nonvital	Vital
Usual area of swelling	Vestibule	Attached gingiva
Pain	Intermittent throbbing	Dull, continuous
Probing	Narrow, isolated defect	Generalized defect
Sinus tract location	Mucosa	Attached gingiva, sulcus
Radiograph	Localized bone loss	Generalized bone loss of area
Local factors	Variable	Calculus
Etiology	Deep caries or restoration	Possibly nonrestored

2. **The correct answer is D.** The recession does not extend to the mucogingival junction (MGJ) and no bone loss exists. Miller class I defects are the most predictable for root coverage. Review the chart below.

Miller 1	Recession not extending to the MGJ and no bone loss
Miller 2	Recession extending to or beyond the MGJ and no bone loss
Miller 3	Recession extending to or beyond the MGJ and some bone loss
Miller 4	Recession extending to or beyond the MGJ and extensive bone loss or tooth malposition

3. **The correct answer is B.** The recession extends to the MGJ and there is some bone loss. Complete (100%) coverage of this root would not be anticipated.

4. **The correct answer is C.** The underlying lamina propria of the connective tissue of the donor graft will be the source of the final tissue result in a free gingival graft. Epithelium is 0.75 mm on average, hence it is better to harvest grafts over 0.75 mm to ensure an underlying connective tissue base.

Figure 7-3. Before a free gingival graft #26.

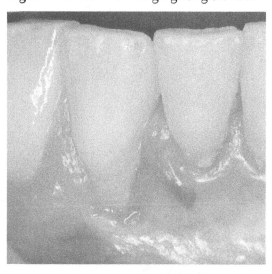

Figure 7-4. After a free gingival graft #26.

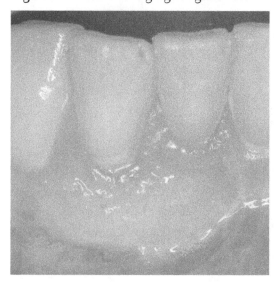

The source of attached tissue was derived from the underlying connective tissue.

5. **The correct answer is C.** Normal values for a nondiabetic person are 4% to 6%. Glycosylated hemoglobin is a test that indicates how much sugar has been in a person's blood during the past 2 to 4 months. It is used to monitor the effectiveness of diabetes treatment. The amount bound reflects how much glucose has been in the blood during the past average 120-day lifespan of red cells. Diabetes treatment should achieve glycosylated hemoglobin levels of less than 7.0%. Uncontrolled diabetes is a risk factor for periodontitis.

6. **The correct answer is A.** When treating a patient with osseous surgery, the surgeon should ramp the bone toward the palate. The following are reasons for a palatal approach to osseous surgery: Palatal embrasures are wider, allowing for better access to osseous surgery. More cancellous bone palatally, therefore better healing. More keratinized tissue. Tongue allows for better hygiene palatally. Better esthetics.

7. **The correct answer is D.** Numerous enzymes and cytokines are secreted by the macrophage. These include collagenases, which debride the wound; interleukins and tumor necrosis factor (TNF), which stimulate fibroblasts (produce collagen) and promote angiogenesis; and transforming growth factor (TGF), which stimulates keratinocytes. They also produce hydrolytic enzymes (lysozyme, proteases), small cationic peptides called defensins, enzymes that create reactive forms of oxygen, and enzymes that create reactive forms of nitrogen.

8. **The correct answer is C.** Average dose is 0.3 mg given sublingually, and may be repeated at 5-minute intervals three times. Nitroglycerin is employed sublingually in the management of anginal discomfort. Indications: angina, acute myocardial infarction, and congestive heart failure with pulmonary edema. Contraindications: myocardial infarction with hypotension, hypotension, and glaucoma.

9. **The correct answer is B.** Xenograft: Tissue transferred from one animal species to another (Bio-Oss® bone grafting material is composed of deproteinized, sterilized bovine bone and is categorized as a calcium deficient carbonate apatite). Autograft: Tissue transferred from one position to another within the same individual (iliac crest graft, mandibular block graft). Alloplast: A synthetic or inert foreign body implanted into tissue (hydroxyapatite). Allograft: A graft between genetically dissimilar members of the same species (demineralized freeze-dried bone allograft, DFDBA; freeze-dried bone allograft, FDBA).

10. **The correct answer is C.** Stainless steel has been used for a long time in prefabricated posts. However, it contains nickel that can cause sensitivity in some people. Titanium posts are biocompatible and least corrosive but have low fracture strength. Also, it is difficult to detect on radiographs because of their similar density as gutta percha material. Fiber-reinforced polymers are esthetic and do not corrode and their removal is easier than that of other material if endodontic failure occurs.

11. **The correct answer is A.** Class I: Up to 1 mm of movement in horizontal direction. Class II: Greater than 1 mm of movement in horizontal direction. Class III: Excessive horizontal movement and vertical movement.

12. **The correct answer is E.** Crohn disease can affect all areas of the digestive tract.

13. **The correct answer is A.** Although the post diameter affects the post retention minimally, when it is increased, root fracture is more likely to occur. Therefore, the post width should not exceed $1/3$ of the root, with a minimum of 1 mm of dentin being retained circumferentially in the apical area.

14. **The correct answer is C.** Early loss of a primary second molar can result in mesial migration of permanent molars. If the first permanent molar has already erupted (usually erupts between 6 and 7 years), band-and-loop is recommended. A distal shoe is an appropriate choice if permanent molar has not fully erupted. Nance appliance is a removable appliance that can be used to prevent mesial movement or tipping of the permanent first molar but has a main disadvantage that it is removable.

Periodontics

15. **The correct answer is C.** Primary resistance form features should prevent restoration and tooth from fracturing against occlusal forces. Other features include removing unsupported enamel, box-like preparation, and marginal amalgam of 90 degrees or higher. Preparation of converging vertical walls is one of the features that help amalgam to be mechanically retained in the tooth structure (primary retention form).

16. **The correct answer is A.** Cervical pull headgear is used to correct class II malocclusions with deep bite and produces an extrusive and distal force on maxillary molars. Herbst appliance is a fixed functional appliance that produces growth of mandible in a forward direction. Twin block appliance also treats class II malocclusion through interaction between maxilla and mandible. It is more easily tolerated by patients. Reverse-pull (or protraction headgear, face mask) is used for patients with class III malocclusion by encouraging growth of maxilla by pulling it forward. It has two soft pads that fit onto patient's forehead and chin, and they are connected by an adjustable framework with anterior wire with hooks that can be used to adjust the movement.

17. **The correct answer is C.** Mineral trioxide aggregate is a medicament that can be used appropriately in pulpotomy procedure in replacement of formocresol. However, because of its high cost, it is not often used.

18. **The correct answer is A.** Kennedy classification system—class I is bilateral edentulous area located posterior to the remaining teeth. Class II is unilateral edentulous area located posterior to the present, natural teeth. Class III is unilateral edentulous area with natural teeth both anterior and posterior to the remaining teeth. Class IV is bilateral-bounded anterior partially edentulous area crossing the midline.

19. **The correct answer is B.** Allografts are grafts obtained from other humans and are stored in tissue banks. They show the following characteristics:
    – Osteoinductive: Induce bone formation by recruiting differentiation of host mesenchymal cells

– Osteoconductive: Provide a lattice or scaffold that promotes bone formation
– Demineralized/decalcified: Allografts are often demineralized to expose components of bone matrix bone morphogenetic proteins (BMPs) to facilitate bone formation. An example is DFDBA.

Autografts are not osteogenic because they do not have live osteocytes to produce bone. Only autografts, which are grafts from the same patient, are osteogenic.

20. **The correct answer is D.** Guided tissue regeneration is a surgical procedure that specifically aims to regenerate lost periodontal tissues. Regeneration is reproduction of lost attachment comprising bone, cementum, and periodontal ligament (PDL). Repair is healing of a wound that does not fully restore original periodontal tissue architecture and attachment. The membrane prevents fast growing gingival epithelial cells from contacting the root to allow regeneration of periodontal attachment rather than repair with a long junctional epithelium.

21. **The correct answer is D.** Periodontitis is defined as progressive destruction of bone and periodontal ligament. All other signs are included in gingival inflammation that may be associated with periodontitis. Attachment and bone loss that is not progressing could be diagnosed as gingivitis on reduced periodontium. Some signs of periodontitis are increased probing depths, radiographic bone loss, increasing tooth mobility, and presence of biochemical markers of tissue breakdown.

22. **The correct answer is B.** Crown lengthening would cause increased furcation involvement; therefore, it would not be an indication for treatment. Crown lengthening would be indicated to improve esthetics in cases where there is excess gingiva such as drug-induced gingival overgrowth. It could also be of esthetic value in cases of delayed passive eruption where natural recession has not occurred. Crown lengthening is also indicated in cases where restorative or crown margins violate biological width because of caries, crown fracture, or post/pin perforations.

23. **The correct answer is B.** Answer as per question.

24. **The correct answer is D.** A class IV furcation is a through-and-through furcation that is visible clinically. When a patient has a through-and-through furcation, it is more advantageous to have it clinically visible because the patient has access to keep the area clean. Good hygiene is possible with a class IV furcation, but not with a class III furcation. A Proxabrush is a good aid in cleaning a furcation. A class III furcation leaves a plaque, debris, and food trap. There are several ways to treat a class III furcation. Successful treatment of a class III furcation can lead to a class IV furcation. This would be a clinical success.

25. **The correct answer is D.** The age of the tooth has no prognostic value in determining if a tooth is a candidate for crown lengthening. If the tooth has no mobility, sufficient attached gingiva, and favorable crown-to-root ratio, and the decay has not entered the furcation, the tooth in question is a viable candidate for crown lengthening. The goal of functional crown lengthening is to create a longer clinical crown to fabricate a restoration that will rest on sound tooth structure that is more than 2 mm away from the crestal bone.

26. **The correct answer is B.** A patient who presents 30% or more of attachment loss is classified as "generalized." Anything less than 30% is classified as "localized." The severity is characterized on the basis of the amount of clinical attachment loss—slight: 1 to 2 mm, moderate: 3 to 4 mm, and severe: anything 5 mm or greater.

27. **The correct answer is E.** A connective tissue graft is an autogenous subepithelial graft that is used to gain root coverage to treat gingival recession. This is the most predictable treatment modality for root coverage. It does not aid in pocket reduction.

28. **The correct answer is B.** The most unpredictable regenerative procedure in periodontal surgery is the regeneration of the interdental papillae. The other four choices are predictable objectives of periodontal surgery.

29. **The correct answer is B.** Dental plaque. Answer A is incorrect because enamel is the hardest and the outermost layer of a tooth structure. Answer C is incorrect because saliva is a secretion from salivary glands that moistens and helps in lubricating the food. Answer D is incorrect because dental caries is an infectious microbiologic disease of the teeth that results in localized dissolution and destruction of the calcified tissues.

30. **The correct answer is C.** Refractory periodontitis. Answer A is incorrect because aggressive periodontitis manifests before age 35 and leads to rapid deterioration of tissues. Answer B is incorrect because chronic periodontitis is a progressive loss of bone and soft tissues. Answer D is incorrect because juvenile periodontitis usually occurs in children and young adult, healthy individuals.

31. **The correct answer is C.** The calcifying epithelial odontogenic tumor (CEOT), or Pindborg tumor, radiographically shows a cyst like radiolucency, and it may contain very small foci of calcified material as white flecks. The CEOT has also been described radiographically to have a "driven snow" appearance. The calcifying odontogenic cyst and the adenomatoid odontogenic cyst radiographically would usually show a well-defined unilocular radiolucency associated with an unerupted tooth. Answer D is incorrect because radiographically, a keratocyst has a uni- or multi-locular appearance and is hazy because of the keratin-filled lumen.

32. **The correct answer is A.** Paget disease has increased alkaline phosphatase levels during osteoblastic phases. Answer B is incorrect because hypophosphatasia has low level of serum alkaline phosphatase activity. Answer C is incorrect because cherubism has no systemic abnormalities. Answer D is incorrect because in hyperparathyroidism, levels of alkaline phosphatase are normal.

33. **The correct answer is B.** Range of densities on a radiograph. Uneven density on a radiograph is incorrect because it is defined as radiographic mottle. Overall appearance of the radiographic is defined as image clarity. Overall degree of darkening of the radiograph is defined as radiographic density.

CHAPTER 8

Radiology

1. As digital radiography has becoming more prevalent for use in the dental settings, the common digital detectors used have changed. What is the most common digital detector used currently in dental digital radiography?

   A. Charged-couple device (CCD)
   B. Intensifying screen phosphors (ISP)
   C. Photostimulable phosphor (PSP)

2. A general dentist has been practicing dentistry for 36 years and is currently in the midst of remodeling his office. He would like to switch to digital radiography. The following are advantages of digital radiology technique in comparison to traditional techniques *except* for:

   A. Radiation dose reduction up to 60%
   B. Low cost of sensors
   C. Increased image resolution and contrast as compared to D speed film
   D. Delayed display of images
   E. Increased ability to detect proximal carries in noncavitated teeth

3. What are the components of a dental x-ray tube?

   A. Glass envelope
   B. Cathode
   C. Anode
   D. Tungsten target
   E. All of the above

4. What are the common rules to follow to have an accurate radiographic image formation when taking x-rays?

   A. Using the correct focal spot size
   B. Placing the film close enough to prevent distortion
   C. Cutting down the amount of divergent x-rays reaching the object by using the longest target-film distance
   D. 90-degree angle of the central ray of the x-ray in relation to the film
   E. Film and object should be as parallel as possible
   F. All of the above

5. Most of the incident radiation during x-ray imaging is absorbed by the soft tissue regions of the face.

   A. True
   B. False

6. A dental student would like to obtain a film that is diagnostic for identifying interproximal caries. After much searching on the internet, he comes to the conclusion that interproximal caries are best diagnosed with films that are low in contrast as it allows the clinician to see the subtle differences in tooth density.

   A. True
   B. False

7. A first-year dental student helping out in the clinic for the first time repeatedly obtains x-rays of tooth #14 with a zigzagged pattern. What could have prevented the zigzagged pattern on the radiographic image?

   A. Placing the film incorrectly with the lead portion facing the cone
   B. Telling the patient not to move during the exposure
   C. Bending the film less when placing in position
   D. Using the film only once instead of exposing it multiple times
   E. Decreasing the kilovoltage

8. A periapical film of tooth #9 was obtained in preparation for a root canal and an initial measurement for length of the canal was performed. After initial debridement of the canal was performed, another x-ray was captured with the initial root length measured and it appears that the file is approximately 4 mm from the apex. How could we have obtained a more accurate initial length measurement?

   A. Increasing the vertical angulation of the cone in relation to the film
   B. Decreasing the vertical angulation of the cone in relation to the film

Radiology

C. Decreasing the horizontal angulation of the cone in relation to the film

D. Increasing the horizontal angulation of the cone in relation to the film

9. What is the name of the radiographic technique when the central ray of the cone is directly perpendicular to the object?

A. Paralleling technique
B. Bisecting technique
C. Submentovertex technique

10. A 17-year-old male was referred to an oral surgeon for extraction of an impacted tooth #11 that is located in area apical to teeth #10–#12, which was found on routine x-rays. How would the oral surgeon decide as to where the impacted tooth lay in respect to being either buccal or palatal to teeth #10 and #12?

A. Application of the SLOB rule
B. Use of panoramic radiograph
C. Towne's view x-ray
D. Water's view x-ray
E. Lateral head radiograph

11. What are the triple arrows pointing to in Figure 8-1?

A. Floor of nasal fossa
B. Floor of maxillary sinus
C. Maxillary zygomatic arch
D. Sigmoid notch
E. Zygomatic bone

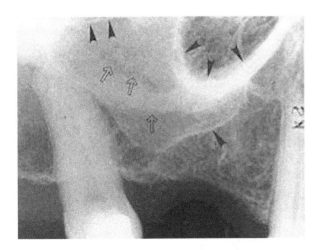

12. What are the double arrows pointing to in Figure 8-1?

A. Floor of nasal fossa
B. Maxillary zygomatic arch
C. Floor of maxillary sinus
D. Zygomatic bone
E. Schneiderian membrane

13. What is the single arrow pointing to in Figure 8-1?

A. Floor of nasal fossa
B. Maxillary zygomatic arch
C. Zygomatic bone
D. Inferior border of maxillary sinus
E. Sigmoid notch

14. What is the single arrow pointing to in Figure 8-2?

A. Lamina dura
B. Periodontal ligament
C. Cementum
D. Enamel
E. Dentin

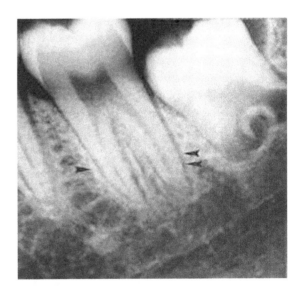

15. What are the double arrows pointing to in Figure 8-2?

A. Periodontal ligament
B. Lamina dura
C. Cementum
D. Enamel
E. Dentin

16. What structures are contained within the radiopaque structure surrounded by the three arrows in Figure 8-3?

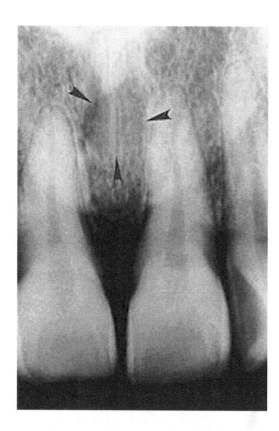

A. Inferior alveolar neurovascular bundle
B. Sphenopalatine neurovascular bundle
C. Infraorbital nerve
D. Facial nerve
E. Nasopalatine neurovascular bundle

17. #4 is referring to what structure in Figure 8-4?

A. Floor of maxillary sinus
B. Infraorbital margin
C. Zygomatic arch
D. Pterygomaxillary fissure
E. Floor of nasal fossa
F. Hard palate

18. #2 is referring to what structure in Figure 8-4?

A. Floor of maxillary sinus
B. Pterygomaxillary fissure
C. Zygomatic arch
D. Infraorbital margin
E. Floor of nasal fossa
F. Hard palate

19. #6 is referring to what structure in Figure 8-4?

A. Floor of maxillary sinus
B. Zygomatic arch
C. Hard palate
D. Pterygomaxillary fissure
E. Floor of nasal fossa
F. Nasal septum

20. #12 is referring to what structure?

A. Styloid process
B. Mandibular condyle
C. Occipital bone
D. Coronoid notch
E. Sphenoid bone
F. Cervical vertebrae

21. What is the main ingredient of the developing solution that serves to convert the exposed silver salts on the emulsion film into silver metallic ions?

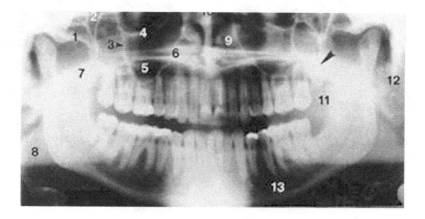

A. Sodium carbonate
B. Potassium bromide
C. Sodium sulfite
D. Hydroquinone
E. Acetic acid

22. What are the components of a developing solution?

A. Clearing agent, antioxidant preservative, acidifier, hardener
B. Developing agent, acidifier, antioxidant preservative, hardener
C. Developing agent, accelerator, restrainer
D. Clearing agent restrainer, accelerator, acidifier

23. In trying to reduce the amount of low-quality, long-wavelength x-rays from exiting the cone, what is commonly added to the cone for added filtration?

A. Aluminum disks
B. Tin disks
C. Thicker glass
D. Different color plastics

24. All of the following cells in the body are relatively resistant to damage by radiation *except*:

A. Muscle cells
B. Mucosal cells
C. Nerve cells
D. Mature bone

25. A 55-year-old female with a history of laryngeal cancer who underwent a prolong course of radiation and chemotherapy presents with pain to her left mandible for 3 weeks. Patient has also noticed a white material appearing through her mucosa. On examination, exposed alveolar bone is noted in teeth #19–#21 area and no erythema or purulence noted in the area. Teeth #19–#21 are without decay. What is likely the first choice in treatment?

A. Antibiotics
B. Daily sodium peroxide rinses
C. Hyperbaric oxygen therapy
D. Extraction of teeth #19–#21
E. Resection of left mandible with reconstruction
F. Saline rinses

26. Which positioning error would most likely cause a reverse occlusal plane curve on a Panorex?

A. Chin tilted too far upward
B. Chin tilted too far downward
C. Head turned slightly laterally

27. Which projection is best for examining zygomatic arch fractures?

A. Waters projection
B. Submentovertex projection
C. Reverse Towne projection
D. Lateral cephalometric projection

28. All of the following are advantages of a panoramic radiograph *except*:

A. It shows areas that may not be visible on a bitewing or periapical
B. It shows both arches on the same film
C. It gives better detail and definition than PAs
D. It is more comfortable for the patient because it eliminates the gagging reflex
E. It requires less time than a full mouth series

29. A phenomenon caused by a relatively lower x-ray absorption on the mesial or distal of a tooth between the edge of the enamel and the adjacent crest of the alveolar ridge is called

A. Apical burnout
B. Cervical burnout
C. Coronal burnout
D. Root burnout

30. Which intra-oral radiographs are the most useful in detecting interproximal caries?

A. Periapical x-rays
B. Bitewing x-rays
C. Occlusal x-rays

31. The period between radiation exposure and the onset of symptoms is called the

A. Latent period
B. Period of cell injury
C. Recovery period

Radiology

32. Removing parts of the x-ray spectrum by using absorbing materials in the x-ray beam is called:

    A. Elimination
    B. Filtration
    C. Collimation
    D. Reduction

33. X-ray fixer contains all of the following *except*:

    A. A clearing agent
    B. An antioxidant preservative
    C. An accelerator
    D. An acidifier
    E. A hardener

34. All are advantages of digital radiography *except*:

    A. Digital subtraction
    B. The ability to enhance the image
    C. Size of the intraoral sensor
    D. Patient education

35. The process of obtaining a digital image similar to scanning a photograph to a computer screen is called:

    A. Indirect digital imaging
    B. Direct digital imaging
    C. Storage phosphor imaging
    D. CMOS/APS

36. Which solid-state detector(s) is/are necessary to capture direct digital x-rays?

    A. CCD (charged-coupled device)
    B. CMOS/APS (complementary metal oxide semiconductor/active pixel sensor)
    C. CID (charge injection device)
    D. All of the above

37. Digital x-rays require less radiation than conventional x-rays because:

    A. The sensor is larger
    B. The exposure time is increased
    C. The sensor is more sensitive to x-rays
    D. The pixels sense transmitted light quickly

38. Which of the following errors in technique would be the most likely reason for an image to appear elongated?

    A. Too much vertical angulation
    B. Too little vertical angulation
    C. Incorrect horizontal angulation
    D. Beam not aimed at the center of the film

39. Foreshorting where the teeth appear too short is caused by:

    A. Too much vertical angulation
    B. Too little vertical angulation
    C. Incorrect horizontal angulation
    D. Beam not aimed at the center of the film

40. Elongation (the most common error) can be caused by:

    A. Too little vertical angulation
    B. The film is not parallel to the long axis
    C. The occlusal plane is not parallel to the floor
    D. All of the above

41. What is the major disadvantage of the paralleling technique?

    A. The image formed on the film will not have dimensional accuracy
    B. Because of the amount of distortion, periodontal bone height cannot be accurately diagnosed
    C. An increase in exposure time is necessary because of the use of a long cone
    D. An increase in exposure time is necessary because of the use of a short cone

42. Which cells are considered the most radioresistant?

    A. Immature reproductive cells
    B. Young bone cells
    C. Mature bone cells
    D. Epithelial cells

43. What is the recommended distance (in feet) that the operator should stand from the patient while taking radiographs?

    A. 2 feet
    B. 4 feet
    C. 6 feet
    D. 8 feet

44. The larger the focal spot the:

    A. The greater the loss of the definition and sharpness of the image

B. The lesser the loss of the definition and sharpness of the image
C. There is no effect

45. Copper is used to house the anode because:

A. It is a good thermal conductor
B. It dissipates heat from the tungsten target
C. It reduces the risk of melting the target
D. All of the above

46. The radiation generated at the anode of the x-ray tube is called:

A. Primary radiation
B. Scattered radiation
C. Potential radiation
D. Reverse radiation

47. X-rays have:

A. More energy than light
B. Less energy than light
C. The same energy as light

48. The yearly MPD (maximum permissible dose) for a nonoccupationally exposed person is:

A. 0.1 REM
B. 0.5 REM
C. 1.0 REM
D. 2.0 REM

49. The yearly MPD (maximum permissible dose) for someone who works near radiation is:

A. 1.0 REM
B. 2.0 REM
C. 3.5 REM
D. 5.0 REM

50. The most effective means in reducing the time of exposure, the amount of radiation reaching the patient and the amount of radiation scattered to the dentist is:

A. A lead apron
B. Ekta-speed film
C. Lead diaphragms
D. Increasing target-film distance

51. The use of metal plates, slots, etc., to confine and direct radiation to a specific region and/or to discriminate against radiation from unwanted directions such as scattered radiation is called:

A. Discrimination
B. Collimation
C. Filtration
D. Coning

52. Filtration:

A. Reduces patient dose
B. Decreases contrast
C. Decreases the density of the film
D. All of the above

53. The herringbone effect will appear on the processed film when:

A. The film is bent
B. The film is placed backwards in the mouth
C. An improper vertical angulation is used
D. An improper horizontal angulation is used

54. Image magnification may be minimized by:

A. Using a short cone
B. Placing the film as far from the tooth as possible
C. Using a long cone
D. Shortening the exposure time

55. The rules for producing the most accurate image formation when taking x-rays are the following *except*:

A. Using the largest focal spot
B. Using the longest source–film distance
C. Placing the film as close as possible to the object
D. Directing the central ray as close to a right angle to the film as anatomical structures will allow:
E. Keeping the film as parallel as possible to the object

56. The size of the focal spot influences radiographic definition and sharpness because they are:

A. Inversely proportional
B. Directly proportional
C. Not related

57. The one aspect of radiography the operator cannot control is:

    A. The source–film distance
    B. The object–film distance
    C. The size of the focal spot
    D. The angulation of the cone beam

58. A short cone (20 cm/8 inches):

    A. Exposes more tissue by producing a more divergent beam
    B. Exposes less tissue by producing a less divergent beam
    C. Produces a sharper image

59. A long cone (41 cm/16 inches):

    A. Exposes more tissue by producing a more divergent beam
    B. Exposes less tissue by producing a less divergent beam
    C. Produces a sharper image
    D. Both B and C

60. Osteoradionecrosis is more common:

    A. In the mandible
    B. In the maxilla

61. The image of the coronoid process of the mandible often appears in periapical x-rays of:

    A. The incisor region of the mandible
    B. The molar region of the mandible
    C. The incisor region of the maxilla
    D. The molar region of the maxilla

62. Which of the following is not a disadvantage of the bisecting technique?

    A. Image on x-ray film may be dimensionally distorted
    B. Increased exposure time
    C. If using a short cone, the image may be distorted
    D. May not be able to determine correct alveolar bone height

63. Which of the following projections is the best for evaluating the maxillary sinus?

    A. Lateral jaw projection
    B. Reverse Towne projection
    C. Waters projection
    D. Submentovertex projection

64. Which of the following projections is the best for evaluating midface fractures?

    A. Lateral jaw projection
    B. Reverse Towne projection
    C. Waters projection
    D. Submentovertex projection

65. Which of the following projections is the best for evaluating the condyles?

    A. Waters projection
    B. Transcranial projection
    C. Townes projection
    D. Submentovertex projection

66. Foreshortening and elongation are produced by:

    A. Incorrect horizontal angulation
    B. Incorrect vertical angulation
    C. Either of the above

67. X-ray developer contains all of the following *except*:

    A. A developing agent
    B. An antioxidant preservative
    C. A clearing agent
    D. An accelerator
    E. A restrainer

68. The functions of the developer and the fixer are:

    A. The developing solution reduces the silver halide crystals to black metallic silver while the fixing solution stops the development and removes the remaining unexposed crystals
    B. The developing solution stops the development and removes the remaining unexposed crystals while the fixing solution reduces the silver halide crystals to black metallic silver

69. After your film has been processed, you notice it appears brown in color. The most likely cause is:

    A. Solutions are too strong
    B. Solutions are too weak
    C. Fixing time was not long enough
    D. Fixing time was too long
    E. Film was underdeveloped

70. After your film has been processed, you notice it appears too dark in color. The least likely cause is:

    A. The film is overdeveloped
    B. The temperature of the solutions was too hot
    C. The temperature of the solutions was too cold

71. After your film has been processed, you notice it appears too light in color. The least likely cause is:

    A. The film was left in the solution for too short of a time
    B. The temperature of the solutions was too cold
    C. The solution was too weak
    D. The solution was too old
    E. None of the above

72. The unit for measuring the absorption of x-rays is called:

    A. REM
    B. RAD

C. Roentgen
D. QF

73. The unit used to measure the equivalent dose that relates the absorbed dose of the human tissue to the effect of the biological damage caused by the radiation is called:

    A. REM
    B. RAD
    C. Roentgen
    D. QF

74. Increasing Peak kilovoltage (kVp) causes the x-ray to have:

    A. Decreased density
    B. More latitude
    C. A shorter scale of contrast
    D. A longer scale of contrast

75. It is best to retain dental x-rays for:

    A. 2 years
    B. 4 years
    C. 6 years
    D. Indefinitely

Radiology

1. **The correct answer is A.** The digital receptor is the device that intercepts the x-ray beam after it has passed through the patient's body and produces an image in digital form, a matrix of pixels, each with a numerical value. Charged-couple device detectors, the most common digital receptor used in dentistry, consist of a chip of pure silicon with an active area that is divided into a two-dimensional array of elements called pixels. CCD detectors generally have a smaller active surface area which approximate intraoral film in size. Intensifying screen phosphor detectors produce an image via the creation of an optical signal when a light is emitted from the incident x-radiation against the phosphor screen. Photo-stimulable phosphor receptors (PSP) work differently from ISP. X-ray photons excite the electrons in the phosphors and light is produced but a significant amount of electrons are trapped. The image is produced when a laser in the read-out unit stimulates the trapped electrons to produce an emitted blue light that is detected by a photomultiplier tube and the output of the tube is digitized to form the image. They are the most widely used detectors in medical radiology.

2. **The correct answer is B.** Advantages of digital technique include radiation dose reduction up to 60% compared with D-speed films, immediate display of images, and ability to enhance image (changes in contrast, gray scale, and brightness). High initial cost of sensors is a disadvantage. Digital-image resolution and contrast is decreased compared with D-speed film. Digital radiology allows us to have immediate display of images. Ability to detect proximal carries in noncavitated teeth via digital radiology is only comparable and not increased with the newer direct digital-imaging techniques.

3. **The correct answer is E.** Dental x-ray tube consists of a glass that houses a vacuum. Inside this vacuum environment is the cathode, anode, and a tungsten target. X-ray is produced when the cathode is heated up to emit electrons, an electrical potential is then created between the cathode and anode with tungsten target in the middle.

When the electrons strike the tungsten target, X-rays are produced.

4. **The correct answer is F.** All of the above and as per the answers.

5. **The correct answer is B.** Subject contrast is the range of characteristics of the subject that influences the radiographic contrast. Dense regions of the face such as the bone and teeth and bones absorb most of the incident radiation. Less dense regions of the face such as the soft tissue profile transmit most of the radiation. Subject contrast is also influenced by the energy of the x-ray beam, such as when the kVp is increased, the overall density of the image also increases, and when it is decreased, the subject contrast increases. A fine balance has to be struck with the kVp and exposure time to obtain an image where subtle changes can be observed and be diagnostic.

6. **The correct answer is B.** Film contrast describes the ability of a radiographic film to reveal differences in the subject's contrast, meaning the variations in the intensity of the remnant beam that strikes the film. A high contrast film reveals small differences in the subject's contrast more clearly than a low-contrast film. Proper exposure of a film will have more contrast than underexposed, light, films. Proper processing is another factor as mishandling of the film will result in incomplete or excessive development will result in diminished contrast of the anatomic structures.

7. **The correct answer is A.** The zigzagged pattern is the result of incorrectly placing the film with the exposed portion facing away from the cone and the lead portion facing the cone causing the herringbone effect. A blurred image is caused when a patient moves during exposure. Overbent films will appear as black semilunar radiopacities or cracks in the film image. Multiple images will appear on the same film if it is exposed more than once. Poor contrast results when the kilovoltage is set too high and not a herringbone image.

8. **The correct answer is B.** Foreshortening is characterized by the film image appearing squashed or shortened in the vertical, caused by too much vertical angulation of the cone in relation to the film. Elongation is the opposite in that the image appears stretched in the vertical caused by too little angulation of the cone to the object. Changing the horizontal angulation of the cone in relation to the film will not change the length of the image.

9. **The correct answer is A.** For the paralleling technique to be accurate in the image capture, the film must be parallel to the long axis of the tooth and the target to film distance must be optimum. Bisecting technique is the technique when a film is placed against the tooth with the central ray perpendicular to the bisecting line made from the angle of the film to the tooth. Disadvantages of this technique include distortion when the angulation is increased and the necessity of a short cone that increases the amount of divergent x-rays. Submentovertex technique is used to provide information on the zygoma, zygomatic arches, and mandible. The occlusal film is placed on the occlusal plane with the emulsion facing the chin and the central x-ray placed perpendicular to the film.

10. **The correct answer is A.** The SLOB rule, or the 'Same side lingual, opposite side buccal' rule can be applied when multiple periapical x-rays are taken in an area. To do this, a reference point must first be assigned with a single PA (such as the root tip of tooth #12). Then, another periapical x-ray is taken, except, this time, the central ray is off-set mesially by 60 degrees. If the impacted tooth #11 appears to move in the same direction of the x-ray tube, then the object (tooth #11) is lingual to the reference point. If the impacted tooth #11 appears to move opposit to the cone, then the object (tooth #11) is buccal to the reference point. The panoramic radiograph can be used as a survey for initial screening for pathology of the maxilla and mandible and offers views of the condylar head and ramus of the mandible. The lateral cephalometric radiograph is used in cephalometric analysis and evaluation of craniofacial growth. The Towne's view is a reverse tilted AP projection that shows the occipital

bone, foramen magnum, mandibular condyles and the midfacial skeleton. The Water's view is an angled PA radiograph of the skull that shows the orbits and maxillary sinuses.

11. **The correct answer is C.** The maxillary zygomatic process forms a radiopaque U-shaped structure from which the zygoma extends posteriorly.

12. **The correct answer is A.** The thin horizontal radiopaque line represents the floor of the nasal fossae.

13. **The correct answer is D.** The inferior border of the maxillary sinus projects downwards.

14. **The correct answer is A.** The bone lining the tooth socket is the lamina dura.

15. **The correct answer is A.** The roots of the tooth are separated from the lamina dura of the socket by the periodontal ligament.

16. **The correct answer is E.** The radiopaque structure being demarcated by the arrows is the incisive foramen. Contained within the nasopalatine foramen is the nasopalatine nerve, artery, and vein.

17. **The correct answer is B.** As per answer.

18. **The correct answer is B.** As per answer.

19. **The correct answer is C.** As per answer.

20. **The correct answer is A.** As per answer.

21. **The correct answer is D.** Hydroquinone is the main ingredient in the developing agent. It converts the exposed silver salts on the emulsion film into silver metallic ions while unexposed silver salts are left unaffected. Sodium Carbonate is an alkali salt in the developing solution that maintains the alkaline pH of the solution as well as provides ideal conditions for reactions to occur. Potassium bromide controls the action of the developing agent such that the unexposed silver salts on the emulsion film are not removed. Sodium sulfite serves to prevent the fixer from spontaneous oxidative processes. Acetic Acid is in the fixer solution and serves to neutralize any

alkaline developing agent carried over and also serves to buffer the solution.

22. **The correct answer is C.** Components of a developing solution include the developing agent, accelerator, restrainer, and antioxidant preservative. The developing agent converts the exposed silver salts on the emulsion film into silver metallic ions. The accelerator maintains the alkali pH of the solution to provide the ideal condition for the reaction to occur. The restrainer prevents the unexposed silver salts from being removed from the emulsion film. The clearing agent, antioxidant preservative, acidifier, and hardener are components of the fixer solution.

23. **The correct answer is A.** For added filtration, additional aluminum disks are placed in the cone to filter the lower grade radiation. Inherent filtration of the beam is accomplished by the glass or plastic cones.

24. **The correct answer is B.** Radiosensitive cells are cells in the body that undergo rapid mitosis or meiosis in the body and include cells such as mucosal cells, hair cells, reproductive cells, lymphocytes, and bone marrow. Radioresistant cells typically do not undergo rapid mitosis or meiosis and are less susceptible to the damage caused by radiation and include cells such as muscle, nerves, and mature bone.

25. **The correct answer is F.** Patients with previous exposure to radiation therapy to head and neck area can develop osteoradionecrosis of the bone. The mandible is the most common site as it is less vascular than the maxilla. The period in between the initial exposure and the first clinical sign of damage is known as the "latency period." Treatment for osteoradionecrosis is primarily supportive and includes superficial debridement of the wound, saline rinses, and nutritional support. Antibiotics are only used if there is definite secondary infection. Hyperbaric oxygen therapy has been advocated but is controversial and results have been inconclusive. Unless the teeth are unrestorable, they should not be extracted.

26. **The correct answer is B.** If the chin is tilted too upward, the occlusal plane on the radiograph may appear flat or inverted. If the chin is tilted too far downward, the teeth become severely overlapped and the symphyseal region of the mandible may be cut off the film. Head slightly turned laterally will cause either depending on the direction of the turned head to be unequally magnified.

27. **The correct answer is B.** The submentovertex view demonstrates the base of the skull, the sphenoid sinuses, the lateral wall of the maxillary sinuses, the curvature of the mandible, and the curvature of the zygomatic arches. The water's view is a slight variation of the PA view and it is useful for evaluating the maxillary sinuses, the frontal and ethmoid sinuses, the orbits, the zygomaticofrontal suture, and the nasal cavity. The reverse Towne's projection is used to evaluate for a condylar fracture, especially a medially displaced condyle. The lateral cephalometric projection is used to survey the skull and bones of the face for abnormalities.

28. **The correct answer is C.** Panoramic radiographs are useful for evaluating problems that require broad coverage of the mandible and maxilla. It is useful as the initial survey film that will provide insight into the need for other more specific films such as intraoral periapical films.

29. **The correct answer is B.** This phenomenon may cause intact mesial or distal tooth surfaces to appear carious on the radiograph when it is not. A true carious lesion can be differentiated by the absence of an image of the tooth edge and by the appearance of a diffuse inner border where the tooth substance has been lost.

30. **The correct answer is B.** Posterior bitewings are useful for evaluating for caries in the distal third of the canine, and the interproximal and occlusal surfaces of the premolars and molars. Periapical x-rays are useful for detecting changes in the periapical and interradicular bone. Occlusal radiographs display a large area of a dental arch and may include either the palate or the floor of the mouth. This is useful in examining for precise locations of roots, supernumerary or unerupted teeth, foreign objects in floor of the mouth, evaluating maxillary sinuses and for

patients with trismus that can only open a few millimeters.

31. **The correct answer is A.** Latent period is the time between exposure to radiation and the appearance of a delayed effect. Period of cell injury is when a cell is exposed to radiation and is affected by it either through direction interaction where a cell's macromolecule such as protein or DNA are hit by the ionizing radiation which affects the cell as a whole or through indirect interaction when the radiation energy is deposited in the cell and the radiation interacts with the cellular water rather than with macromolecules within the cell. Recovery period is used to refer to the period after radiation therapy when the body replaces the malignant cells with normal cells.

32. **The correct answer is B.** Filtration is the mechanism where the low-quality, long-wavelength x-rays are absorbed by the exiting beam. Collimation refers to the control of the size and shape of the emitted beam through the use of shaped cones to reduce the total area exposed to radiation. Elimination and reduction are terms not used in radiation physics.

33. **The correct answer is C.** X-ray fixer consists of clearing agent, antioxidant preservative, acidifier, and hardener.

34. **The correct answer is C.** The size of the intraoral sensor tends to be three to four times the size of an intraoral film. Advantages to using digital radiography include the ability for digital subtraction, immediate display of images, ability to enhance images, and radiation dose of up to 60%. It is easier for patient education as you can enlarge the image on the computer screen to demonstrate the findings to the patient.

35. **The correct answer is A.** Radiographic film is used as the image receiver and the image is subsequently digitized from signals created by a video device or scanner that views the radiograph. Radiographic image is acquired by a CCD or complementary metal oxide semiconductor that is sensitive to electromagnetic radiation. In storage phosphor imaging, phos-phor screens are exposed to ionizing radiation, which excites the BaFBR/EU+2 crystals in the screen storing the image. A computer-assisted laser then promotes the release of energy from the crystals in the form of blue light that is subsequently scanned to reconstruct the image digitally. CMOS stands for complementary metal oxide semiconductor, which is one of the detectors used for direct digital imaging.

36. **The correct answer is D.** Charged-couple device consists of a chip or pure silicon with an active area called pixels. After exposure to radiation, charges stored by the pixels are sequentially removed electronically and an output signal is created. Charge injection device is an image sensor in that the image points are accessed in reference to their horizontal and vertical coordinates. Complementary metal oxide semiconductor/active pixel sensor is an image sensor consisting of an integrated circuit containing an array of pixel sensors, each pixel containing a photodetector and amplifier.

37. **The correct answer is C.** Sensors used in digital radiography are more efficient than film in detecting radiation. Sensors used in digital radiography tend to be larger and bulkier compared to plain films but size is not the reason as to why it requires less radiation. Exposure time in digital radiography is decreased compared with plain films as the sensors are more sensitive. Pixels sense transmitted electromagnetic energy in the range of x-rays and not visible light.

38. **The correct answer is B.** When the beam of the x-ray is not perpendicular to the bisector plane, the length of the projected image of the tooth can change. If the central beam is directed at too much vertical angulation, the tooth can appear foreshortened and when there is too little vertical angulation, it appears elongated. Horizontal angulation does not cause elongation or foreshortening of the image on film.

39. **The correct answer is A.** When the beam of the x-ray is not perpendicular to the bisector plane, the length of the projected image of the tooth can change. If the central beam is directed at too much vertical angulation, the tooth can appear

foreshortened and when there is too little vertical angulation, it appears elongated. Horizontal angulation does not cause elongation or foreshortening of the image on film.

40. **The correct answer is D.** If the central beam is directed at too little vertical angulation, the resultant radiographic image will appear elongated. Elongation of a radiographic image occurs when the central ray is perpendicular to the object but not the film. When the occlusal plane is not parallel to the floor, the tooth and film is likely not perpendicular to the central x-ray causing elongation.

41. **The correct answer is C.** The paralleling technique uses a long cone to increase the focal spot-to-object distance and as a result of the increased distance, an increase in exposure time is necessary. The paralleling technique is the preferred method for intraoral radiographs as it allows for minimal image distortion and more accurate imaging, such as assessing periodontal bone height. There is slight image magnification because to achieve the parallel orientation, the practitioner must often place the film toward the middle of the oral cavity away from the teeth.

42. **The correct answer is C.** The most radiosensitive cells are cells with high mitotic rates, undergo many future mitoses, and are most primitive in differentiation such as immature reproductive cells, young cells, and epithelial cells.

43. **The correct answer is C.** The radiation received by the person taking the x-ray comes from the scatter. The strength of the radiation hitting any unit area falls off geometrically depending on the distance from the source of scatter. A person standing 6 feet away from the target receives one-ninth as much scatter radiation as person standing 2 feet away from the target.

44. **The correct answer is A.** The focal spot is the area on the target where the focusing cup directs the electrons from the filament. The sharpness and definition of the image decreases as the size of the focal spot increases. The heat generated per unit target area becomes decreased as the focal spot increases in size.

45. **The correct answer is D.** The anode consist of a tungsten target embedded in a copper stem and the purpose of the target in an x-ray tube is to convert the kinetic energy of the electrons generated from the filament into x-ray photons. The thermal conductivity of the target is relatively low and as a result is typically embedded in a large copper block. Copper is a good thermal conductor that dissipates heat from the tungsten target to reduce the risk of melting the target.

46. **The correct answer is A.** Primary radiation is emitted directly from the anode in the x-ray tube toward the object. Scattered radiation arises from the interactions of the primary radiation beam with the atoms in the object being image and deviates from the straight line between the x-ray focus and the image receptor.

47. **The correct answer is A.** X-radiation is a form of electromagnetic radiation with wavelengths in the range of 10–0.01 nm with frequencies in the range of 30 PHz to 30 EHz and energies in the range from 12 eV to 120 KeV. Visible light consists of photons with energies from 1.6 eV (red light) up to 3.4 eV (violet light).

48. **The correct answer is B.** The maximum permissible dose of radiation for a nonoccupationally exposed worker in a calendar year is 0.5 REM.

49. **The correct answer is D.** The maximum permissible dose of radiation for radiation workers in a calendar year is 5 REM.

50. **The correct answer is B.** Film speed can be an important aspect in determining the amount of radiation exposure received by a patient. The greater the film speed, the lesser the radiation exposure received by the patient.

51. **The correct answer is B.** A collimator is a device for use to narrow waves or particles toward a specific region. Filtration in radiology is used to absorb the lower-energy photons emitted by the tube before they reach the targets. Use of filter

produces a cleaner image by absorbing the lower energy x-ray photons that tend to scatter more.

52. **The correct answer is D.** Filtration in radiology is used to absorb the lower-energy photons emitted by the tube before they reach the targets. Use of filter produces a cleaner image by absorbing the lower energy x-ray photons that tend to scatter more.

53. **The correct answer is B.** When the film is placed backwards in the mouth, the image of the foil which is in a herringbone fashion would appear on the processed film. Overlapped contacts of interproximal surfaces of teeth will superimpose over each other if the direction of the x-rays is misdirected in the horizontal plane. A shortened image or elongated image will appear if too much vertical angulation is used or not enough vertical angulation is used, respectively.

54. **The correct answer is C.** A long cone results in greater definition and less image magnification. A short cone is used to take x-rays with the bisecting-angle technique. The resultant image is somewhat larger than when using the long cone. Placing the film away from the tooth results in distortion and image magnification. Shortening the exposure time will not change size of the image but clarity of film.

55. **The correct answer is A.** The increase in the source–film distance increases the sharpness of the image. To get the most accurate image, the smallest focal spot should be used. The distance between the film and object should be as close as possible and the film should be parallel. To decrease the distortion, the x-ray should be as close to a right angle to the film as possible.

56. **The correct answer is A.** As the size of the focal spot decreases, the radiographic definition, and sharpness increases.

57. **The correct answer is C.** Size of the focal spot is set on the anode of the x-ray by the manufacturer and cannot be changed by the operator.

58. **The correct answer is A.** A short cone is used to take x-rays with bisecting angle exposure tech-

niques. The target-film distance is usually 8 inches and the beam is more divergent causing more tissue to be exposed. The resulting image x-ray is also somewhat larger than the long cone. Image is also less sharp compared to a long cone.

59. **The correct answer is D.** The x-ray source to object distance should be as long as possible. This will enable the x-ray photons to emerge in a straighter line in a less divergent beam, therefore producing more accurate shadow. The straighter the x-ray photon line, the less divergent the beam with a resulting image that is more accurate.

60. **The correct answer is A.** Osteoradionecrosis is a complication of surgery or trauma in a previously irradiated bone. Radiation-induced vascular insufficiency rather than infection causes bone death and occurs most commonly in the mandible after head and neck irradiation. Condition is painful, debilitating, and may result in significant bone loss. The recommended treatment guidelines include irrigation, antibiotics, hyperbaric oxygen therapy, and surgical techniques, including hemimandibulectomy and graft placements.

61. **The correct answer is D.** In the periapical x-rays of the maxilla, the image of the coronoid process of the mandible often appears.

62. **The correct answer is B.** Exposure time is similar between the bisecting technique and parallel technique determined by film speed. But images resulting from the bisecting technique maybe dimensionally distorted and may not be able to determine the correct alveolar bone height depending on the angulation of the x-ray.

63. **The correct answer is C.** Waters projection is an x-ray technique used to show the maxilla, maxillary sinuses, and zygomatic bones. Lateral Jaw projection is useful to examine the posterior region of the mandible and this radiographic projection is also called the lateral oblique view. Reverse Townes projection is a tilted mandibular posterior anterior projection to shows the frontal view of those portions of the mandible that can only be visualized laterally in the panoramic film. Submentovertex projection helps to

identify the position of the condyle, visualize base of the skull, and evaluate fractures of the zygomatic arch. This projection also demonstrates the sphenoid and the ethmoid sinuses and lateral wall of maxillary sinus.

64. The correct answer is C.

65. The correct answer is C. Townes projection is a reverse tilted anterior–posterior technique of the skull used for the visualization of the foramen magnum, petrous ridges, internal auditory canal, mandibular condyle, and articulating fossa. Waters projection is an x-ray technique used to show the maxilla, maxillary sinuses, and zygomatic bones. Transcranial projection is a technique used to evaluate the condylar head anatomy and position in relation to the fossa from a lateral aspect. Submentovertex projection helps to identify the position of the condyle, visualize base of the skull, and evaluate fractures of the zygomatic arch. This projection also demonstrates the sphenoid and the ethmoid sinuses and lateral wall of maxillary sinus.

66. The correct answer is B. A shortened image or elongated image will appear if too much vertical angulation is used or not enough vertical angulation is used, respectively. Overlapped contacts of interproximal surfaces of teeth will superimpose over each other if the direction of the x-rays is misdirected in the horizontal plane.

67. The correct answer is C. Components of a developing solution include the developing agent, accelerator, restrainer, and antioxidant preservative. The developing agent converts the exposed silver salts on the emulsion film into silver metallic ions. The accelerator maintains the alkali pH of the solution to provide the ideal condition for the reaction to occur. The restrainer prevents the unexposed silver salts from being removed from the emulsion. Clearing agent, antioxidant preservative, acidifier, and hardener are components of the fixer solution.

68. The correct answer is A. As per answer. The role of the developing solution is to reduce the silver halide crystals to black metallic silver while the fixing solution stops the devel-

opment and removes the remaining unexposed crystals.

69. The correct answer is C. When solutions are too weak or if it is excessively fixed or when the film is underdeveloped, a light radiograph results. If it appears brown in color, it can be because of multiple causes such as fixing time that is not long enough, depleted fixer, insufficient washings, or contaminated solutions. When solutions are too strong, the radiograph becomes very dark.

70. The correct answer is C. When a dark radiograph results it is because of processing errors such as overdevelopment with too high a temperature or too long a time in the developer, inadequate fixation, accidental exposure to light, or improper safelighting. A dark radiograph can also result due to overexposure from excessive milliamperage, excessive peak kilovoltage excessive time, or too short a film to source distance. When a solution is to cold, underdevelopment of the radiograph results and a light radiograph is the result.

71. The correct answer is E. A light radiograph is the result of processing errors and underexposure. Processing errors such as underdevelopment with too low a processing temperature or too short a time, depleted developer diluted, or contaminated developer or excessive fixation will cause a light radiograph. Underexposure from insufficient milliamperage, insufficient peak kilovoltage, insufficient time, too great a fill to source distance or reversed film packet in mouth are also causes of a light radiograph.

72. The correct answer is B. Absorbed dose is a measure of the amount of energy absorbed by any ionizing radiation per unit mass of any type of matter. RAD, radiation absorbed dose, is the traditional unit. The SI unit is gray, Gy, and 1 Gy is equal to 1 J/kg. Roentgen equivalent man, REM, is the traditional unit of equivalent dose. The equivalent dose is used to compare the biologic effects of different types of radiation on a tissue. Roentgen, R, is the traditional unit used to measure radiation quantity, the capacity of radiation to ionize air. Quality factor, QF, is a variable that takes into account the different degrees of biological damage produced by equal doses of different types of radiation.

73. **The correct answer is A.** Roentgen equivalent man, REM, is the traditional unit of equivalent dose. The equivalent dose is used to compare the biologic effects of different types of radiation on a tissue. Absorbed dose is a measure of the amount of energy absorbed by any ionizing radiation per unit mass of any type of matter. RAD, radiation absorbed dose, is the traditional unit. The SI unit is gray, Gy, and 1 Gy is equal to 1 J/kg. Roentgen, R, is the traditional unit used to measure radiation quantity, the capacity of radiation to ionize air. Quality factor, QF, is a variable that takes into account the different degrees of biological damage produced by equal doses of different types of radiation.

74. **The correct answer is D.** As the kilovoltage is increased, the energy of the x-ray beam is increased and the scale of contrast is decreased. A low contrast image allows for the visualization of smaller differences in density within an object and a longer scale of contrast results. Higher kilovoltage images are useful for periodontal diagnosis where minute changes in bone can be detected. Lower kVp images are useful when analyzing large differences in density within an object such as caries or soft tissue calcifications.

75. **The correct answer is D.** Ideally, records and x-rays should be maintained and kept accessible indefinitely as it is the patient's treatment history. But, regulations for record retention do exist and are mostly regulated by individual state regulations. HIPAA mandates a 6-year requirement to keep records, but offices should abide by the state requirements.

Radiology

CHAPTER 9

Pathology

1. An otherwise healthy 19-year-old female was admitted to the pediatric ward with longstanding, multiple painful oral ulcers on her buccal mucosa and ventral tongue. She was underweight and reported severe oral pain. An examination revealed lesions on her skin similar to those in her mouth. She was placed on acyclovir. The lesions persisted and showed no signs of improvement. Ophthalmologic and pelvic examination revealed no lesions. Which of the following is the most likely diagnosis?

   A. Pemphigus vulgaris
   B. Benign mucous membrane pemphigoid (BMMP)
   C. Erythema multiforme (EM)
   D. Recurrent aphthous stomatitis
   E. Herpes simplex

2. A 45-year-old male smoker presents with a slightly elevated, asymptomatic 2 mm × 1 cm white plaque on the posterior lateral tongue extending onto the ventral surface. The lesion was picked up on routine head and neck examination and the patient was unaware of its existence. Adjacent to this area, a molar with a fractured distolingual cusp is present. What is the most appropriate action to be taken?

   A. Inform the patient that this is a high-risk area for oral cancer and biopsy immediately.
   B. Make a note of the lesion in the chart describing its size and appearance and re-evaluate at a 3-month recall visit.
   C. Inform the patient that this is due to trauma from biting his tongue and is nothing to be concerned about.
   D. Remove any suspected etiology and biopsy in 2 weeks if still present and not improving.

3. There are many types of odontogenic tumors, both benign and malignant. Treatment for these neoplasms varies from simple procedures such as curettage to more extensive surgery, including resections. Knowing the prevalence, prognosis, and associated features of these lesions will help with both patient education and in determining a more predictable treatment plan and outcome. What is the most common clinically significant odontogenic tumor?

   A. Adenomatoid odontogenic tumor (AOT)
   B. Cementoblastoma
   C. Ameloblastoma
   D. Calcifying epithelial odontogenic tumor (CEOT)
   E. Hemangioma
   F. Odontogenic myxoma

4. A routine panoramic examination revealed the following finding in 17-year-old male. All of the teeth in the quadrant were vital and the patient was asymptomatic. Intraorally, there was obliteration of the vestibule on the affected side. Which of the following is the most likely diagnosis?

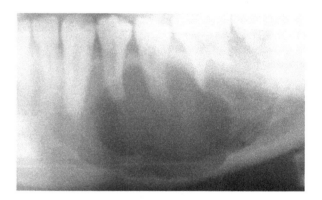

   A. Dentigerous cyst
   B. Osteosarcoma
   C. Periapical cyst
   D. Buccal bifurcation cyst
   E. Ameloblastoma

5. A 45-year-old male of Southeast Asian descent presents to the dentist with a chief complaint of staining of his teeth and difficulty opening his mouth to chew. Upon clinical examination, it is noted that the patient has a maximum opening of 27 mm. Diffuse white lesions are seen bilaterally on his buccal mucosa, lateral borders of tongue, and labial mucosa. Further inspection of his buccal mucosa reveals what is seen in this picture. Subsequent manipulation of this mucosa did not change the appearance of the

lesion. He reports no pain associated with any of the intraoral findings. His social history is significant for 20 pack-years smoking and occasional alcohol drinking. What is the most likely diagnosis of the lesions in this patient's mouth?

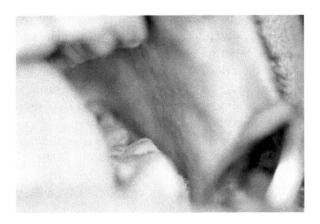

A. Smoker's melanosis
B. Oral submucous fibrosis
C. Morsicatio buccarum
D. Oral hairy leukoplakia (OHL)
E. Leukoedema

6. A 38-year-old otherwise healthy male presents with a crusted-over ulcer on his left upper lip. He states that he noticed a tingling 9 days ago and little "blisters" 8 days ago. He reports having had lesions like this before and is positive that he has never had any intraoral lesions in the past. What is the best plan of treatment for his current lesion?

A. Re-evaluate in 2 weeks
B. Topical antivirals
C. Systemic antivirals
D. Biopsy the lesion
E. Refer to ophthalmologist

7. A 33-year-old otherwise healthy male presents to the clinic with a 5-mm diameter painless ulcer on his left upper lip that has been present for 3 weeks. He reports sexual encounters with multiple partners over the past 3 months and has no other symptoms. What is the most likely diagnosis of this lesion?

A. *Histoplasma capsulatum* infection
B. *Herpes simplex* infection
C. *Cryptococcus neoformans* infection

D. *Neisseria gonorrhoeae* infection
E. *Treponema pallidum* infection

8. A 43-year-old male presents for routine dental care. He is asymptomatic and intraoral and extraoral examinations are all within normal limits. All teeth in the lower right quadrant were vital. A panoramic radiograph was taken. What is the most likely diagnosis?

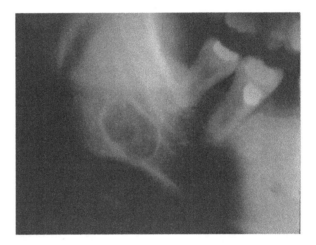

A. Dentigerous cyst
B. Metastatic lesion
C. Stafne bone cyst
D. Calcifying odontogenic cyst
E. Periapical cyst

9. A 40-year-old female presents to the dental clinic with the following appearance of her lateral tongue. She is asymptomatic and a former intravenous (IV) drug user. She also reports a 25-pack-year history of smoking. A cytologic smear was positive for candida organisms and the lesion was treated with antifungals. A follow-up examination 2 weeks later showed some resolution of the lesion, but white patches were still present and were subsequently biopsied. The biopsy demonstrated chromatin beading of the superficial epithelial cells that was consistent with Oral hairy leukoplakia (OHL). She reports no lesions elsewhere and that she is in good health. What is the next step in the management of this patient?

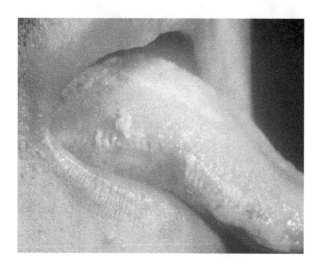

A. Watch the lesion at subsequent follow-up visits and biopsy if there is a change.
B. Referral to her primary care physician for HIV testing.
C. Do nothing and continue routine dental.
D. Excise the lesion with margins.
E. Treat the lesion with topical steroids.

10. A 65-year-old man presents with painless cervical lymphadenopathy. He notes gradual enlargement over the past year. A routine radiographic examination revealed no abnormalities in any bones. He is asymptomatic and the rest of his physical examination is unremarkable. Biopsy of the neck mass demonstrated binucleated ("owl-eye") and multinucleated cells with prominent nucleoli. These findings are consistent with a diagnosis of which of the following?

A. Burkitt's lymphoma, African type
B. Burkitt's lymphoma, North American type
C. Multiple myeloma
D. Ewing's sarcoma
E. Hodgkin's lymphoma

11. A 14-year-old male presents with diffuse, boggy, nontender enlargement of maxillary and mandibular gingiva. His parents report no significant prior medical history and that he has never been on any kind of long-term medication. Scaling was performed and no resolution was noted at a 2-week re-evaluation. A biopsy was performed and the tissue showed infiltration of normal tissue by sheets of poorly differentiated cells with myelomonocytic characteristics. These findings are most consistent with a diagnosis of which of the following disorders?

A. Leukemia
B. Thrombocytopenia
C. Neutropenia
D. Multiple myeloma
E. Anemia

12. A 63-year-old nonsmoking African American female presents with a 3-cm preauricular single nodular mass. She states that the lesion has been slowly growing over the past 13 years. She is asymptomatic and wants it removed for cosmetic reasons. Examination reveals that the nodule is freely mobile and not fixed to underlying tissue. The most likely diagnosis for this lesion is which of the following?

A. Warthin's tumor
B. Hodgkin's lymphoma
C. Adenoid cystic carcinoma
D. Pleomorphic adenoma
E. None of the above

13. A 24-year-old male presents at a clinic for routine dental care. A panoramic radiograph is taken and a 2 × 2 cm multilocular radiolucency is noticed in the right posterior mandible. The patient is asymptomatic, and there is no clinical expansion noted. An incisional biopsy is performed and the specimen shows focal areas of giant cells clustered around areas of hemorrhage. The background stroma consists of plump,

ovoid-shaped cells. What is the next step in the management of this patient?

A. Assess circulating platelet levels
B. Assess serum calcium levels
C. Enucleation of the lesion
D. Intralesional steroid injections
E. Partial mandibular resection

14. A 12-year-old healthy male presents for routine dental care during December vacation from school. Upon examination, you notice that he has coryza, cough, and red, watery, photophobic eyes. He is slightly febrile and has significant lymphadenopathy. His mother reports that he has been symptomatic for the past 2 days. Intraorally, he has multiple areas of erythema bilaterally on his buccal mucosa. Within these erythematous areas, numerous small, painless, blue-white macules are noted. No other lesions were noted elsewhere on his body. What is the most likely diagnosis?

A. Rubeola
B. Mumps
C. Secondary herpes simplex
D. Hand-foot-and-mouth disease
E. None of the above

15. A 45-year-old female presents with multiple osteomas, odontomas, and supernumerary teeth. She reports a history of intestinal polyps. What syndrome does this patient most likely have?

A. Gorlin syndrome
B. Ascher syndrome
C. Gardner syndrome
D. Klinefelter's syndrome

16. A 49-year-old HIV+ male with a CD4+ count of 120 presents with a long-standing indurated, ulcerated lesion on the right lateral border of his tongue. A biopsy was performed and a fungal organism was detected. A special stain (mucicarmine) was positive and provided positive identification of the fungal organism. Which of these fungal organisms has a mucopolysaccharide capsule that is mucicarmine-positive?

A. *Blastomyces dermatitidis*
B. *Paracoccidioides brasiliensis*
C. *Histoplasma capsulatum*
D. *Cryptococcus neoformans*

17. A mass in the right mandibular buccal vestibule of a 60-year-old female has been slowly enlarging over the past few months. Upon biopsy, sheets of amorphous, glassy pink material are noted subjacent to the surface epithelium. Which of the following disorders is consistent with this finding?

A. Hodgkin's lymphoma
B. Multiple myeloma
C. African-type Burkitt's lymphoma
D. Ewing's sarcoma

18. A 27-year-old male presents for evaluation of gingival discoloration. The discoloration appears as a bluish line along the marginal gingiva. Gray areas are also noted on the buccal mucosa and tongue. Upon protrusion of his tongue, a visible tremor is noted. Radiographs reveal advanced periodontal disease. Salivary flow tests indicate excessive salivation. These findings are most consistent with which of the following?

A. Plumbism
B. Acrodynia
C. Argyria
D. Arsenic poisoning

19. A 15-year-old male with a history of epilepsy and grand mal seizures presents for routine dental care. His medical history is otherwise unremarkable. Upon examination, he is noted to have generalized moderate gingival hyperplasia. Which of the following drugs is the most likely cause of his gingival hyperplasia?

A. Sodium valproate
B. Cyclosporine
C. Verapamil
D. Nifedipine

20. An otherwise healthy 10-year-old male presents for routine dental care. Upon examination, multiple teeth (both deciduous and permanent) are noted to be mobile. Bitewings and periapical films are taken. Moderate to severe bone loss is noted in all four quadrants. No other radiographic changes are noted and the patient is normocephalic. Examination of the ventral surface of the hands reveals palmar keratosis. While questioning, the patient reveals similar findings on the soles of his feet. No other skin lesions are noted. On the basis of this information, what is the most likely diagnosis of this patient?

    A. Nevoid basal cell carcinoma syndrome
    B. Apert syndrome
    C. Ascher syndrome
    D. Papillon–Lefèvre syndrome

21. A 50-year-old female with no significant medical history presents for evaluation of "sores on her gums." Upon inspection, several areas of Desquamative gingivitis are noted. There are also some blistering areas on the buccal mucosa. Applying firm lateral pressure on an unaffected area induces a bulla and pain. A biopsy is taken and sent for direct immunofluorescence. The pattern of deposition of antibodies shows a "chicken wire" appearance. The diagnosis and appropriate management of this patient are which of the following?

    A. BMMP and referral to ophthalmologist.
    B. BMMP and treatment with topical steroids.
    C. Pemphigus vulgaris and referral to a vesiculobullous specialist.
    D. Pemphigus vulgaris and treatment with topical steroids.

22. A 60-year-old female presents with a firm, movable, 1-cm swelling in his right upper lip. He reports that it has been slow growing "for a while." Other than occasionally biting on it and traumatizing it, the lesion is asymptomatic. The overlying mucosa is normal in color. Which of the following is the most likely diagnosis?

    A. Monomorphic adenoma
    B. Mucocele
    C. Peripheral ameloblastoma
    D. Ranula
    E. Stafne cyst

23. A 10-year-old male presents for evaluation of a missing mandibular right permanent first molar. A panoramic radiograph is taken and the tooth is seen displaced apically toward the inferior border of the mandible. Coronally, there is a well-circumscribed, unilocular radiolucent defect with a significant amount of calcified material with the radiodensity of tooth structure. The crown of the tooth is present within the defect. Which of the following is the most likely diagnosis?

    A. Odontogenic keratocyst (OKC)
    B. Cementoblastoma
    C. Radicular cyst
    D. Ameloblastic fibro-odontoma

24. An incisional biopsy of a palatal swelling in a 30-year-old male patient reveals necrosis of salivary gland acini with preservation of overall lobular architecture, squamous metaplasia of the salivary ducts, and overlying pseudoepitheliomatous hyperplasia. What is the appropriate management of this patient?

    A. Refer this patient to a head and neck surgeon.
    B. Excise the remaining portion of this lesion down to bone.
    C. Assure the patient he has nothing to worry about and monitor the lesion every 2 weeks. Biopsy again in 6 weeks if no improvement.
    D. Refer the patient to begin chemotherapy and/or radiation therapy.
    E. Refer the patient to ophthalmology to rule out ocular lesions.

25. A 30-year-old female presents with a nonexpansile multilocular radiolucency in the left posterior body of the mandible. The lesion is apical to the teeth in the area (they are not involved) and extends from the distal of second molar to the distal of the ipsilateral canine. Inferiorly, the lesion extended to just superiorly to the inferior alveolar nerve canal. Prior to biopsy, aspiration of the lesion is performed. A white, cheese-like material is obtained upon first aspiration. The second aspiration returns more of the same material, this time with a slight reddish hue. Which of the following is the most likely diagnosis?

A. Dentigerous cyst
B. Static bone cyst
C. Traumatic bone cyst
D. Odontogenic keratocyst (OKC)

26. A 50-year-old man is referred by his primary care physician for "multiple blood-filled blisters" in his mouth. Bilaterally on his buccal mucosa, you note large dome-shaped, red-blue raised lesions that are fluctuant. Multiple smaller petechiae are noted on the dorsal surface of his tongue and gingiva. Medium-sized lesions are noted on his lateral tongue. The patient reports that they wax and wane and he sometimes tastes blood. He reports that he is a heavy drinker and frequently takes acetaminophen for headaches. Which of the following is the most likely cause of these lesions?

A. Kidney disease
B. Liver disease
C. Crohn's disease
D. Hodgkin's disease

27. A 3-year-old female presents with Stickler syndrome. Upon examination, she is noted to have the following abnormalities: posterior displacement of her tongue, cleft palate, and mandibular micrognathia. This triad of anomalies is well recognized and is seen isolated and in association with other syndromes. What is this triad of anomalies more commonly known as?

A. Klinefelter sequence
B. Apert sequence
C. Pierre Robin sequence
D. Gorlin sequence
E. Gardner sequence

28. A 60-year-old male presents for evaluation of a nonhealing ulcer (>2 months) on the lateral border of his tongue. He reports a 60-pack-year history of smoking and is a heavy drinker. The lesion is 1 cm by 1 cm. It is painless and indurated. Adjacent to the tooth is a fractured tooth. In order to rule out a traumatic etiology, the tooth is smoothed out and the patient is re-evaluated in 2 weeks. The lesion persists and the decision is made to perform a biopsy. Which of the following is the most appropriate method of performing the procedure?

A. Perform an incisional biopsy that samples both the ulcerated component and the adjacent normal mucosa.
B. Perform an excisional biopsy.
C. Perform an incisional biopsy on tissue that is taken from the central, ulcerated portion of the lesion.
D. Sample tissue from normal mucosa adjacent to the lesion.

29. A 24-year-old Caucasian female dental student recently visited Africa to participate in a dental outreach program. After spending 4 weeks performing routine dental procedures, she returned home. While volunteering to allow one of her professors to demonstrate a procedure to the class on her, it was noticed that she had a diffuse, symmetrical, brown-black pigmentation covering most of her palate. At an examination just prior to leaving, she had no pigmentation at all. She is asymptomatic. What is the most likely cause of this dental student's palatal pigmentation?

A. Amalgam tattoo
B. Racial pigmentation
C. Melanoma
D. Drug-related pigmentation

30. A 50-year-old man presents for evaluation of a darkly pigmented area of the facial gingiva apical to his maxillary left lateral incisor. He reports having been to the dentist regularly before and that the spot was a lot smaller when he started. It has gradually increased in size and gotten darker. The only restoration in the patient's mouth is an all-ceramic crown on his mandibular right second molar. He is asymptomatic and otherwise healthy. What is the proper management for this patient?

A. Remove the lesion purely for cosmetic reasons and perform a periodontal procedure for esthetics.
B. Biopsy the lesion and submit for histopathological examination.
C. Have the patient return in 3 months for re-evaluation.
D. Inform the patient he has nothing to worry about, but if it gets bigger he should return.

31. A 56-year-old woman presents with a chief complaint of pain in her mandibular right second molar. Her medical history is significant for breast cancer (6 years ago) and she subsequently had a total left-sided mastectomy. The tooth that was bothering her was deemed nonrestorable and requires extraction. Which of the following should the dentist be most concerned about regarding this patient's extraction?

    A. Osteoradionecrosis
    B. Xerostomia secondary to chemotherapeutics
    C. Hypoglycemia
    D. Potential IV bisphosphonate therapy

32. A 25-year-old male is given a broad-spectrum antibiotic to combat a streptococcal pharyngitis. After a few days of taking the antibiotic, he develops several erythematous patches on his posterior hard palate that burn. The patient informs you that aside from the strep throat, he is unaware of any other medical conditions he may have. How should this patient be managed?

    A. Discontinue the antibiotic immediately. Prescribe a liquid steroid such as dexamethasone to swish and spit.
    B. Treat the patient with an antifungal and continue until antibiotic therapy is complete.
    C. Refer to oral surgeon to biopsy as soon as possible.
    D. Explain to the patient that it is probably unrelated and to come back in 3 months for follow-up.

33. An 8-year-old female presents for initial examination. She comes in with her parents who say she has a number of abnormalities. They mention she has missing clavicles, is short in stature, and has a large head with prominent frontal bossing. Because of her missing clavicles, she is able to approximate her shoulders in front of her chest. On skull films, sutures demonstrate delayed closing. Intraorally, she has a narrow, high-arched palate. A panoramic film is taken. What is most likely to be seen on a panoramic radiograph of this patient?

    A. Multiple osteomas
    B. Multiple OKCs

    C. Multiple giant cell lesions
    D. Multiple supernumerary teeth

34. A 20-year-old male presents for initial examination. Although his overall hygiene is good, you notice generalized loss of tooth structure. This loss includes incisal edges and occlusal surfaces. The lingual of the anterior maxillary teeth and the labial of the anterior mandibular teeth are also affected. Large, flat wear facets are seen. He reports that he has been grinding his teeth for years. What type of tooth wear is this patient suffering from?

    A. Attrition
    B. Abrasion
    C. Abfraction
    D. Erosion

35. A 30-year-old female lawyer presents with hyperelasticity of the skin and cutaneous fragility. In areas of prior trauma (i.e., knees), she has scars that resemble crumpled cigarette paper. She also has hypermobility of the joints and bruises easily. Other than the scarring, she has no other lesions on her skin. She reports no other medical problems. These findings are most consistent with which of the following?

    A. Osler–Weber–Rendu syndrome
    B. Tuberous sclerosis
    C. Ehlers–Danlos syndrome
    D. Sturge–Weber angiomatosis

36. A 60-year-old woman presents with stiff, shiny fingers. The fingers are permanently flexed and resemble a claw. Her fingers and toes also experience blanching when exposed to cold and can take up to 5 minutes to regain their color after warming. Intraorally, she has multiple petechiae on the lateral borders of her tongue and buccal mucosa bilaterally. Further examination reveals painless, movable, subcutaneous nodules of her skin. These findings are most consistent with which of the following?

    A. Ehlers–Danlos syndrome
    B. Tuberous sclerosis
    C. CREST syndrome
    D. Osler–Weber–Rendu syndrome

37. A 60-year-old female presents with herpes zoster of the face and external auditory canal. The lesions on her face are crusted over and follow the course of the V_2 branch of the trigeminal nerve stopping at the midline. There is also involvement of the facial and auditory nerves of the same side. She reports facial paralysis, hearing deficits, and vertigo. These findings are consistent with which of the following syndromes?

   A. Exanthema subitum
   B. Chronic fatigue syndrome
   C. Zoster sine herpete
   D. Ramsay Hunt syndrome

38. A 60-year-old female presents with bilateral white lesions on her buccal mucosa. She says she has not noticed them before and they are asymptomatic. She states that she has never smoked and drinks a glass of wine once a week. Clinically, the lesions appear striated and extend into the mandibular vestibule bilaterally. After ruling out any other etiology, an incisional biopsy is performed. The biopsy shows keratinized mucosal epithelium overlying fibrous connective tissue. At the epithelial-connective tissue interface, a dense band of lymphocytes is noted. Degeneration of the basal cell layer and saw-tooth rete ridge formation is also seen. What is the diagnosis?

   A. Leukoplakia
   B. Lichen planus (LP)
   C. Squamous cell carcinoma
   D. Leukoedema

39. A 40-year-old male presents with an asymptomatic, unilocular, mixed radiolucent–radiopaque lesion in the right posterior mandible that extends from the distal of the first molar into the ramus. Inferiorly, it extends to just above the inferior border of the mandible. There is no paresthesia reported. All three molars are erupted and have become more and more mobile over the past year. Slight buccal expansion is noted. Which of the following is the most consistent with this radiographic presentation?

   A. Calcifying epithelial odontogenic tumor (CEOT)
   B. OKC

C. Dentigerous cyst
D. Ameloblastoma

40. A 45-year-old male presents with a red, nodular lesion on the anterior hard palate. He states that it is tender to touch and bleeds easily. He does not know how long it has been present. He was diagnosed 15 years ago with the human immunodeficiency virus. His CD4+ count has subsequently fallen below 200. What is the most likely diagnosis?

   A. Pleomorphic adenoma
   B. Necrotizing sialometaplasia (NS)
   C. Kaposi's sarcoma (KS)
   D. Mucoepidermoid carcinoma

41. A 15-year-old boy presents with symptomatic submandibular lymphadenopathy for the past 2 weeks. Intraoral and extraoral examinations were unremarkable except for the previously mentioned lymphadenopathy. A fine needle aspiration was performed and *Bartonella henselae* organisms were isolated. These findings are consistent with which of the following?

   A. Cat-scratch disease
   B. Mumps
   C. Rubeola
   D. Rubella

42. A 50-year-old male presents with recurring oral ulcers for the past 3 months. He currently has a 2-cm ulcer on his left buccal mucosa and a similar sized one on his right lateral tongue. His anterior maxillary gingiva is eroded from canine to canine. Skin lesions are evident and appear as tiny vesicles that rupture. An incisional biopsy is performed and the histology picture consists of detached epithelium and mildly inflamed connective tissue. The epithelial detachment is suprabasilar and the basal cells remain attached to the underlying connective tissue. What is the diagnosis?

   A. Benigh mucous membrane pembhigoid (BMMP)
   B. Pemphigus vulgaris
   C. Erythema multiforme (EM)
   D. Erosive LP

43. A 25-year-old male presents with a 0.3-cm nodular mass on his right maxillary attached gingiva in the area of the cuspid and first premolar. It was submitted for biopsy and the report came back as following: Multiple sections show stratified squamous epithelium overlying a cellular lesion composed of haphazardly arranged, plump, uniform, fibroblasts set in an immature collagenous stroma. Metaplastic calcifications are noted throughout the lesion. What is the diagnosis?

   A. Mucocele
   B. Peripheral ossifying fibroma
   C. Peripheral giant cell granuloma (PGCG)
   D. Pyogenic granuloma (PG)

44. A 20-year-old male presents with a multilocular radiolucency in his right posterior mandible. The lesion extends from the distal of the ipsilateral canine into the ramus. Teeth are displaced, as is the inferior border of the mandible. There is considerable expansion of the buccal cortex. No paresthesia is reported. The lesion is aspirated and a straw-colored fluid is obtained. Tissue is removed and submitted for histopathological examination. The report is as follows: Multiple sections show fragments of fibrous connective tissue containing a tumor composed of islands and cords of odontogenic epithelium. The epithelium is composed of basal cells with hyperchromatic nuclei that exhibit reverse polarity and subnuclear vacuolization. Within the islands, a central edematous area resembling stellate reticulum is seen. In areas, prominent juxtaepithelial hyalinization is present adjacent to the tumor cells. What is the diagnosis?

   A. Ameloblastoma
   B. OKC
   C. Odontogenic myxoma
   D. Central giant cell granuloma

45. Mr. Smith has hemophilia A and is planning on having children. He along with his wife presents to a genetic counselor and blood tests are performed on the female to determine if she has hemophilia or is a carrier. It was determined that she neither has hemophilia nor carries the trait for it. He inquires about future children. The genetic counselor says to him, "Mr. Smith, if you and your wife have children, they will have a ____% chance of inheriting hemophilia." What percent chance do the Smiths have of having a child with hemophilia?

   A. 0%
   B. 25%
   C. 50%
   D. 100%

46. A 15-year-old female presents with a 1.5-cm neck swelling. The lesion is in the midline and at approximately the level of the hyoid bone. It is asymptomatic, fluctuant, and movable. Upon swallowing, the swelling moves superiorly. This superior movement of the swelling is also noted when the patient protrudes her tongue. What is the most appropriate clinical diagnosis?

   A. Cat-scratch disease
   B. Metastatic disease
   C. Branchial cleft cyst
   D. Thyroglossal duct cyst

47. A 40-year-old male presents with a diffuse, boggy swelling of his gingiva. His entire gingiva is bluish-green and is hyperplastic. The facial and lingual surfaces of most of his teeth are covered by this hyperplastic gingiva. The patient reports bruising easily, constant urinary tract infections, and states that overall he "just doesn't feel healthy." A biopsy of an affected area of the gingiva shows diffuse infiltration of normal tissue by sheets of poorly differentiated cells with myelomonocytic features. It is diagnosed as a granulocytic sarcoma. Which malignancy is granulocytic sarcoma associated with?

   A. Hodgkin's lymphoma
   B. Multiple myeloma
   C. Leukemia
   D. Ewing's sarcoma

48. A 35-year-old male presents for routine dental care. During a head and neck examination, it is noted that he has a redundant fold of tissue on the mucosal side of his upper lip. When questioned about it, he says that he has had it for approximately 2 years. During the examination, you also notice that he has drooping upper eyelids and a larger-than-normal thyroid gland. He states that his upper eyelid problems started

around the same time as his lip problem began. No other significant findings are noted. On the basis of this information, which of the following syndromes does this man have?

A. Gardner syndrome
B. Papillon–Lefèvre syndrome
C. Gorlin syndrome
D. Apert syndrome
E. Ascher syndrome

49. A 70-year-old female presents with herpes zoster on the left side of her face. The distribution is along the maxillary branch of the trigeminal nerve. There is involvement of the tip of her nose. Her medical history is noncontributory. What should be the next step in the management of this patient?

A. Administration of systemic steroids.
B. Administration of systemic antiviral medication and application of topical steroids.
C. Administration of systemic antiviral medication.
D. Administration of systemic antiviral medication and referral to ophthalmologist.

1. **The correct answer is A.** Pemphigus vulgaris is a rare autoimmune disease in which the body produces antibodies against desmoglein 3 and desmoglein 1. These proteins are components of desmosomes (intercellular adhesion structures between epithelial cells). When these desmosomes are disrupted, epithelial cells are no longer able to bond to each other and a split develops within the epithelium (causing a blister). The average age is 50 (this patient was a bit younger) and there is no sex predilection. Oral lesions are distributed haphazardly and appear as superficial, ragged erosions and ulcerations. Oral lesions usually precede cutaneous lesions, sometimes by a year or more. Patients with pemphigus demonstrate a positive Nikolsky sign (induction of bulla by firm, lateral pressure). Diagnosis can be made histopathologically by seeing suprabasilar cleavage of epithelial cells, but is confirmed by direct immunofluorescence. Treatment consists mainly of immunosuppressive agents (corticosteroids, azathioprine, etc.). Left untreated, pemphigus vulgaris is fatal.

Benign mucous membrane pemphigoid (BMMP), while in the same differential for the intraoral lesions, typically does not present with skin lesions. The ulcers are, instead, limited to the mucous membranes (oral mucous, eyes). Desquamative gingivitis is a common finding in patients with BMMP. This patient had multiple skin lesions, which are not seen in classic BMMP.

Erythema multiforme (EM) tends to have an explosive onset and is self-limiting. Characteristic appearances of EM include crusting of the lips and ulceration of the periphery of the tongue. Targetoid lesions, though pathognomonic for EM, are rarely seen. This patient had longstanding lesions and no crusting of her lips. EM minor is often caused by a prior recurrent herpetic episode and oftentimes responds to antiviral treatment (as is also seen in major recurrent aphthous stomatitis).

Recurrent aphthous stomatitis fits with this patient except for the duration of the disease (most aphthous heal in 10–14 days) and the skin lesions. Patients who have major aphthous stomatitis may have large, painful lesions that take a while to heal (weeks to months), but skin involvement is not seen. Acyclovir may play a role in treating stubborn lesions that result from prior herpetic outbreaks (as is also seen in EM).

Primary and recurrent herpes simplex virus infections are self-limiting in immunocompetent patients and usually resolve in 10 to 14 days. Also, recurrent intraoral herpes is seen only on attached mucosa (gingiva and hard palate). This patient had lesions on her buccal mucosa and ventral tongue. Skin lesions outside of the perioral region are not seen in herpes simplex virus (HSV) infections. Acyclovir, while not indicated for treatment of established herpetic lesions, did not prevent this patient from getting new lesions.

2. **The correct answer is D.** All leukoplakias require a diagnosis. If trauma is suspected, the etiology should be removed. In this case, the fractured cusp should be remedied and the patient should be re-evaluated in 2 weeks. Nightguards can also be fabricated in suspected cases of trauma. Any white lesion present for more than 2 weeks without improvement needs a scalpel biopsy to rule out epithelial dysplasia, neoplasm, etc. It is important to note that obvious traumatic lesions (linea alba, morsicatio) can usually be diagnosed clinically. In cases of atypical presentation or change in appearance over time, further investigation (scalpel biopsy) is required.

Immediate biopsy is rarely indicated in cases of leukoplakias. Removing suspected etiology and waiting 2 weeks to re-evaluate is perfectly acceptable treatment. There will be a significant amount of lesions that will resolve after inciting factors are removed. This will result in patients not having to undergo unnecessary procedures. Any lesion present after 2 weeks with no signs of improvement requires a scalpel biopsy.

Noting a suspicious lesion and waiting 3 months to evaluate it is below the standard of care and not acceptable treatment. Although all lesions should be measured and described (a photograph of the lesion is an excellent idea), 2 weeks is the recommended re-evaluation time for suspicious lesions, not 3 months.

Although this lesion is adjacent to a fractured tooth, there is no way to definitively know that this lesion is due to trauma. Because of this, it is recommended to remove the suspected etiology (address the fractured tooth) and re-evaluate in 2 weeks. Biopsy is indicated if lesion is still present and not improving.

3. **The correct answer is C.** Ameloblastoma is by far the most common odontogenic tumor. Its frequency equals the combined total of all the other odontogenic tumors (excluding odontomas that some classify as hamartomas). The preferred site for ameloblastoma is the posterior mandible (approximately 66% of total). Overall, mandibular lesions are more frequent than maxillary lesions in their respective bony locations (posterior, middle, anterior).

Adenomatoid odontogenic tumors (AOTs) account for 3% to 7% of all odontogenic tumors. They have a striking predilection for the anterior jaws and maxillary lesions are two-thirds as common as mandibular lesions. Two-thirds of AOTs occur in teenage females and are oftentimes associated with an impacted tooth (usually a canine).

Cementoblastomas account for less than 1% of odontogenic tumors. When they do occur, 75% occur in the mandible with a striking predilection for the molar and premolar region. Fifty percent involve the first permanent molar. Patients are typically in their 2nd and 3rd decades.

Calcifying epithelial odontogenic tumor (CEOT) (also known as a Pindborg Tumor) is a rare odontogenic tumor accounting for less than 1% of odontogenic tumors. Two-thirds occur in the posterior mandible. Patients are typically middle-aged.

Hemangiomas, while seen quite commonly in soft tissue (and less frequently centrally), are not odontogenic in origin.

Odontogenic myxomas are rare tumors of odontogenic ectomesenchyme. The average age for their occurrence is 25 and they may occur anywhere in the jaws.

4. **The correct answer is E.** This lesion is radiolucent and has smooth borders with some scalloping of the inferior border of the mandible.

On the basis of the significant intraoral swelling (due to expansile nature of this tumor) and the multilocularity of the lesion, ameloblastoma is the most likely answer. Ameloblastomas are tumors of odontogenic epithelium and are the most common clinically significant odontogenic tumor. They occur over a wide age range and can develop de novo or arise from the lining of an odontogenic cyst. Radiographically, they can appear as uni- or multilocular radiolucencies. Ameloblastomas can be locally destructive and treatment and prognosis are determined by the extent of the lesion.

Dentigerous cysts, by definition, are associated with the crown of an impacted tooth, usually mandibular third molars. Although any tooth can be affected, frequent sites (other than mandibular third molars) include maxillary canines, maxillary third molars, and mandibular second premolars. Dentigerous cysts are rarely seen involving unerupted deciduous teeth. Odontogenic tumors and other types of cysts can arise from the epithelium lining a dentigerous cyst.

Osteosarcoma can present as a radiolucent, radiopaque, or mixed lesion. When opacities are present, they tend to appear as "sunburst" appearance. Swelling and pain are common symptoms. This patient had swelling, but was asymptomatic. In addition, this lesion is well defined, and has smooth borders. Although there is still a possibility for this radiograph to represent an osteosarcoma, a benign lesion would be much more likely.

Periapical cysts, by definition, are associated with the apical area of nonvital teeth. Although the apices of the teeth in this radiograph are involved, it was noted in the history that all teeth were vital. On the basis of this information, periapical cyst can be excluded. It is also important to note that it is impossible to distinguish a periapical cyst from a periapical granuloma or a fibrous scar radiographically.

Buccal bifurcation cysts typically develop on the buccal aspect of a permanent mandibular first molar. It is that cervical enamel projection in the furcation is responsible for the development of this cyst. Occasionally, these lesions can be seen bilaterally. Radiographically, they are sometimes hard to visualize on a periapical film due to the tendency to expand perpendicularly to the buccal cortex. A mandibular occlusal film is best used to diagnose these. With this patient, there is no involvement of the furcation of any teeth.

5. **The correct answer is B.** Oral submucous fibrosis is a chronic, progressive disease that inevitably results in oral cancer. It is seen in higher frequency in populations of Indian and Southeast Asian descent. A mixture of nuts, tobacco, and sweeteners are wrapped in a betel quid leaf and sucked on. Chemicals released from this mixture are responsible for the clinical findings. Dense collagenous bands (evident in the picture) form and limit the opening of mouth in these patients. Teeth almost always exhibit some form of staining, and the leukoplakic areas are almost universally dysplastic (premalignant) due to the tobacco component. Despite cessation of this habit, the changes that have taken place do not revert. These patients become a challenge to treat both dentally (because of decreased opening) and surgically (to release fibrous bands and excise dysplastic lesions).

Although this patient does have a significant smoking history, smoker's melanosis typically affects the anterior facial gingiva. Smoker's melanosis is also darker in color due to an increase in melanin production by melanocytes in the basement membrane of the oral mucosa. The lesions in this patient's mouth were white in nature.

Morsicatio buccarum, or chronic cheek chewing, results from excessive nibbling of the buccal mucosa, usually in the anterior portions. It is quite common and most people are aware that they are doing it. Lesions occur along the occlusal plane (just like linea alba) and may extend slightly above or below it. In the case of this patient, lesions are present high in the vestibules (an impossible area to bite) and a definitive fibrous band can be seen on the buccal mucosa. The lesions in this patient also appear smooth and not ragged, as one would expect in a lesion secondary to chewing. The excessive staining of this patient's teeth may also hint that something else may be going on.

Oral hairy leukoplakia (OHL) is an entity that occurs exclusively on the lateral borders of the tongue. It is caused by Epstein–Barr virus infection of epithelial cells. It is seen almost exclusively in HIV+ patients, but can be seen in other immunocompromised states. Very rarely, it can be seen in immunocompetent patients. This diagnosis does not fit this case because of the widespread nature of the disease process in question.

Leukoedema is an extremely common finding in darker-skinned patients. It is considered a variant of normal. Normally, it is seen bilaterally on the buccal mucosa with occasional extension onto the labial mucosa. On rare occasion, it can be seen on the floor of the mouth. These lesions characteristically disappear when the mucosa is stretched. In this case, the lateral tongue was affected and the buccal mucosa tissue did not change in appearance upon stretching.

6. **The correct answer is A.** This is a classic presentation of recurrent herpes labialis. A tingling prodrome, vesicle formation and coalescence, and eventual crusting over and healing are typical with these lesions. Although he mentions that he has never had intraoral lesions in the past (a question asked to determine if he had had primary herpetic gingivostomatitis), only approximately 10% of patients experience any clinical symptoms during primary infection. All of this information coupled with the patient stating that he has had these before leads to the diagnosis of recurrent herpes. Treatment for herpes during the prodrome is antivirals (topical or systemic), but antiviral therapy is not indicated once lesions are well established and crusted over. Left on their own, herpetic ulcers resolve in 10 to 14 days without scarring in immunocompetent patients. Herpetic ulcers that last longer are suspicious of immunosuppression and should be investigated as needed.

Topical antivirals are only effective during the prodrome and are not indicated once a lesion is established. A prescription may be written for application during prodrome of next outbreak.

Systemic antivirals are only effective during the prodrome and are not indicated once a lesion is established. The exception to this rule is in an immunocompromised patient, where new lesions have the potential to develop and the host's immune system cannot effectively deal with them.

Once a strong suspicion of herpes is evident, this lesion can be left alone. If, upon follow-up in 2 weeks, the lesion is still present, and incisional biopsy is indicated.

Recurrent herpes labialis has no ocular manifestations and thus an ophthalmologic referral is not warranted.

7. **The correct answer is E.** *Treponema pallidum* is a gram-negative spirochete that causes syphilis, a sexually transmitted disease. The patient in this question is exhibiting a classical chancre of primary syphilis. These chancres occur at the site of inoculation 3 to 90 days after contact. They are characteristically painless and take 3 to 8 weeks to heal. Although the majority of chancres occur in the genital region, the most common oral site for these lesions is the upper lip. Treatment for primary syphilis is penicillin G. Left untreated this lesion could progress to the disseminated secondary syphilis and eventually to the life-threatening tertiary syphilis and neurosyphilis.

Histoplasmosis is the most common systemic fungal infection in the United States. It is endemic to the Ohio and Mississippi River Valleys. The vast majority of cases produce little or no clinical symptoms. When patients are symptomatic, the lungs are the most commonly affected sites. Immunocompromised patients can experience disseminated histoplasmosis, which is a serious complication. Treatment for histoplasmosis consists of systemic antifungals. This patient had an isolated ulcer, was immunocompetent, and had no pulmonary symptoms.

Recurrent herpes labialis (caused by herpes simplex virus type 1 or type 2) is painful and heals in 10 to 14 days in immunocompetent patients. This patient was otherwise healthy, had an ulcer present for 3 weeks, and reported no pain associated with it.

Cryptococcosis is a fungal infection that usually causes no symptoms in immunocompetent patient. HIV+ patients are very susceptible to cryptococcal infection. As with histoplasmosis, cryptococcosis is seen primarily in the lungs and can experience dissemination. This patient was immunocompetent and had no pulmonary symptoms. Treatment for cryptococcosis is systemic antifungals therapy.

Gonorrhea is the most common reportable bacterial infection in the United States. It is a sexually transmitted disease and is usually limited to genital involvement, though oral involvement has been seen. When a patient has oral manifestations, the most commonly affected site is the oropharynx. Although usually asymptomatic, erythema and sore throat can be present. Tonsils may be erythematous and edematous. Left untreated, most cases spontaneously resolve. Treatment is appropriate antibiotic therapy and is indicated to reduce the potential spread of the disease.

8. **The correct answer is C.** A Stafne bone cyst (Stafne defect, static bone defect) is not a true cyst. It represents a developmental defect in which the submandibular gland causes a depression on the lingual aspect of the mandible. This depression either contains a portion of submandibular salivary gland tissue or fibrous tissue and muscle. These lesions classically present as an asymptomatic radiolucency near the angle of the mandible and below the level of the mandibular canal. Literature states that 80% to 90% of Stafne lesions occur in male patients and, once recognized, require no treatment.

Dentigerous cysts, by definition, are associated with the crown of an impacted tooth. There is no tooth associated with this radiolucency.

Although certain malignant lesions do metastasize to the jawbones, their radiographic appearance tends to be ill-defined, indicating a destructive process. This lesion is well defined with a sclerotic border around it. In this particular case, a metastatic lesion should be considered low on the differential.

Calcifying odontogenic cyst is an uncommon lesion. They can occur in both the maxilla and mandible and approximately 65% of them are found in the incisor and canine region. Lesions can be unilocular and well defined, and often exhibit calcifications within the lesion. Although this lesion could, theoretically, represent a calcifying odontogenic cyst (COC), there are other lesions that this is more likely to be.

Periapical or radicular cysts are associated with the apex of a nonvital tooth. Besides the fact that these teeth were stated to be vital, this lesion does not appear to be associated with the apex of a tooth in any way.

9. **The correct answer is B.** OHL is seen almost exclusively in HIV+ patients. Its prevalence increases once a patient's CD4 count drop below 200. This is a benign lesion in and of itself, but it serves as an indicator of a patient's immune status. This patient stated that she was healthy (unaware of her immune status) but given her history of IV drug use and the presence of this lesion, her HIV status needs to be assessed. Once diagnosed, this lesion requires no further treatment. OHL is caused by the inclusion of the Epstein–Barr virus (HHV-4) in the nuclei of superficial epithelial cells and causes a phenomenon known as chromatin beading. Any patient who has a diagnosis of OHL needs to have an HIV test. Routine dental care can proceed as indicated. Although some patients choose to have this lesion excised for cosmetic reasons, it tends to recur. The best treatment for this condition is to do nothing. Topical steroids are indicated only if the patient becomes asymptomatic. Frequently, these lesions become suprainfected with candida and require treatment with an antifungal.

10. **The correct answer is E.** Hodgkin's lymphoma is a malignant lymphoproliferative disorder composed of Reed–Sternberg cells (bi- and multinucleated) in enlarged lymph nodes. The most common sites of initial presentation are the cervical and supraclavicular lymph nodes (70–75% of cases). A bimodal pattern with respect to patient's age is also noted: between 15 and 35 years, and another peak after age 50. Overall, a male predilection is observed. Treatment depends on stage but usually consists of radiation therapy, chemotherapy, or a combination of the two.

African-type Burkitt's lymphoma is a type of B-cell lymphoma. It was originally reported in African children and has a predilection for the jawbones. More than 90% of tumor cells show expression of Epstein–Barr virus nuclear antigen. Peak prevalence is 7 years of age. These lesions are extremely aggressive and can grow in size in short period of time. Treatment generally consists of aggressive chemotherapy.

North American-type Burkitt's lymphoma is similar to the African type but usually initially presents as an abdominal mass.

Multiple myeloma is a malignancy of plasma cells that typically affects older patients (median age between 60 and 70). It represents the most common hematologic malignancy among black persons in the United States. Bone pain is the most common symptom. Punched-out radiolucencies can be seen in the skull, jawbones, vertebrae, and other bones. Treatment consists of chemotherapy and overall prognosis is poor. Additionally, with regards to dental care of these patients, it should be stated that these patients are typically placed on IV bisphosphonate therapy.

Ewing's sarcoma is a malignancy of bone composed of small, undifferentiated round cells of uncertain lineage. Peak prevalence is in the second decade and the vast majority of those affected are white. Long bones, pelvis, and rib are most affected. Pain is common and soft-tissue invasion adjacent to affected bone can be seen. Treatment consists of surgery, radiation, and chemotherapy.

11. **The correct answer is A.** Leukemic cells can infiltrate soft tissues and cause a diffuse, nontender swelling. This is most frequent with the myelomonocytic types of leukemia acute myelogenous leukemia (AML), chronic myelogenous leukemia (CML). Tissues affected are most commonly gingiva, with diffuse gingival enlargement that can mimic drug-related gingival hyperplasia. Occasionally, the gingiva can take on a dark green to black appearance. This is known as a granulocytic sarcoma or extramedullary myeloid tumor.

Thrombocytopenia is a term used to refer to a decrease in the number of circulating platelets. It is often a sign of an underlying disease. Thrombocytopenia can be caused by either an increased destruction of thrombocytes (platelets) or a decreased production. Clinically, patients exhibit signs of inability to achieve hemostasis (spontaneous gingival hemorrhage, petechiae, and ecchymoses, and inability to stop bleeding after dental treatment, etc.).

Neutropenia is a term that refers to a decrease in the number of circulating neutrophils. This can be caused by either an increased destruction of neutrophils or a decreased production. Clinically, patients present with bacterial infections. Orally, ulcerative lesions of the gingival mucosa are common. Treatment consists of treating the underlying condition and antibiotics for infections.

Multiple myeloma is a malignancy of plasma cells that typically affects older patients (median age between 60 and 70). It represents the most common hematologic malignancy among black persons in the United States. Bone pain is the most common symptom. Punched-out radiolucencies can be seen in the skull, jawbones, vertebrae, and other bones. Treatment consists of chemotherapy and overall prognosis is poor. Additionally, with regards to dental care of these patients, it should be stated that these patients are typically placed on IV bisphosphonate therapy.

Anemia is a generic term that refers to either a decrease in volume of red blood cells (hematocrit) or in the concentration of hemoglobin. It can be caused by an increased destruction of erythrocytes (red blood cells), a decreased production of erythrocytes, or sequestration of erythrocytes in the spleen. Anemia is often a sign of an underlying disease. Symptoms include tiredness, headache, and lightheadedness. Treatment consists of treating the underlying disease.

12. **The correct answer is D.** Pleomorphic adenoma (benign mixed tumor) is the most common neoplasm of salivary gland origin. They are most frequently encountered in the parotid but can also occur intraorally (the most common site being the palate). There is a female predilection and the average age of diagnosis is 43 years. Clinically it presents as a slow-growing, asymptomatic, discrete mass in the superficial (lateral) lobe of the parotid, although it can also occur in the deep lobe. Treatment for these lesions usually consists of superficial parotidectomy with preservation of the facial nerve.

Warthin's tumor presents as a painless, sometimes fluctuant mass in the parotid gland. It is the second most common benign parotid salivary gland tumor. Warthin's tumor has an extremely low frequency among black patients (approximately 2.5%). In addition, older studies have demonstrated a male predilection for Warthin's tumor. Smoking also seems to increase the risk of

developing this tumor. Newer studies still show a male predilection, but not as lopsided as the previous numbers (M:F 26:1 vs. M:F 1.6:1). This may be due to an increased number of women smokers. Because this patient is a nonsmoking, black female, it is unlikely that this represents a Warthin's tumor.

Hodgkin's lymphoma is a malignant lymphoproliferative disorder composed of Reed–Sternberg cells in enlarged lymph nodes. The most common sites of initial presentation are the cervical and supraclavicular lymph nodes (70–75% of cases). A bimodal pattern with respect to patient's age is also noted: between 15 and 35 years, and another peak after age 50. Overall, a male predilection is observed. Treatment depends on stage but usually consists of radiation therapy, chemotherapy, or a combination of the two.

Although adenoid cystic carcinomas do occur in the parotid gland, they are vastly outnumbered by pleomorphic adenomas. Adenoid cystic carcinomas can also present as painless, discrete masses, but often patients complain of tenderness, pain, and facial nerve paralysis due to the propensity of adenoid cystic carcinomas to invade nerve. It is also worthy to note that larger lesions usually become fixed to the skin or deeper surrounding tissues. Although certainly possible, it is much more likely that this patient has a pleomorphic adenoma.

13. **The correct answer is B.** Patients who are suffering from hyperparathyroidism have elevated levels of serum calcium and present with lesions known as brown tumors. These lesions are histologically identical to central giant cell granulomas. If this patient has normal serum calcium levels, this lesion represents a central giant cell granuloma and should be treated appropriately. If he has elevated levels of serum calcium, his underlying hyperparathyroidism needs to be addressed. Resolution of brown tumor occurs after balance is restored.

Circulating platelet levels have no relevance in the differentiation of a central giant cell granuloma from a brown tumor of hyperparathyroidism.

Definitive treatment of any pathologic finding should not be initiated until a diagnosis has been made. This histology of this lesion is consistent with both a central giant cell granuloma and a brown tumor of hyperparathyroidism. Treatment should be deferred until it is determined whether or not the patient has hyperparathyroidism. Treatment for brown tumor consists of treatment of the underlying condition. Resolution of the lesion occurs after the metabolic imbalance is corrected.

14. **The correct answer is A.** Rubeola (measles) is produced by a paramyxovirus. Because of the MMR vaccine, measles incidence is low, but the clinical signs and symptoms still need to be recognized. The incubation period is 10 to 12 days. Significant lymphoid hyperplasia is noted. In this case, the patient is in Stage 1. Stage 1 is characterized by the 3Cs: (coryza, cough, and conjunctivitis). Intraorally, lesions known as Koplik's spots are noted bilaterally on the buccal mucosa. Stage 2 shows fading of Koplik's spots and development of a maculopapular rash. Stage 3 shows the end of the fever and resolution of skin rash. Each stage is approximately 3 days long.

Mumps (epidemic parotitis) is also caused by a paramyxovirus. Clinical features include significant salivary gland changes. These changes include discomfort and swelling in the preauricular region extending down the posterior, inferior border of the mandible. Another common finding in males is epididymoorchitis, which is rapid testicular swelling with pain and tenderness. This patient had none of these findings.

Recurrent intraoral herpes is seen only on attached mucosa (gingiva and hard palate) in immunocompetent patients. This patient's lesions were on his buccal mucosa and they were asymptomatic. Herpetic lesions are exquisitely painful.

Hand-foot-and-mouth disease is caused by an enterovirus. Because this patient had no lesions outside of his mouth, this diagnosis should be excluded.

15. **The correct answer is C.** Gardner syndrome is an autosomal dominant syndrome that is part of the spectrum of diseases including familial colorectal polyposis. Patients present with multiple osteomas of the jaws 90% of the time and can demonstrate benign cysts and tumors of the skin. Supernumerary teeth, odontomas, and im-

pacted teeth are also common findings. Of particular importance is the presentation of colonic polyps that ultimately transform into adenocarcinoma (usually before the age of 30). Females also demonstrate a 100-fold increase of thyroid carcinoma. It is because of the malignant manifestations of this syndrome that patients need to be referred to their primary care physician for evaluation of colon and thyroid gland.

Gorlin syndrome (also known as nevoid basal cell carcinoma syndrome) is an autosomal dominant syndrome caused by a mutation in the PTCH tumor suppressor gene on chromosome 9. It is characterized by multiple basal cell carcinomas and multiple odontogenic keratocysts.

Ascher syndrome is characterized by the following three features: double lip, blepharochalasis (edema of the upper eyelids), and nontoxic thyroid enlargement.

Klinefelter's syndrome is the most common sex chromosome disorder that affects males. These individuals are 47, XXY. Although these patients are affected with disorders related to abnormal hormone production (hypogonadism, gynecomastia, etc.), the dental abnormalities in the patient described earlier do not fit with Klinefelter's. Also, the fact that this patient is a female eliminates Klinefelter's as a reasonable choice.

16. **The correct answer is D.** *Cryptococcus neoformans* is uncommon and usually causes no problems in immunocompetent people. It is associated with pigeons (living in their excrement) and can grow in soil. It produces a mucopolysaccharide capsule that protects it from host immune defenses. This capsule is visualized using a mucicarmine stain. It is acquired by inhalation of spores. Most infections are limited to the lungs, but dissemination of disease is common in immunocompromised patients.

Blastomyces dermatitidis grows in rich, moist soil. Geographically, it is seen in the eastern half of the United States. It is also found north into the provinces of Canada surrounding the Great Lakes. Blastomycosis is a rare fungal infection that is acquired by inhalation of spores and is normally no problem in immunocompetent people. In certain cases, it becomes hematogenously disseminated. The Blastomyces organisms do not have a capsule.

Paracoccidioides brasiliensis is the causative agent of *Paracoccidioidomycosis* (South American Blastomycosis). It is seen in people who live in South America and has features similar to Blastomycosis. The organism is unencapsulated.

Histoplasmosis is the most common systemic fungal infection in the United States. It grows as both yeast and a mold. It is endemic to the Ohio and Mississippi River Valleys. It is acquired by inhalation and usually produces no symptoms in immunocompetent patients. Disseminated disease can be found in immunocompromised patients. These Histoplasma organisms are unencapsulated.

17. **The correct answer is B.** Multiple myeloma is a malignancy of plasma cells that typically affects older patients (median age between 60 and 70). It represents the most common hematologic malignancy among black persons in the United States. Bone pain is the most common symptom. Punched-out radiolucencies can be seen in the skull, jawbones, vertebrae, and other bones. Patients with multiple myeloma can also show focal deposits of acellular protein known as amyloid. These deposits can be found in internal organs, as well as skin and mucosal surfaces. Histologically, it appears as an amorphous, glassy pink material.

Hodgkin's lymphoma is a malignant lymphoproliferative disorder composed of Reed–Sternberg cells (bi- and multinucleated) in enlarged lymph nodes. The most common sites of initial presentation are the cervical and supraclavicular lymph nodes (70–75% of cases). A bimodal pattern with respect to patient's age is also noted: between 15 and 35 years, and another peak after age 50.

African-type Burkitt's lymphoma is a type of B-cell lymphoma. It was originally reported in African children and has a predilection for the jawbones. More than 90% of tumor cells show expression of Epstein–Barr virus nuclear antigen. Peak prevalence is 7 years of age. These lesions are extremely aggressive and can grow in size in short period of time. Treatment generally consists of aggressive chemotherapy.

Ewing's sarcoma is a malignancy of bone composed of small, undifferentiated round cells of uncertain lineage. Peak prevalence is in the second decade and the vast majority of those affected are white. Long bones, pelvis, and rib are most affected. Pain is common and soft-tissue invasion adjacent to affected bone can be seen. Treatment consists of surgery, radiation, and chemotherapy.

18. **The correct answer is A.** Plumbism, or lead poisoning, has widespread systemic effects, including anemia, fatigue, renal dysfunction, and musculoskeletal pain. Oral manifestations include ulcerative stomatitis, gingival lead line (Burton's line), and grayish discoloration of buccal mucosa and tongue. Additional manifestations of lead poisoning include tremor of tongue upon thrusting, excessive salivation, and advanced periodontal disease.

Acrodynia is the result of chronic exposure to mercury. Oral changes noted include metallic taste, ulcerative stomatitis, inflammation and enlargement of the salivary lands, gingiva, and tongue.

Argyria is the result of systemic silver intoxication, which can result in coma, pleural edema, hemolysis, and bone marrow failure. Diffuse gray discoloration is noted in sun-exposed areas of skin. A blue-silver line may also appear along the gingival margins.

Arsenic poisoning has widespread effects on numerous organ systems. Diffuse macular hyperpigmentation and palmar and plantar hyperkeratosis are noted. Long-term exposure can result in basal cell carcinoma and cutaneous squamous cell carcinoma. Oral manifestations are rare.

19. **The correct answer is A.** Sodium valproate (valproic acid) is an anticonvulsant used to treat neurological disorders such as epilepsy. Its use has been associated with gingival hyperplasia.

Cyclosporine, while one of the major drugs implicated in drug-induced gingival hyperplasia, is an immunosuppressant agent used in the treatment of transplant patients, rheumatoid arthritis, and psoriasis. This patient has no history of anything other than epilepsy and thus would not be taking cyclosporine.

Verapamil is a calcium-channel blocker and is also implicated in the occurrence of drug-related gingival hyperplasia. This patient has no history of anything other than epilepsy and thus would not be taking verapamil.

Nifedipine is a calcium-channel blocker and is also implicated in the occurrence of drug-related gingival hyperplasia. This patient has no history of anything other than epilepsy and thus would not be taking nifedipine.

20. **The correct answer is D.** Papillon–Lefèvre syndrome is an autosomal recessive syndrome that is characterized by palmar–plantar keratosis and dramatically advanced periodontitis in both deciduous and permanent dentitions.

Gorlin syndrome (also known as nevoid basal cell carcinoma syndrome) is an autosomal dominant syndrome caused by a mutation in the PTCH tumor suppressor gene on chromosome 9. It is characterized by multiple basal cell carcinomas, multiple odontogenic keratocysts, palmar/plantar pitting, calcification of the falx cerebri, and rib abnormalities.

Apert syndrome is a rare condition similar to Crouzon syndrome and is characterized by craniosynostosis (premature closing of the cranial sutures). Patients typically have cranial malformations that result in abnormal-shaped heads (tower skull, cloverleaf skull). Affected individuals also have a hypoplastic midface and syndactyly of the second, third, and fourth digits of the hand. Mental retardation is common.

Ascher syndrome is characterized by the following three features: double lip, blepharochalasis (edema of the upper eyelids), and nontoxic thyroid enlargement.

21. **The correct answer is C.** Pemphigus vulgaris is an autoimmune disorder that is diagnosed by direct immunofluorescence that shows a characteristic "chicken wire" deposition of antibodies between epithelial cells. The induction of a bulla secondary to firm, lateral pressure on mucosa is known as a positive Nikolsky sign. These patients need to be treated by someone with experience. Left untreated, pemphigus vulgaris is fatal.

Although BMMP has a similar appearance clinically and referral to an ophthalmologist is appropriate treatment, the result of the immunofluorescence rules it out. BMMP shows a linear deposition of antibodies subjacent to the basement membrane. BMMP is normally not fatal, but blindness may result if left untreated.

BMMP can sometimes be managed by topical steroids, but should only be done by someone with experience with the disease. As with the previous explanation, this patient does not have BMMP.

Pemphigus vulgaris is the correct diagnosis, but the treatment here is wrong. These patients need to be seen by someone who is well versed in treating patients with this specific malady.

22. **The correct answer is A.** Monomorphic adenomas are benign salivary gland tumors. They are sometimes classified into one of two categories: canalicular adenoma or basal cell adenoma. They can be found in minor glands and major glands. The canalicular type is found almost exclusively in the upper lip. It presents as a slow-growing, painless swelling in older adults. Literature states that there is approximately a 2:1 female predominance lesion. This is the most appropriate clinical diagnosis of the choices presented here.

Mucoceles are the result of extravasation of mucin into surrounding tissues secondary to a disruption in the continuity of a duct (usually caused by trauma). Although mucoceles are quite common in the lower lip, they are exquisitely rare in the upper lip and should not be near the top of a differential.

Ameloblastomas are the most common odontogenic tumor. Although they do occur in extraosseous locations (peripherally), they are confined to the gingiva and alveolar mucosa. Ameloblastoma would not be an appropriate lesion for a swelling of the upper lip.

A ranula is a mucocele of the floor of the mouth. By definition, this lesion cannot represent a ranula.

A Stafne bone cyst (Stafne defect, static bone defect) is not a true cyst. It represents a developmental defect in which the submandibular gland causes a depression on the lingual aspect of the mandible. This depression either contains a portion of submandibular salivary gland tissue or fibrous tissue and muscle. These lesions classically present as an asymptomatic radiolucency near the angle of the mandible and below the level of the mandibular canal. Literature states that 80% to 90% of Stafne lesions occur in male patients and, once recognized, require no treatment.

23. **The correct answer is D.** Ameloblastic fibro-odontomas are odontogenic tumors usually encountered in children. They are most common in the posterior jaws with mandible favored over maxilla. They are frequently encountered when radiographs are taken to determine why a tooth has not erupted. The radiographic features described earlier are classic for ameloblastic fibro-odontomas. The degree of calcification can range from very little to a solid mass of calcified material. Treatment is generally conservative, as these do not behave as classic ameloblastomas do.

Odontogenic keratocysts (OKCs) are developmental cysts that have a high rate of recurrence. They can appear uni- or multilocular and have a predilection for the posterior mandible. They can be found as one of the oral manifestations of nevoid basal cell carcinoma syndrome. Lesion size ranges from quite small to large enough to fill entire ramus. Calcifications are rarely (if ever) seen radiographically.

Cementoblastomas are rare neoplasms that have a mandibular predilection and occur in the molar/premolar region. Radiographically, this lesion appears as a radiopaque mass fused to one or more tooth roots and surrounded by a radiolucent rim. The patient in this question had a mass coronal to the impacted tooth, not attached to the root(s).

Radicular (periapical) cysts are found at the apex of nonvital teeth.

24. **The correct answer is C.** This histological appearance is classic of necrotizing sialometaplasia. Necrotizing sialometaplasia (NS) is a reactive phenomenon thought to be caused by ischemic injury to a portion of the palate. It is more common in males and once a diagnosis is rendered (via incisional biopsy), no further treatment is required. Lesions spontaneously heal in 5 to 6 weeks. If lesion does not seem to be healing, another biopsy is warranted.

NS spontaneously resolves and requires no further intervention once a diagnosis is made.

Referral to ophthalmology is required in patients diagnosed with BMMP.

25. **The correct answer is D.** OKCs are developmental cysts that have a high rate of recurrence. They can appear uni- or multilocular and have a predilection for the posterior mandible. They can be found as one of the oral manifestations of nevoid basal cell carcinoma syndrome. Lesion size ranges from quite small to large enough to fill entire ramus. Upon aspiration, they typically produce a cheese-like substance (keratin). The reason the second aspiration was slightly reddish was because there was hemorrhage in the area due to prior aspiration. Treatment of these lesions is controversial and ranges from marsupialization to resection.

Dentigerous cysts, by definition, are associated with the crown of an impacted tooth, usually mandibular third molars. Although any tooth can be affected, frequent sites (other than mandibular third molars) include maxillary canines, maxillary third molars, and mandibular second premolars. The lesion described in this case was not associated with any teeth.

A Stafne bone cyst (Stafne defect, static bone defect) is not a true cyst. It represents a developmental defect in which the submandibular gland causes a depression on the lingual aspect of the mandible. This depression either contains a portion of submandibular salivary gland tissue or fibrous tissue and muscle. These lesions classically present as an asymptomatic radiolucency near the angle of the mandible and below the level of the mandibular canal. Literature states that 80% to 90% of Stafne lesions occur in male patients and, once recognized, require no treatment.

Traumatic bone cysts (simple bone cysts) are not true cysts. They are not lined by conventional epithelium, but rather by a compressed fibrous tissue. Upon surgical exploration, these lesions are found to be empty. Aspiration may return a slightly serosanguinous fluid. Treatment is to induce bleeding during biopsy and allow the lesion to fill up with blood. Cause of these lesions was once thought to be due to trauma (hence, the name), but some seem to be idiopathic.

26. **The correct answer is B.** The liver is responsible for producing the vitamin K-dependent clotting factors (II, VII, IX, X). Liver disease can result in the decreased production of these factors and place the patient in a hypocoagulated state. In addition to the other answers not compatible with this question, this patient is a heavy drinker (alcohol is a known risk factor for liver disease). If that was not enough, this patient reported frequent acetaminophen use. One of the metabolites of acetaminophen is hepatotoxic in high doses (and even more so in a liver suffering the effects of alcohol).

Patients with acute or chronic renal failure can rarely demonstrate oral manifestations known as uremic stomatitis. Although rare, it is mostly seen in acute rather than chronic disease. Clinically, white plaques appear on buccal mucosa, tongue, and floor of mouth. The onset of these plaques is often abrupt. There may also be an odor of ammonia or urine on the patient's breath. Lesions resolve once the underlying kidney disease is treated.

The oral manifestations of Crohn's disease (an inflammatory disease affecting the distal small bowel and proximal colon) include nodular swelling, cobblestone appearance of oral mucosa, and deep, granulomatous-appearing ulcers. These findings were not seen in this patient. Abdominal pain, nausea, diarrhea, and weight loss may also be seen.

Hodgkin's lymphoma is a malignant lymphoproliferative disorder composed of Reed–Sternberg cells in enlarged lymph nodes. The most common sites of initial presentation are the cervical and supraclavicular lymph nodes (70–75% of cases). A bimodal pattern with respect to patient's age is also noted: between 15 and 35 years, and another peak after age 50. Overall, a male predilection is observed. Treatment depends on stage but usually consists of radiation therapy, chemotherapy, or a combination of the two.

27. **The correct answer is C.** The Pierre Robin sequence is characterized by posterior displacement of his tongue, cleft palate, and mandibular micrognathia. The retruded mandible results in the posterior displacement of the tongue, and also in lack of support of the tongue musculature and airway obstruction. This sequence is seen in Stickler and velocardiofacial syndromes most commonly, but has been reported in others.

Klinefelter's syndrome is the most common sex chromosome disorder that affects males. These individuals are 47, XXY. Although these patients are affected with disorders related to abnormal hormone production (hypogonadism, gynecomastia, etc.), the dental abnormalities in the patient described earlier do not fit with Klinefelter's. The fact that this patient is a female also eliminates Klinefelter's as a reasonable choice.

Apert syndrome is a rare condition similar to Crouzon syndrome and is characterized by craniosynostosis (premature closing of the cranial sutures). Patients typically have cranial malformations that result in abnormal-shaped heads (tower skull, cloverleaf skull). Affected individuals also have a hypoplastic midface and syndactyly of the second, third, and fourth digits of the hand. Mental retardation is common.

Gorlin syndrome (also known as nevoid basal cell carcinoma syndrome) is an autosomal dominant syndrome caused by a mutation in the PTCH tumor suppressor gene on chromosome 9. It is characterized by multiple basal cell carcinomas, multiple OKCs, palmar/plantar pitting, calcification of the falx cerebri, and rib abnormalities.

Gardner syndrome is an autosomal dominant syndrome that is part of the spectrum of diseases including familial colorectal polyposis. Patients present with multiple osteomas of the jaws 90% of the time and can demonstrate benign cysts and tumors of the skin. Supernumerary teeth, odontomas, and impacted teeth are also common findings. Of particular importance is the presentation of colonic polyps that ultimately transform into adenocarcinoma (usually before the age of 30). Females also demonstrate a 100-fold increase of thyroid carcinoma. It is because of the malignant manifestations of this syndrome that patients need to be referred to their primary care physician for evaluation of colon and thyroid gland.

28. **The correct answer is A.** This is a suspected malignancy. Given the patient's age, sex, and social history, he is a prime candidate for oral

cancer. Compounding this is the fact that this lesion is large, persistent, painless, and indurated. Suspected malignancies should have an incisional biopsy performed. This biopsy should include both the ulcerated portion and adjacent normal mucosa. Sutures may be used to orient the pathologist.

Suspected malignancies should have an incisional biopsy performed. If the clinical diagnosis is appropriate (i.e., malignant), further surgical intervention will be warranted. Removing the clinical lesion may hinder efforts to evaluate it in the future.

Performing a biopsy of an ulcer without adjacent tissue leads to a diagnostic dilemma. In some cases, a diagnosis may still be made. In other cases, a diagnosis of "nonspecific ulcer" will be rendered and another biopsy will be needed. When biopsying ulcers, always take adjacent normal mucosa (this is especially important for vesiculobullous diseases such as pemphigus and BMMP).

Normal adjacent mucosa, while it may contain some diagnostic information, is far inferior to tissue from the lesion itself.

29. **The correct answer is D.** Malaria has a high prevalence in African nations. Subsequently, people traveling there for any length of time are usually administered chloroquine (or another quinine derivative). Quinine is known to cause dark brown-black pigmentation in patients, most often in the palate. A good correlation between beginning of medication and onset of appearance can be helpful diagnostically.

Amalgam tattoos are pigmented and result from the traumatic implantation of amalgam into the submucosal. They usually present in isolated foci (i.e., not the entire palate) and are not symmetrical. This patient also reports no dental work prior to the onset. Radiographs can sometimes be handy to see if any radiopaque material is present within the lesion.

Racial pigmentation is generally seen on the facial aspect of the gingiva. This patient is a Caucasian and this lesion was not present 2 months prior. All of these reasons rule out racial pigmentation.

Although melanoma is certainly a concern and should be included in the differential for any pigmented lesion on the palate (a high-risk site), they generally take time to evolve (i.e., not appear in 1 month's time). If the patient was symptomatic (or becomes symptomatic), or areas appeared raised, ulcerated, asymmetrical, or changing in color, an incisional biopsy would be indicated.

30. **The correct answer is B.** Although most lesions are given 2 weeks to resolve on their own before biopsy, this "waiting period" can often times be skipped based on clinical information and the biopsy performed immediately (assuming the patient is medically cleared to undergo a surgical procedure). In this particular case, there are a few hints that allow this to be biopsied immediately. First is the location; anterior maxillary gingiva and hard palate are high-risk sites for melanoma. Second is that the lesion has increased in size over time. The last hint is that it has gotten darker. All of these things are pointing toward a premalignant or malignant process. The ABCDs of melanoma are: Asymmetry, Border irregularities, Color variegation, and Diameter greater than 6 mm. All of these have a negative impact on the prognosis of melanoma. Oral mucosal melanoma has a poor overall prognosis.

Although performing a periodontal procedure after removing the lesion may be done, the impetus to remove the lesion should not be cosmesis. Pigmented lesions on the anterior maxillary gingiva and hard palate should be viewed with skepticism, as these are high-risk sites for melanoma. What good does nice looking gingiva do when the patient may require resection for a malignant process?

Waiting 3 months to re-evaluate a pigmented lesion in a high-risk site that has undergone changes in size and color is below the standard of care. This lesion should be biopsied as soon as possible.

Decisions of this nature are not up to the patient. As a licensed medical professional, it is the responsibility of the health care provider to make sure this lesion is managed appropriately. The patient should also not be told he has nothing to worry about, especially when all clinical signs (location, change in size and color) are pointing toward a potentially premalignant or malignant process.

31. **The correct answer is D.** Patients who have a history of breast cancer (and prostate cancer in males) are often placed on IV bisphosphonate therapy to help prevent metastatic disease to bone. It is known that IV bisphosphonates can cause delayed healing and osteonecrosis, especially in the mandible. This should be a major consideration in how this patient should be treated.

Although osteoradionecrosis does occur in the jawbones, it is unlikely that this patient will be affected by it. First off, the scenario did not even mention that she had radiation therapy. If she did, her mandible would most likely not be in the field of radiation. Add this to the fact that her tooth problem was on the contralateral side makes this a relatively low possibility.

Although drug-related xerostomia is a problem on many different levels (patient comfort, caries risk, candidiasis, etc.), it falls low on the list of concerns regarding the actual procedure of the extraction of the tooth.

This is most likely unrelated to breast cancer and should have little to no impact on the actual extraction of the affected tooth. The cause should be determined (is she a diabetic who took her insulin but did not eat?) and remedied. Once the reason is determined, she can have the tooth extracted. In an emergency situation, a patient in a hypoglycemic state can be given oral glycemic agents to raise blood-glucose levels.

32. **The correct answer is B.** Young, healthy patients usually do not get candida infections. They are, however, susceptible to such infections after being on a broad-spectrum antibiotic. The antibiotic wipes out normal oral bacterial flora and allows the native candida organisms (present in approximately 70% of the population) to proliferate. This patient should be given a topical antifungal to use until antibiotic therapy is completed. If the infection returns with no apparent inciting factors, immunosuppression should be ruled out.

Steroids should not be prescribed to patients who have infections. Steroids suppress the host response to the infection and allow the organ-

isms to flourish. It is also important for patients to finish a course of antibiotics once they have been started on them.

This lesion should be easily recognized and identified based on the patient's description and timeline (i.e., onset soon after beginning antibiotic therapy). A cytologic smear may be performed to confirm the diagnosis. Biopsy is not indicated unless the lesion does not resolve following administration of antifungal agents.

Sudden onset of symptoms and clinical signs should never be dismissed. At most, 2 weeks is an acceptable time frame to follow-up on a patient. In this case, the patient was symptomatic and should not be dismissed without appropriate therapy or a plan.

33. **The correct answer is D.** This is a classic presentation of cleidocranial dysplasia. It is caused by a defect in the CBFA1 gene on chromosome 6p21. These patients often have a large number of supernumerary teeth.

Multiple osteomas are seen in Gardner syndrome. It is an autosomal dominant syndrome that is part of the spectrum of diseases including familial colorectal polyposis. Patients present with multiple osteomas of the jaws 90% of the time and can demonstrate benign cysts and tumors of the skin. Supernumerary teeth, odontomas, and impacted teeth are also common findings. Of particular importance is the presentation of colonic polyps that ultimately transform into adenocarcinoma (usually before the age of 30). Females also demonstrate a 100-fold increase of thyroid carcinoma. It is because of the malignant manifestations of this syndrome that patients need to be referred to their primary care physician for evaluation of colon and thyroid gland.

Gorlin syndrome (also known as nevoid basal cell carcinoma syndrome) is an autosomal dominant syndrome caused by a mutation in the PTCH tumor suppressor gene on chromosome 9. It is characterized by multiple basal cell carcinomas, multiple OKCs, palmar/plantar pitting, calcification of the falx cerebri, and rib abnormalities.

Multiple giant cell lesions can be seen in both cherubism and in hyperparathyroidism. Neither of these entities have clinical manifestations as mentioned earlier.

34. **The correct answer is A.** Attrition is loss of tooth structure due to tooth-to-tooth contact during contact and mastication. Bruxing, premature contacts, and poor-quality enamel can accelerate the damage.

Abrasion is the pathologic wearing away of tooth structure secondary to the mechanical action of an external agent. Vigorous tooth brushing with abrasive toothpastes is the most common cause. Patterns can vary depending on cause.

Abfraction is loss of tooth structure secondary to occlusal stress that creates repeated tooth flexure and results in failure of enamel and dentin at a point away from the point of loading. This is most frequently seen in the cervical area of teeth and appears as a wedge-shaped defect.

Erosion is loss of tooth structure caused by a nonbacterial chemical process. This can include acidic drinks, certain medications, and reflux of gastric secretions both involuntarily (hiatal hernia) and voluntarily (bulimia). Clinically, tooth loss does not correlate with functional wear patterns. Posterior teeth tend to lose occlusal tooth structure and they can appear cupped out, with the center being dentin and the edges enamel. The palatal and lingual surfaces of anterior teeth may also be affected.

35. **The correct answer is C.** Ehlers–Danlos syndromes (there are at least 10) are inherited connective tissue disorders. The symptoms are related to production of abnormal collagen, the main structural component of connective tissue. The symptoms this patient exhibits are consistent with the classical type, which is inherited in an autosomal dominant fashion.

Osler–Weber–Rendu syndrome (hereditary hemorrhagic telangiectasia) is an autosomal dominant syndrome with clinical features including frequent episodes of epistaxis and multiple telangiectasias in the nasal, oral, and oropharyngeal mucosa. Patients also have telangiectasias on their hands and feet, gastrointestinal, genitourinary, and conjunctival mucosa.

Tuberous sclerosis is a syndrome characterized by mental retardation, seizure disorders,

and angiofibromas of the skin. These symptoms do not match those of the patient mentioned earlier.

Sturge–Weber angiomatosis (encephalotrigeminal angiomatosis) is a nonhereditary developmental condition characterized by vascular proliferations involving the brain and face. Patients are born with a capillary vascular malformation of the face known as port wine stain.

36. **The correct answer is C.** CREST syndrome is rare and may represent a variant of systemic sclerosis. Patients are affected with the following: *C*alcinosis cutis, *R*aynaud's phenomenon, *E*sophageal dysfunction, *S*clerodactyly, and *T*elangiectasia. This patient exhibited four of these symptoms (esophageal dysfunction is oftentimes only detected by barium radiological studies).

Ehlers–Danlos syndromes (there are at least 10) are inherited connective tissue disorders. The symptoms are related to production of abnormal collagen, the main structural component of connective tissue. The symptoms include hyperelasticity of skin, hypermobility of joints, papyraceous scarring, and easy bruising. The hypermobility of the skin seen in Ehlers–Danlos syndrome is opposite to the tightness of the skin in the patient mentioned earlier.

Tuberous sclerosis is a syndrome characterized by mental retardation, seizure disorders, and angiofibromas of the skin. These symptoms do not match those of the patient mentioned earlier.

Osler–Weber–Rendu syndrome [hereditary hemorrhagic telangiectasia (HHT)] is an autosomal dominant syndrome with clinical features including frequent episodes of epistaxis and multiple telangiectasias in the nasal, oral, and oropharyngeal mucosa. Patients also have telangiectasias on their hands and feet, gastrointestinal, genitourinary, and conjunctival mucosa. Although the patient mentioned earlier does, indeed, have telangiectasias, none of her other symptoms fit with HHT.

37. **The correct answer is D.** Ramsay Hunt syndrome classically presents with the symptoms mentioned earlier. Herpes zoster is caused by

the human herpesvirus 3 (HHV-3, or varicella-zoster virus).

Exanthema subitum (roseola) is caused by human herpesvirus 6 (HHV-6). It is usually contracted at a young age and is asymptomatic. Occasionally, an erythematous macular eruption with slightly elevated papules may appear.

Chronic fatigue syndrome is a controversial symptom complex thought to be caused by human herpesvirus 4 (HHV-4, or Epstein–Barr virus). Patients report nonspecific symptoms of chronic fatigue, fever, pharyngitis, myalgia, and headaches. These symptoms are inconsistent with the findings in the patient mentioned earlier.

Zoster sine herpete (zoster without rash) is when a patient experiences a recurrence of a zoster outbreak but shows no vesiculation of the skin or mucosa. Affected patients experience severe pain and an abrupt onset. The patient mentioned earlier has visible healing vesicles and thus would not be diagnosed as zoster sine herpete.

38. **The correct answer is B.** This histological description is classic for lichen planus (LP). LP is an autoimmune, dermatologic entity that can present in the mouth. The two most common forms in the mouth are the reticular form (which the patient mentioned earlier has) and the erosive form. The erosive form is commonly found on the anterior gingiva, but may be seen in other patients. These lesions do not need to be treated if asymptomatic, but should be followed up on every 6 months. Symptomatic lesions can be treated with corticosteroids.

Leukoplakia is a clinical term only. It is a term used for a white lesion in the mouth that cannot be rubbed off and has no diagnosis. Once a diagnosis is made (i.e., via histology), the term leukoplakia no longer applies. *Note:* The clinical term leukoplakia should not be confused with the entity of OHL, which is caused by human herpesvirus-4 and is most frequently seen in HIV+ patients.

Squamous cell carcinoma of the buccal mucosa, while it does occur, is quite rare. The fact that this patient also has symmetrical, bilateral lesions also puts it extremely low on the differential diagnosis. The histology of squamous cell carcinoma consists of islands or cords of neoplastic epithelial cells invading the connective tissue. Transition from dysplastic epithelium is often seen. Invasive lesions can be seen infiltrating muscle, gland, and vasculature. The histology mentioned earlier does not work with a diagnosis of squamous cell carcinoma.

Although leukoedema may, in some cases, clinically resemble LP, the histology given is that of LP.

39. **The correct answer is A.** CEOT (Pindborg tumor) is a rare odontogenic neoplasm. It presents as mentioned earlier and may also involve an impacted tooth. Although the lesion may be totally radiolucent, scattered calcifications are frequently seen. This is the only diagnostic choice that may contain calcifications.

OKCs are developmental odontogenic cysts that exhibit a specific histology. They are important because they can be aggressive in nature and have a high rate of recurrence. They can occur anywhere but are most common in the posterior jaws, with the mandible favored over the maxilla. They can be associated with impacted teeth (but do not have to be) and do not have a radiopaque component to them. Multiple OKCs are seen in nevoid basal cell carcinoma syndrome (Gorlin syndrome).

Dentigerous cysts, by definition, are associated with the crown of an impacted tooth, usually mandibular third molars. Although any tooth can be affected, frequent sites (other than mandibular third molars) include maxillary canines, maxillary third molars, and mandibular second premolars. Dentigerous cysts are rarely seen involving unerupted deciduous teeth. Odontogenic tumors and other types of cysts can arise from the epithelium lining a dentigerous cyst. All of this patient's molars were erupted (i.e., he had no impacted teeth) and thus dentigerous cyst should be excluded as a potential diagnosis. Also, calcifications are not seen in dentigerous cysts.

Ameloblastoma is by far the most common odontogenic tumor. Its frequency equals the combined total of all the other odontogenic tumors (excluding odontomas that some classify as hamartomas). The preferred site for ameloblastoma is the posterior mandible (approximately

66% of total). Overall, mandibular lesions are more frequent than maxillary lesions in their respective bony locations (posterior, middle, anterior). Ameloblastomas, however, do not present as mixed radiolucent–radiopaque lesions. It is for this reason that ameloblastoma should be excluded from the differential diagnosis.

40. **The correct answer is C.** Kaposi's sarcoma (KS) is a malignant vascular neoplasm that is divided into four types. One of the types is the AIDS-related type. This patient is HIV+ and has a CD4+ count below 200; this places him into the AIDS category. KS is associated with human herpesvirus 8 (HHV-8) and although any site may be affected, the palate and gingiva are the most commonly involved. Clinically, it can appear as a raised, dark-red enlargement of tissue.

Pleomorphic adenomas are the most common benign salivary gland neoplasm and they most commonly occur in the parotid. When they do occur intraorally, they are most common on the posterior hard palate and soft palate. The anterior one-third of the hard palate does not contain salivary glands; therefore, this would be an inappropriate choice to include in a differential diagnosis.

NS is thought to result from ischemic necrosis of salivary glands. The anterior one-third of the hard palate does not contain salivary glands; therefore this would be an inappropriate choice to include in a differential diagnosis.

Mucoepidermoid carcinomas are the most common malignant salivary gland tumor. The anterior one-third of the hard palate does not contain any salivary glands; therefore, this would be an inappropriate choice to include in a differential diagnosis.

41. **The correct answer is A.** The isolation of the organism *Bartonella henselae* gives this diagnosis away. Cat-scratch disease is a bacterial infection that begins in the skin but spreads to the lymph nodes. It is the most common cause of chronic regional lymphadenopathy in children. The lymphadenopathy can occur after the cutaneous lesion has healed. A careful history can often aid in the diagnosis.

Mumps (epidemic parotitis) is also caused by a paramyxovirus. Clinical features include significant salivary gland changes. These changes include discomfort and swelling in the preauricular region extending down the posterior, inferior border of the mandible. Another common finding in males is epididymoorchitis, which is rapid testicular swelling with pain and tenderness.

Rubeola (measles) is caused by a paramyxovirus. Because of the MMR vaccine, measles incidence is low, but the clinical signs and symptoms still need to be recognized. The incubation period is 10 to 12 days. Significant lymphoid hyperplasia is noted in addition to an erythematous, maculopapular rash.

Rubella (German measles) is an infection caused by a togavirus. Because of the MMR vaccine, rubella incidence is low, but the clinical signs and symptoms still need to be recognized. Lymphadenopathy is the most common clinical feature. An exanthematous rash of the face and neck is also seen.

42. **The correct answer is B.** Pemphigus vulgaris is a rare autoimmune disease in which the body produces antibodies against desmoglein 3 and desmoglein 1. These proteins are components of desmosomes (intercellular adhesion structures between epithelial cells). When these desmosomes are disrupted, epithelial cells are no longer able to bond to each other and a split develops within the epithelium (causing a blister). The average age is 50 (this patient was a bit younger) and there is no sex predilection. Oral lesions are distributed haphazardly and appear as superficial, ragged erosions and ulcerations. Oral lesions usually precede cutaneous lesions, sometimes by a year or more. Patients with pemphigus demonstrate a positive Nikolsky sign (induction of bulla by firm, lateral pressure). Diagnosis can be made histopathologically by seeing suprabasilar cleavage of epithelial cells, but is confirmed by direct immunofluorescence. Treatment consists mainly of immunosuppressive agents (corticosteroids, azathioprine, etc.). Left untreated, pemphigus vulgaris is fatal.

BMMP, while in the same differential for the intraoral lesions, typically does not present with skin lesions. The ulcers are, instead, limited to the mucous membranes (oral mucous, eyes). Desquamative gingivitis is a common finding in patients with BMMP. This patient had multiple skin lesions, which are not seen in classic BMMP.

Erythema multiforme (EM) tends to have an explosive onset and is self-limiting. Characteristic appearances of EM include crusting of the lips and ulceration of the periphery of the tongue. Targetoid skin lesions, though pathognomonic for EM, are rarely seen. This patient had longstanding lesions, no crusting of his lips, and skin lesions that were not targetoid in appearance.

Although erosive LP can present in a similar fashion to the patient above, the histopathologic picture described earlier is not that of LP. LP is a dermatologic disease and can thus have cutaneous involvement. The cutaneous manifestations of LP are not vesicular in nature, but rather a flat, itchy rash.

43. **The correct answer is B.** The histology described earlier is that of a peripheral ossifying fibroma. It occurs exclusively on the gingiva and presents as a nodular mass usually emanating from the interdental papilla. They can be mistaken for other lesions clinically and thus should be included in the differential with pyogenic granuloma (PG), peripheral giant cell granuloma (PGCG), and irritation fibroma. Excision is the treatment of choice. A small recurrence rate has been reported (8–16%).

Mucoceles do not occur on the gingiva, as the gingiva contains no salivary glands. In addition, the histology given is not that of a mucocele.

Clinically, PGCG is an appropriate choice to include in the differential. The reason that it is not is based on the histology given. The histology of a PGCG consists of a proliferation of multinucleated giant cells set in a background of plump ovoid and spindle-shaped mesenchymal cells. Hemorrhage is often seen within these lesions. PGCGs occur exclusively on the gingiva. Treatment is excision and up to 10% of lesions have been reported to recur.

PG is also an appropriate choice to include in a clinical differential. PGs can occur anywhere on the body. Intraorally, the gingiva is the most frequent site. Histologically, PGs consist of

a vascular proliferation resembling granulation tissue. Endothelium-lined vessels are also seen and are arranged in a lobular pattern. There is a mixed inflammatory infiltrate of neutrophils, plasma cells, and lymphocytes.

44. **The correct answer is A.** This is a classic presentation both clinically and histologically of ameloblastoma. Ameloblastoma is by far the most common odontogenic tumor. Its frequency equals the combined total of all the other odontogenic tumors (excluding odontomas that some classify as hamartomas). The preferred site for ameloblastoma is the posterior mandible (approximately 66% of total). Overall, mandibular lesions are more frequent than maxillary lesions in their respective bony locations (posterior, middle, anterior).

OKCs are developmental cysts that have a high rate of recurrence. They can appear uni- or multilocular and have a predilection for the posterior mandible. They can be found as one of the oral manifestations of nevoid basal cell carcinoma syndrome. Lesion size ranges from quite small to large enough to fill entire ramus. OKCs tend to grow in an anterior–posterior direction rather than expand in a buccal–lingual direction. The histology presented in this case does not fit and thus OKC is an incorrect diagnosis.

Odontogenic myxomas are rare tumors of odontogenic ectomesenchyme. The average age for their occurrence is 25 and they may occur anywhere in the jaws. Again, the histology present is classic for ameloblastoma and thus odontogenic myxoma can be ruled out.

Central giant cell granulomas can occur anywhere in the jaws and be uni- or multilocular. Special care should be taken in evaluating the patient for hyperparathyroidism if they have a central giant cell lesion. The histology mentioned earlier is not that of a central giant cell granuloma.

45. **The correct answer is A.** Hemophilia is an x-linked recessive disorder. The only scenarios in which a male hemophiliac may have a child with hemophilia are if the mother is a carrier (Xx) or a hemophiliac (xx) herself. If the mother is a carrier and the father is affected, 50% of the male offspring will have hemophilia (XY, xY).

Fifty percent of the female offspring in this situation will either have hemophilia (xx) or be a carrier of the trait (Xx). The only way a male offspring can have hemophilia is if his mother is affected (xx; in which case he has a 100% chance of having hemophilia) or carries the trait (Xx; in which case he has a 50% chance of having hemophilia). Male hemophiliacs do not pass an affected allele to any male offspring. In the case presented earlier, the mother is neither affected nor a carrier and hence cannot produce a male offspring with hemophilia. By the same token, since all female offspring will have a dominant X allele from their mother and a recessive x allele from their affected father, 100% of female offspring will be carriers.

46. **The correct answer is D.** Thyroglossal duct cyst is a developmental cyst that results from a persistence of epithelium of the thyroglossal duct, an embryonic structure that connects the foramen cecum to the final position of the thyroid in the anterior neck. The thyroid gland begins development in the ventral floor of the pharynx and descends to the anterior neck via the thyroglossal duct. This duct usually undergoes atrophy, but can persist and give rise to a cyst. This cyst may occur anywhere along the tract. It is intimately associated with the hyoid bone and thus the swelling moves with movement of the hyoid (i.e., upon swallowing or tongue protrusion).

Cat-scratch disease is an infection caused by the organism *Bartonella Henselae* that begins in the skin but spreads to the lymph nodes. It is the most common cause of chronic regional lymphadenopathy in children. The lymphadenopathy can occur after the cutaneous lesion has healed. A careful history can often aid in the diagnosis. It would be unusual for cat-scratch disease present as a fluctuant swelling in the anterior midline of the neck.

Although this patient is only 15, it is not unheard of for young patients to have metastatic disease. That being said, metastatic disease to a neck node would be in the lateral neck and firm, not fluctuant.

Branchial cleft cysts are developmental cysts of the lateral neck that develop from remnants of the branchial clefts.

47. **The correct answer is C.** Granulocytic sarcoma (chloroma, extramedullary myeloid tumor) is the result of diffuse infiltration of the gingiva by leukemic cells. It is more common with the myelomonocytic type of leukemia (AML, CML). Patients who present with this should be referred back to their primary physician for further management of a known condition or for treatment of a previously unknown disease process.

Hodgkin's lymphoma is a malignant lymphoproliferative disorder composed of Reed–Sternberg cells (bi- and multinucleated) in enlarged lymph nodes. The most common sites of initial presentation are the cervical and supraclavicular lymph nodes (70–75% of cases). A bimodal pattern with respect to patient's age is also noted: between 15 and 35 years, and another peak after age 50.

Multiple myeloma is a malignancy of plasma cells that typically affects older patients (median age between 60 and 70). It represents the most common hematologic malignancy among black persons in the United States. Bone pain is the most common symptom. Punched-out radiolucencies can be seen in the skull, jawbones, vertebrae, and other bones. Patients with multiple myeloma can also show focal deposits of acellular protein known as amyloid. These deposits can be found in internal organs, as well as skin and mucosal surfaces. Histologically, it appears as an amorphous, glassy pink material.

Ewing's sarcoma is a malignancy of bone composed of small, undifferentiated round cells of uncertain lineage. Peak prevalence is in the second decade and the vast majority of those affected are white. Long bones, pelvis, and rib are most affected. Pain is common and soft-tissue invasion adjacent to affected bone can be seen. Treatment consists of surgery, radiation, and chemotherapy.

48. **The correct answer is E.** Ascher syndrome is characterized by the following three features: double lip, blepharochalasis (edema of the upper eyelids), and nontoxic thyroid enlargement. In general, no treatment is necessary. Occasionally, the drooping eyelids impair vision and require surgical correction. The double lip may be excised for esthetics or function.

Gardner syndrome is an autosomal dominant syndrome that is part of the spectrum of diseases including familial colorectal polyposis. Patients present with multiple osteomas of the jaws 90% of the time and can demonstrate benign cysts and tumors of the skin. Supernumerary teeth, odontomas, and impacted teeth are also common findings. Of particular importance is the presentation of colonic polyps that ultimately transform into adenocarcinoma (usually before the age of 30). Females also demonstrate a 100-fold increase of thyroid carcinoma. It is because of the malignant manifestations of this syndrome that patients need to be referred to their primary care physician for evaluation of colon and thyroid gland.

Papillon–Lefèvre syndrome is an autosomal recessive syndrome that is characterized by palmar–plantar keratosis and dramatically advanced periodontitis in both deciduous and permanent dentitions.

Gorlin syndrome (also known as nevoid basal cell carcinoma syndrome) is an autosomal dominant syndrome caused by a mutation in the PTCH tumor suppressor gene on chromosome 9. It is characterized by multiple basal cell carcinomas, multiple OKCs, palmar/plantar pitting, calcification of the falx cerebri, and rib abnormalities.

Apert syndrome is a rare condition similar to Crouzon syndrome and is characterized by craniosynostosis (premature closing of the cranial sutures). Patients typically have cranial malformations that result in abnormal-shaped heads (tower skull, cloverleaf skull). Affected individuals also have a hypoplastic midface and syndactyly of the second, third, and fourth digits of the hand. Mental retardation is common.

49. **The correct answer is D.** Systemic antivirals are indicated for patients with herpes zoster (HHV-3), especially in elderly patients who have age-related immunosuppression. The treatment regimen should also include palliative measures (analgesics) and antipyretics if the patient if febrile. Zoster involving the tip of the nose warrants a referral to an ophthalmologist, since this is most often a sign of involvement of the nasociliary branch of the trigeminal nerve. This is turn, can lead to ocular infection and potential blindness.

Steroids, be they systemic or topical, are contraindicated in viral infections. If administered, they will delay the host response and prolong the duration of disease and discomfort.

Although administration of systemic antiviral medication is indicated in herpes zoster infections, involvement of the tip of the nose requires mandatory referral to ophthalmology to make sure there is no ocular infection.

CHAPTER 10

Patient Management, Public Health, Ethics, and Biostatistics

1. Which of the following behaviors would be considered unethical with regards to a physician–patient relationship?

    A. Dating or engaging in a sexual relationship with one of your patients.
    B. Refusing to date or engage in any sexual relationship with your patients.
    C. Returning a call from one of your patients who called you to complain of pain from the tooth you worked on yesterday.
    D. Requesting to drop off or transfer a patient from your treatment list to a different provider due to his/her persistent multiple sexual advances directed toward you.

2. What is the golden rule that could be used to broadly define all ethical behaviors with regards to patient treatment?

    A. Be nice only to the patients who are nice to you.
    B. Administer palatal injections to any patient who annoys you, even though you are treating mandibular teeth.
    C. Physicians are expected to respect and treat patients as they would like to be treated, using the best of their knowledge and ability, excluding any modifiers or outside bias.
    D. Treat patients the way you would like to be treated except if they are noncompliant with your instructions.

3. Which of the following scenarios would be considered a type of unethical behavior that might justify an ethical board to recommend immediate licensure suspension?

    A. Mistakenly extracting the wrong tooth on a patient, but informing the patient immediately afterward and offering an apology
    B. Refusing to extract a wisdom tooth that is near the inferior alveolar nerve, but referring the patient to an oral surgeon for evaluation and further treatment
    C. Extracting a tooth on a patient taking Coumadin with an INR of 1.7, resulting in the patient's admission to the hospital for 4 days to control excessive bleeding from the

extraction socket. The patient is eventually discharged from the hospital in stable condition.
    D. Gross negligence or severe overtreatment and deviation from standard of care, resulting to an injury or death of a patient

4. Which of the following situations illustrate unethical behavior of a dental student?

    A. Explaining all the risks and benefits of a procedure to patients before obtaining their signature in an informed consent form for extraction of teeth
    B. Creating a root canal during an operative procedure to meet a clinical requirement and graduate on time
    C. Accepting a Christmas present from a patient
    D. Refusing to offer free treatment to a low-income, cash-paying patient

5. All of the following statements as regards to ethical framing are true *except* one:

    A. Ethical framing can lead to conflicts, because different people have different frames of reference based on their environments, religious or professional backgrounds, and moral values.
    B. Ethical framing means one's perspective of ethics may be different from others.
    C. Personal ego and financial interest are some of the many factors that influence ethical framing, which often leads to rationalization of an ethical decision with attempts to find support for a predetermined conclusion.
    D. There is usually one black-and-white answer to every ethical situation, which meets commonly held ethical standards, and does not lead to conflicts or different ethical interpretations.

6. If a patient of record has been out of town for 10 months and returns to your office to have a temporary crown made by another dentist recemented, you may:

    A. Remove and recement the crown if there is compensation prior to treatment.

B. Remove the crown and recement it with permanent cement.

C. Remove the crown and recement it with temporary cement.

D. Remove the crown, recement it with temporary cement, and refer the patient back to the dentist who made the crown.

7. When laboratory procedures are required, the dentist should prescribe treatment for HMO and private pay patients equally; all patients deserve the same quality of treatment.

A. First statement is true and second is false.

B. Both statements are true.

C. First statement is false and second is true.

D. Both statements are false.

8. If Mr. Smith calls the office saying he just moved to town and needs a cleaning and dental prophylaxis, with whom should the appointment be scheduled?

A. The hygienist

B. The assistant so that the necessary radiographs can be taken

C. The dentist

D. It does not matter with whom the patient is scheduled.

9. The PREAMBLE in the ADA's document on ETHICS states that our primary goal when treating patients should be to benefit:

A. The dental profession

B. Mankind

C. Ourselves

D. The patient

E. All of the above

10. If a dentist does not keep up with CE courses and current trends or advances in dentistry, which of the following principles of ethics is being broken?

A. Veracity

B. Justice

C. Beneficence

D. Nonmaleficence

E. Autonomy

11. Technical assault or battery and maligning a patient are forms of:

A. Civil law

B. Contract law

C. Tort law

D. Negligence

12. As dental professionals, we are ethically bound to guarantee patients:

A. Nothing

B. The appropriate standard of care

C. Successful results

D. Professionalism

13. All of the following are correct in regard to the patient records *except* which one?

A. Records are kept for 1 year.

B. Records must include updated medical histories.

C. Records must be recorded in ink or electronically.

D. Records include radiographs of the patient.

14. When treating a patient, whose value system is of the most importance?

A. The dentist

B. The patient

C. Both are of equal importance

D. Value systems should not affect dental treatment

15. If Mrs. Jones shares with you that she has been diagnosed with breast cancer what ethical principle must you uphold?

A. Justice

B. Confidentiality

C. Beneficence

D. Veracity

Patient Management, Public Health, Ethics, and Biostatistics

16. Your brother is in the office to have a deep restoration placed on tooth #19. While you are waiting for the effect of the anesthetic, he states that his back is still bothering him greatly and that the only effective medication is Vicodin. He asks you to write this prescription for him. What do you do?

    A. Write the prescription for just 10 tablets.
    B. Give him a prescription for a month of Vicodin, to be taken as needed for pain.
    C. Give him some samples of Vicodin that you happen to have in the office.
    D. Refer him back to his physician or orthopedist to obtain the prescription.

17. You have taught your staff members how to monitor nitrous oxide analgesia; you are confident that they are all comfortable performing this, but your assistant (although registered) still has not taken the nitrous oxide certification course. A patient presents with a problem for which nitrous oxide analgesia is indicated. You get called from the room but not wanting to turn off the nitrous and have to turn it back on again, you tell the assistant to sit with the patient. She is instructed that if the patient has any deleterious effects, "lower the nitrous just a little." When relating this to a fellow colleague, you are informed that this was not the correct thing to do; you disagree since you were "only in the next room." The two of you get into a discussion about this. Is this an ethical issue or an ethical dilemma?

    A. This is an ethical dilemma.
    B. This is an ethical issue.
    C. This is not an ethical problem at all. Your actions were justified.

18. In your private office, you keep MSDS (medical safety data sheets); you have one of your staff members in charge of monitoring and updating them. At monthly meetings, you also have this person inform the staff of any recent OSHA or HIPAA directives. In this situation, MSDS paperwork falls under the guidance of which of the following agencies?

    A. Occupational Safety and Health Administration (OSHA)
    B. Health Insurance Portability and Accountability Act of 1996 (HIPAA)
    C. State Law
    D. Joint Commission on Accreditation of Healthcare Organizations (JCAHO)

19. There are improvements in the following trends in oral health *except* for:

    A. Edentulism and periodontitis among seniors
    B. Prevalence of dental caries, tooth retention, and periodontitis among adults
    C. Prevalence of dental caries and dental sealants among youths and adolescents
    D. Dental caries in primary teeth among children aged 2 to 5 years
    E. None of the above

20. Which of the following statement best described the caries burden among children?

    A. Approximately 80% of tooth decay is found in approximately 25% of children.
    B. Tooth decay is evenly distributed among different racial and socioeconomic groups.
    C. Approximately 90% of tooth decay is found in approximately 10% of children.
    D. None of the above

21. What percentage of adults have tooth decay (treated or untreated)?

    A. Approximately 35% of adults aged 20 to 39 years have coronal decay.
    B. Approximately 52% of adults aged 20 to 39 years have coronal decay.
    C. Approximately 87% of adults aged 20 to 39 years have coronal decay.
    D. All adults aged 20 to 39 years have coronal decay.

22. What percentage of the U.S. population is plagued by moderate to severe periodontitis?

    A. Approximately 1% to 20%, depending on the age groups
    B. Approximately 20% to 40%, depending on the age groups
    C. Approximately 40% to 60%, depending on the age groups
    D. None of the above

23. What is the incidence of oral and pharyngeal cancer (i.e., new oral and pharyngeal cancer cases) each year?

    A. Approximately 10,000 new cases of oral and pharyngeal cancer each year
    B. Approximately 35,000 new cases of oral and pharyngeal cancer each year
    C. Approximately 50,000 new cases of oral and pharyngeal cancer each year
    D. None of the above

24. What is/are the measure(s) of central tendency in statistical methods?

    A. Mean
    B. Median
    C. Mode
    D. All of the above

25. Currently, nine states mandate the installation of amalgam separators in the dental office. Which of the following is/are among the nine states?

    A. California
    B. Massachusetts
    C. Alaska
    D. South Carolina
    E. A and B

26. What is the most effective community-based intervention to control dental decay?

    A. School-based dental sealant programs
    B. Community health centers with dental clinics
    C. Fluoridation of drinking water
    D. Introduction of sugarless chewing gums

27. Up to 800,000 percutaneous injuries occur annually among all U.S. healthcare workers. After percutaneous injury with a contaminated sharp instrument, the risks of infection are as follows:

    i. Average rate of anti–hepatitis C virus (HCV) seroconversion after percutaneous exposure to HCV-infected blood is 1.8% (range, 0–7%)
    ii. Average transmission rate is 0.3% after percutaneous exposure to human immunodeficiency virus (HIV)-infected blood.

    iii. Average rate of hepatitis B virus (HBV) transmission to susceptible healthcare workers after percutaneous exposure to HBV-infected blood is 6% to 30%

    Which statements are correct?

    A. Only i and iii are correct.
    B. Only ii is correct.
    C. All are correct.
    D. None is correct.

28. The portion or percentage of individuals having a disease at a given time is:

    A. Frequency
    B. Incidence
    C. Prevalence
    D. Mortality

29. Specificity is the proportion of truly diseased persons who are identified as being diseased. False-positive result identifies individuals as having a disease, but in reality they do not.

    A. Both statements are true.
    B. Both statements are false.
    C. The first statement is true, the second statement is false.
    D. The first statement is false, the second statement is true.

30. After a needlestick or cut exposure, the pathogen with the highest risk of infection is:

    A. HBV
    B. HIV
    C. HCV
    D. *Mycobacterium tuberculosis*

31. Latex allergies can result in which of the following reactions:

    i.   Type I
    ii. Type II
    iii. Type III
    iv. Type IV

    A. ii and iii
    B. ii and iv
    C. i and ii
    D. i and iv

32. The mechanism of action of povidone iodine is:

    A. Irreversible inactivation of deoxyribonucleic acid and proteins via alkylation
    B. Heat inactivation of critical enzymes
    C. Pore formation within the bacterial cell wall, resulting in cellular leakage
    D. Oxidization of free sulfhydryl groups

33. Which of the following statements is correct concerning sterilization of dental instruments?

    A. Gentle washing with bleaching and soaking for 10 minutes in the bleach is required before putting instruments in the autoclave.
    B. ADA recommends biological monitors being used once a month
    C. Biological indicators contain spores of a heat-resistant bacterium *Eikenella corrodens*.
    D. Chemical indicators are sterilizer specific.

34. You just bought a sterilization machine from a retiring dentist for your new office, and then your staff tells you that the machine just "failed" the test. What measures should you take right after taking sterilization out of service?

    i.   Review the sterilization process being followed in the office to rule out operator error.
    ii. Check electrical outputs from the wall, since this may alter the performance of the sterilization machine.
    iii. Biological indicator tests should be conducted during three consecutive empty-chamber sterilization cycles.
    iv. After three consecutive empty-chamber testing, another three consecutive tests should be run using only chemical indicators before resterilizing instruments.

    A. i and ii
    B. i and iii
    C. i, ii, and iii
    D. ii, iii, and iv
    E. ii and iv

35. You performed a crown prep on tooth #28 on this gentleman with moderate to poor oral hygiene. Now, he is back for cementation of his PFM crown. You decided to use Glass Ionomer Cement. Please choose the INCORRECT statement concerning Glass Ionomer Cement:

    A. Glass ionomer has a high modulus of elasticity.
    B. Fluoride is released from the glass powder at the time of mixing and lies free within the matrix.
    C. Fluoride released has no effect on cariogenic bacteria but will harden only the tooth's enamel.
    D. Glass ionomer is known for little shrinkage and good marginal seal.

36. A 6-year-old healthy boy presented to your office for the first time. His mother said he has never been to a dentist and has never had a radiograph taken. Intraoral examination revealed that his permanent molars are erupted. The patient has no clinically evident dental problems. What kind of screening radiographic examination will you perform?

    i.   Occlusal radiographs
    ii. Periapical radiographs
    iii. Panorex radiographs
    iv. Posterior bitewing radiographs

    A. i and ii
    B. i and iii
    C. ii and iii
    D. iii and iv
    E. iii only

1. **The correct answer is A.** It is unprofessional, unethical, and morally inappropriate for a physician to abuse his/her position of public trust and engage in any form of sexual relationship with one of his/her patients. A physician's involvement with a patient sexually will compromise his/her ability to offer good services to the patient, thereby creating an ineffective and abnormal physician–patient relationship. Physicians should carefully and tactfully transfer a patient in their care to a different provider, if multiple attempts to redirect their sexual gestures away from the physician failed. Choices B and C are completely ethical and appropriate.

2. **The correct answer is C.** Physicians are expected to treat every patient with courtesy and respect, using the best of their knowledge without any prejudice or bias. Partial or total deviation from this golden rule would be considered unethical. All patients should be treated with respect irrespective of whether they are nice or not, or noncompliant with their medications. Inflicting unnecessary pain to patient by administering palatal injections while extracting mandibular teeth is unethical and unprofessional.

3. **The correct answer is D.** Gross negligence resulting in severe injury or patient's death is a gross deviation for standard of care and might lead to licensure suspension or withdrawal. The appropriate thing to do if the wrong tooth is extracted on a patient is to inform your supervisor or attending, and the patient should be informed immediately and an apology offered. Options A and C are not the best expected outcomes, but they would not be considered a type of unethical behavior that might justify an ethical board to recommend immediate licensure suspension. It is appropriate to refer a patient to a different provider with better experience or training to manage a patient with a problem that is beyond your scope of practice. Treating a patient with a problem beyond your level of training, leading to an unexpected outcome or harm to the patient, is considered malpractice.

4. **The correct answer is B.** Despite the pressure to fulfill all requirements prior to graduation, dental students are held to the highest moral and professional standard. So intentionally converting a class I amalgam restoration into a root canal therapy on a patient to meet the graduation requirement is unethical. It is appropriate for a dental student to accept a gift from a patient, as long as it is not in exchange to providing a free treatment to the patient, and the practice is allowed by the dental school. Dental students are expected to explain all the risks, benefits, alternatives, and complications to all patients and obtain a signed informed consent form prior to any dental procedure, including dental extractions.

5. **The correct answer is D.** There is usually NO black-and-white answer to an ethical situation that meets commonly held ethical standards without conflicts or different ethical interpretations. Ethical framing means one's perspective of ethics based on the frames of reference, environment, religious or professional background, moral values, personal ego, or financial interest, which often leads to rationalization of an ethical decision with attempts to find support for a predetermined conclusion.

6. **The correct answer is D.** It would be unethical to not treat the patient but the sole responsibility should lie with the dentist who initially made the crown.

7. **The correct answer is B.** Both HMO patients and private paying patients should receive the same quality of care and treatment. The dental profession holds a special position of trust with society. The ADA Code of Ethical Principles is a written expression of this "contract." Note: Dentist's ethical considerations often exceed legal duties and business obligations, factors that do not excuse them from putting the patient's welfare first.

8. **The correct answer is C.** The dentist should see the patient first to "diagnose" the condition

and dental needs of the patient. The hygienist is not allowed to diagnose. Therefore, if the patient requires further treatment following a "prophy," the dentist must be consulted. The assistant cannot perform a "prophy" on a patient in most states, and the radiographs would need to be prescribed by the dentist. It does make a difference who sees the patient first, and that must be the physician to diagnose and prescribe treatment.

9. **The correct answer is D.** The patient's needs come first, and we must offer the patient a choice of the appropriate treatments available. All risks, benefits, alternatives, and complications of the possible treatment options must be explained to the patient as part of the informed consent process. The primary goal in treating patients should have nothing to do with the dental profession or mankind but the patients themselves. We should not treat patients to benefit ourselves since the patient's needs come first.

10. **The correct answer is D.** Nonmaleficence means not causing harm to be inflicted on anyone. By taking CE courses, you are providing the patient with the choices of the most effective and current available treatment. By keeping up with current advances in dentistry, one will not cause undue harm to the patient. This principle is part of the Hippocratic Oath ("Primum non nocere" — "First, do no harm"). Veracity is truthfulness. Justice is treating patients fairly. Beneficence has to do with the benefit to the patient by meeting their particular needs. Autonomy has to do with the final decision being made by the patient.

11. **The correct answer is C.** Tort law is a form of civil law that involves a civil wrong or injury to another person, whereas civil law involves a crime against a person with actions that cause harm to that individual. The civil law suit is filed with a private attorney. Contract law is a form of civil law that involves a breach of contract. Negligence is synonymous with malpractice; it is carelessness without the intent to harm a patient. Negligence occurs when the appropriate standard of care is NOT met and some damage results.

12. **The correct answer is B.** We must meet the minimum standards of care when treating patients. Guaranteeing nothing implies a lack of interest in patient welfare. We are obligated to meet the minimum standards of care. No one can predict, promise, or guarantee successful results, but one can state risks and benefits for a variety of treatments. We are not obligated to guarantee professionalism, but we should show the patient respect and should act in a professional manner.

13. **The correct answer is A.** Records must be kept for as long as the individual State Dental Practice Act dictates or the length of the statute of limitations within that state. Treatment records must include updated medical histories and radiographs of patients. They must also be recorded in ink (not pencil) and electronically.

14. **The correct answer is B.** Patients' value system is what is of the most importance. We should not judge patients by their values. The only value system that matters is that of patients'. The practitioners' values might be very different from those of patients but must be set aside in favor of patients.

15. **The correct answer is B.** Regardless of how you feel, any information shared with you professionally by patients must be kept confidential. Justice involves the tenet of treating individuals fairly; giving patients their due or what is owed them. The principle of beneficence can be illustrated with the statement "the action is moral if it is good and helps to enhance patient welfare." Veracity involves truthfulness or speaking the truth.

16. **The correct answer is D.** A dentist may prescribe a medication only for a dentally related problem.

17. **The correct answer is B.** An auxiliary must have a nitrous oxide certification course to monitor or discontinue nitrous oxide. If there is a state or federal statute mandating something, it then becomes an ethical issue. If there is no state or federal statute mandating something, then it is just an ethical dilemma with no right or wrong answer.

18. **The correct answer is A.** Occupational Safety and Health Administration (OSHA) has to do with infection control and the Health Insurance Portability and Accountability Act of 1996 (HIPAA) has to do with privacy issues. The OSHA is an agency of the U.S. Department of Labor. State Law is the Dental Practice Act governing the practice of licensed dental professionals in each state. The Joint Commission (JCAHO) is a private, not-for-profit organization that operates accreditation programs for hospitals and healthcare organizations. It is not a requirement that all private dental offices undergo evaluation by the JCAHO; however, it is a requirement that all dental offices be OSHA compliant.

19. **The correct answer is D.** These results for trends in oral health in the United States between 1988 to 1994 and 1999 to 2004 are from the National Health and Nutrition Examination Survey (NHANES), which showed an increase in dental caries in primary teeth among 2- to 5-year-olds.

20. **The correct answer is A.** The differential caries burden among children is such that 80% of dental caries are borne by 25% of persons younger than 19 years.

21. **The correct answer is C.** This information about the prevalence of decay among young adults (aged 20–39 years) was obtained from NHANES 1999 to 2002.

22. **The correct answer is A.** This information regarding the prevalence of moderate to severe periodontitis was obtained from NHANES 1999 to 2004. Moderate periodontal disease is defined as two or more interproximal sites with 4 mm or more clinical attachment loss (CAL), or two or more interproximal sites with 5 mm or more probing pocket depth (PPD). Severe disease is defined as two or more interproximal sites with 6 mm or more CAL and one or more interproximal sites with 5 mm or more PPD.

23. **The correct answer is B.** According to the National Cancer Institute's Surveillance Epidemiology and End Results, in 2009, it was estimated that there will be 35,720 (25,240 men and 10,480 women) newly diagnosed cases of oral and pharyngeal cancer and 7,600 deaths from it.

24. **The correct answer is D.** In biostatistics, mean is the average, median is the statistic that separates the upper half of the population from the lower half, and mode is the statistic that is of the highest frequency.

25. **The correct answer is B.** The nine U.S. states that have mercury safety laws are the six New England states (Connecticut, Massachusetts, Maine, New Hampshire, Rhode Island, and Vermont) and New York, New Jersey, and Oregon. Some other states have local mandates or are in the process of phasing in statewide mandates.

26. **The correct answer is C.** Community water fluoridation is cited as one of the top 10 public health achievements of the 20th century.

27. **The correct answer is C.** This information on infection control/percutaneous injuries was obtained from the National Institute for Occupational Safety and Health.

28. **The correct answer is C.** Prevalence is the portion or percentage of individuals having a disease at a given time. Frequency is the number of individuals having a disease at a given time. Incidence is the rate of new cases of disease per time. Mortality is the rate of deaths resulting from a specific disease.

29. **The correct answer is D.** The first statement is false, the second statement is true. Specificity is the proportion of truly nondiseased persons who are identified as such. In a false-positive result, the individual does not have the disease but is identified as having the disease. A true-positive result describes a situation where the individual has the disease and is correctly identified as such. A false-negative result is when the individual has the disease and is incorrectly identified as not having the disease. In a true-negative result, the individual does not have the disease and is correctly identified as such.

30. The correct answer is A. The average risk for infection after needle stick or cut exposure is 6% to 30% for hepatitis B virus, 1.8% for hepatitis C virus, and 0.3% for human immunodeficiency virus. *Mycobacterium tuberculosis* airborne droplet nuclei are generated when infected individuals sneeze, cough, and speak.

31. The correct answer is D. Natural rubber latex proteins may result in a type I (immediate) hypersensitivity reaction. Common presentations include urticaria, rhinorrhea, itchy eyes, and a burning sensation at the point of contact. Severe reactions may result in anaphylactic shock and death. Latex allergies can also result in a type IV (delayed) hypersensitivity reaction as in allergic contact dermatitis. These reactions are usually localized to the contact area and occur over a 12- to 48-hour period.

32. The correct answer is C. All answers describe a legitimate antimicrobial mechanism of action. "Irreversible inactivation of deoxyribonucleic acid and proteins via alkylation" describes the mechanism of action of ethylene oxide gas. "Heat inactivation of critical enzymes" describes the mechanism of action of steam autoclave, dry heat, rapid heat transfer, and unsaturated chemical vapor. "Oxidization of free sulfhydryl groups" describes chlorine compounds (hypochlorite). Povidone iodine causes pore formation within the bacterial cell wall, resulting in cellular leakage.

33. The correct answer is D. According to ADA guideline on sterilization, indicator tapes are sterilizer specific (i.e., tapes for steam sterilizers cannot be used to test chemical vapor sterilizers). The ADA also recommends the weekly use of biological indicators. *Eikenella corrodens* is a slow-growing, facultative, anaerobic, gram-negative bacillus that is part of the normal oral flora and is found in dental plaque. Biological indicators contain spores of a heat-resistant bacterium *Geobacillus stearothermophilus*.

34. The correct answer is B. According to the ADA guidelines, "What to do when results indicate sterilization failure:

If the chemical indicator does not change color or the spore test result is positive, the following steps are recommended:

1. Take the sterilizer out of service.
2. Review the sterilization process being followed in the office to rule out operator error as the cause of failure.
3. Correct any identified procedural problems, and retest the sterilizer using biological, mechanical, and chemical indicators.
4. If the biological indicator test is positive, or the mechanical or chemical test results indicate failure, the sterilizer should not be used until the reason for failure has been identified and corrected.

If no procedural errors are identified or failures persist after procedural errors are corrected, the sterilizer should not be used until the reason for failure has been identified and corrected.

Before the sterilizer can be returned to service, negative results should be returned for biological indicator tests conducted during three consecutive empty-chamber sterilization cycles to ensure that the problem has been corrected.

To the extent possible, reprocess all instruments that were sterilized since the last negative spore test.

Record the positive test results and all actions taken to ensure proper functioning of the sterilizer in the monitoring log."

35. The correct answer is C. According to Qin et al.'s, "Fluoride Inhibition of Enolase: Crystal Structure and Thermodynamics," and van Loveren's, "The Antimicrobial Action of Fluoride and Its Role in Caries Inhibition", fluoride does have bacteriocidal/bacteriostatic effects on oral bacteria.

Glass ionomer is described as having the following properties:

Advantages
   Inherent adhesion to tooth structure
   High retention rate
   Little shrinkage and good marginal seal
   Fluoride release and hence caries inhibition
   Biocompatible

Minimal cavity preparation required, hence easy to use on children and suitable for use even in absence of skilled dental manpower and facilities

Disadvantages

Brittle

Soluble

Abrasive

Water sensitive during setting phase

Some products release less fluoride than conventional GIC

Not inherently radiopaque although addition of radiodense additives such barium can alter radiodensity

Less aesthetic than composite

36. **The correct answer is D.** In a child with a transitional dentition, after eruption of the first permanent tooth, the radiographic examination should be individualized and should consist of posterior bitewings and panoramic examination, or posterior bitewings and selected periapical radiographs.

Jason E. Portnof, DMD, MD

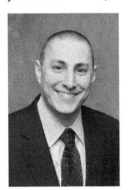

Dr. Portnof is currently full-time faculty of the Oral and Maxillofacial Surgery residency program at Beth Israel Medical Center/Jacobi Medical Center/Albert Einstein College of Medicine. He is Assistant Professor in the Departments of Dentistry and Otorhinolaryngology, Albert Einstein College of Medicine. He completed his undergraduate education at Washington University in St. Louis, Missouri, and received his doctorate in dental medicine (DMD) from Nova Southeastern University in Ft. Lauderdale, Florida. His medical school training (MD) was completed at Weill Cornell Medical College in New York City. He completed a residency in oral and maxillofacial surgery and an internship in general surgery at New York Presbyterian Hospital/Weill Cornell Medical Center, where he also served as Chief Resident in oral and maxillofacial surgery. Dr. Portnof completed a fellowship in pediatric maxillofacial surgery/craniomaxillofacial surgery in the Department of Plastic and Maxillofacial Surgery, Royal Children's Hospital, Melbourne, Australia.

Tim Leung, DMD, MHSc, MD

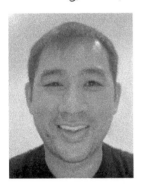

Dr. Leung is presently in private practice oral and maxillofacial surgery in Toronto, Ontario, Canada and New York, NY. He is also a faculty member of the oral and maxillofacial surgery residency program at Jacobi Medical Center Department of Dentistry, Oral and Maxillofacial Surgery, Bronx, NY. He completed a residency in oral and maxillofacial surgery and an internship in general surgery at New York Presbyterian Hospital — Weill Cornell Medical Center, where he also served as Chief Resident in oral and maxillofacial surgery. He received an MD degree from Weill Cornell Medical College, and a DMD from University of Pennsylvania School of Dental Medicine. He earned an MHSc from the University of Toronto. His undergraduate education (BA) was completed at Cornell University.

Melvyn S. Yeoh, DMD, MD

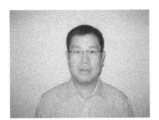

Dr. Yeoh is currently the Chief Resident in oral and maxillofacial surgery at New York Presbyterian Hospital, Cornell Medical Center. He completed an internship in general surgery at New York Presbyterian Hospital — Weill Cornell Medical Center. He received his dental degree from the University of Pennsylvania and his medical degree from Cornell University. His undergraduate education was at Claremont McKenna College in Claremont, California.

INDEX

Note: Page locators followed by f indicates figure.

Printed in the USA
CPSIA information can be obtained
at www.ICGtesting.com
JSHW060434261023
50760JS00019B/279